On Innovation of TREATMENT of CANCER

Cancer Immune treatment combined Chinese with Western medicine

VOLUME II

XuZe XuJie BinWu

authorHOUSE®

AuthorHouse™
1663 Liberty Drive
Bloomington, IN 47403
www.authorhouse.com
Phone: 1 (800) 839-8640

Published by AuthorHouse 12/23/2015

ISBN: 978-1-5049-6506-4 (sc)
ISBN: 978-1-5049-6507-1 (e)

Library of Congress Control Number: 2015920095

Print information available on the last page.

Table of Contents

Pictures

Introduction to Volume II

Volume II of our collection is an unique series of our integrating cancer immune treatment theories which we researched and discovered how central immune organs thymus and bone marrow, immune cells such as T-cell and periphery immune system such as spleen are related to cancer therapy and how we developed our innovating immune regulation medications etc . It is all of our dedicating work of searching the new ways and new medications for cancer therapy. This monograph is full of innovative concepts and contents both on the basis of experimental research and clinical verification which are excellent for cancer patients, especially for the advanced stage of cancer patients, no surgical indication cancer patients.

(1)Dr. XU proposed the comprehensive cancer treatment such as surgery + immune regulation as the main methods; and radiation and chemotherapy as the supplement. The multidisciplinary model for long- term therapy: surgery + biological treatment + immunotherapy and short-term therapy supplemented such as radiotherapy and chemotherapy cannot be long-term and not excessive. The treatment is better to regulate the whole body, but not only kill the cancer cells.

(2).Dr. Xu proposed chemotherapy can be within the target organ vascular chemotherapy.

(3) It is necessary to search and innovate more selective intelligent anticancer drug such as: $XZ_{1, 4}$ are selective drugs. Z-C immune regulation medications protect thymus and increase immune functions.

(4) Many chemotherapy drugs are the absence of chemotherapy sensitivity testing: Dr. Xu Ze recommended to have sensitivity testing (to avoid blindness).

(5) Now the tumor specimens were not cultured for cancer treatment; Dr. Xu Ze proposed that it better to reform to make that the cancer cells are cultured (individual, selective).

(6) Radical surgery should be designed to further research and improvement; Dr. Xu pointed out that the current radical mastectomy are only concerned about the route of lymph node metastasis; however the blood and implant metastasis should be paid attention to because there are several metastasis routes; Dr.Xu Ze proposed that the

technology of designation and operation should be reformed and emphasis **on tumor-free technology** to prevent intraoperative blood cancer cell metastasis.

(7) Thymic atrophy and immune dysfunction is one of pathogenesis of cause of cancer.

(8) Cancer therapy target must be the same time for both tumor and host to establish the comprehensive treatment concept, but not simple to kill the cancer cells to overcome one-sided treatment concept.

(9) Cancer in the body mainly exist in three forms and the third form of cancer is the cells on the metastasis route which should be focused on.

(10) The whole process of cancer development was "two point and one line" theory. Cancer treatment should pay attention to two points and also cut off line; the cancer treatment has three steps and three policies to develop the third field.

In brief, our experimental surgery research explored the cancer etiology, pathogenesis, pathophysiology experimental study since 1985. On animal models and clinics practice level 48 kinds of Chinese medications were selected into our XZ-C $_{1-10}$ immune regulation medications. Out-patient medical records have been kept for more than 20 years, nearly more than 12,000 cases, follow-up and long-term follow-up to establish the patient medical records library and achieve wonderful results.,

Science - is endless frontier.

Our scientific work has followed the scientific concept of development, based on the known science, to look forward. After 28 years of long and hard work, facing the frontiers of science, innovative and forward, we deeply appreciate:

- To overcome cancer, it must come from the clinic, through experimental study, go to the clinic in order to solve practical problems of patients;

- Must be realistic, speak with facts, data; must constantly self-transcendence, self-advancement;

- The research should address the ideological shackles, get rid of the traditional old ideas, based on independent innovation and original innovation.

- Our two decades of research line is to find the problem →ask a question →research questions → solve problems or explain the problem. The road walks out step by step and it is difficult journey. Under the guidance of the concept of development we hope to walk out a Chinese characteristics way with innovation and properity.

- Our oncology research model is based on patient-centered to discover questions from clinical work, then come back to the in-depth animal experiments, and then turn to the clinical application in order to improve overall level of health care and ultimately the patient gets the benefit.

- Experimental surgery is extremely important in the medicine development and is a key to open the medicine box. After lots of animal studies many diseases have achieved stability of results and then is used clinically to promote the development of the medical industry.

A Brief Introduction to the Author

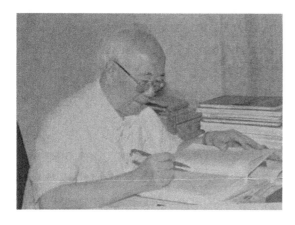

Xu Ze, male, born in Leping County of Jiangxi Province in Oct. 1933, gradated from Tongji Medical University in 1956, successively held the post of director of department of surgery of Affiliated Hospital of Hubei College of Traditional Chinese Medicine, professor, chief physician, tutor of postgraduate and doctoral student, President of Experimental Surgery Restitute Institute of Hubei College of Traditional Chinese Medicine, Director of Abdominal Tumor Surgery Research Room and Director of Anti Carcinomatous Metastasis and Reoccurrence Research Room. in addition, he held concurrent posts of Standing Director of China Medical Association Wuhan Branch, Vice President of Wuhan Micro-circulation Academy, Academic Member of International Liver Disease Research, Cooperation and Exchange Center, Member of International Surgeon Union, Standing Member of 1st, 2nd, 3rd and 4th Editorial Board of China Experimental Surgery Journal, Standing Member of 1st, 2dn and 3rd Editorial Board of Abdominal Surgery Journal. Enjoying Special Allowance of State Council.

He has been engaged in surgery work for 49 years and accumulated rich experience in radical operation of lung cancer, esophageal carcinoma, liver cancer, carcinoma of gallbladder, adenocarcinoma of pancreas, gastric carcinoma and intestinal cancer as well as in clinical therapy with Chinese Traditional Medicine combined with Western Medicine of prevention of reoccurrence and metastasis after operation.

He has been engaged in scientific research of surgery for 15 years and obtained many fruits, among which the task of Experimental Study and Clinical Application of Self-made Type Z-C1 Abdominal Cavity---Vein Flow Turning Unit in Therapy of Chronic Ascites of Hepatic Cirrhosis issued by Science Commission of Hubei Province was awarded Second Prize of Scientific Fruit by People's Government of Hubei Province and was popularized and applied in 38 hospitals in 12 provinces all over the country in 1982. The task "Experimental Study on Physiological Mechanism and Pathogenesis of Schistosome with Method of Experimental Surgery", issued by National Natural Fund

Commission was awarded Second Prize of Scientific Fruit by People's Government of Hubei Province in 1986.

He began to study the tumor experience, established the tumor animal model and metastasis and reoccurrence animal model and probed into the mechanism and rules of carcinomatous metastasis and reoccurrence to find out the method to inhibit the metastasis. 48 kinds of Chinese traditional herbs that could counteract the intrusion, metastasis and reoccurrence were found and selected from a large number of natural herbs. Based on this, he invented and developed China Xu Ze (Z-C) Medicine Treating Malignancy, which had remarkable curative effects through over 10 years' clinical validation of many cases.

He has been engaged in teaching for 40 years and has cultivated many young doctors, 10 masters and 2 doctors. He has released 126 papers, published New Understanding and New Mode of Therapy of Cancer as the editor in charge, participate in writing 8 medical exclusive books including Therapeutics of Liver Disease, Surgery of Liver, Gallbladder and Pancreas and Surgical Operation of Abdomen.

A Brief Introduction to the Second Author

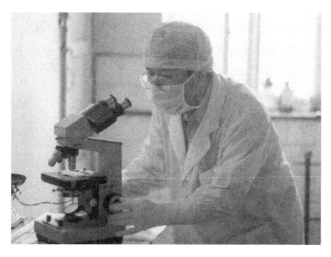

Xu Jie, male, graduated from Department of Traditional Chinese Medicine of Hubei University of Chinese Medicine in 1992 and from Department of Clinical Medicine of Hubei Medical University (now the Medicine School of Wuhan University) in 1996, serving as the associate chief physician of the surgery in Affiliated Hospital of Hubei University of Chinese Medicine, namely Hubei Hospital of Traditional Chinese Medicine and engaged in study on experimental tumor of experimental surgery and the clinical work of general surgery and urinary surgery.

Since 1992, he has participated in study on the experimental tumor in Research Institute of Experimental Surgery of Hubei University of Chinese Medicine, made the transplantation of cancer cells, established the tumor animal model, carried out a series of study on experimental tumor; probed in the mechanism and rules of cancerous reoccurrence and metastasis, screened and studied through the in vivo tumor-inhibiting experiment on the tumor-bearing animal model over 200 kinds of traditional Chinese herbs that may play a role in anticancer and cancer inhibition held by the literature and found and screened 48 kinds of traditional Chinese herbs with the role in preventing cancerous invasion, metastasis and reoccurrence from a large number of natural herbs.

He has participated in the clinical verification of XZ-C Medicine and the follow-up survey, completed the experimental study and clinical verification, data processing, collection and summary of this book.

A Brief Introduction to the Third Author and the Main Translator

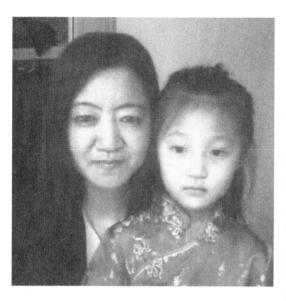

Bin Wu, MD, Ph.D., graduated from College of Yunyang of Tongji University of Medical Sciences for her MD degree; studied her Master degree and her Ph. D degree in Sun Yat-Sen University of Medical Sciences. After she received her Ph.D., she worked as a Post-doctoral Fellow in the Johns Hopkins Medical School and University of Maryland Medical School. She passed all of her USMLE tests and is going to do her residency training in America. She dedicates herself to oncology clinical and research. Her goal is to conquer cancer, which she believes this is great contribution to our health. She has a daughter, Lily Xu.

Preface

These series monographs are not the books which we wrote down only, but things which we accomplished, all of which are from our clinical experiences, lessons, reviews, profound considerations and practices.

The contents in these series are the experimental research results and harvests.

The contents in these series are the true records of the scientific practices from the experiments to clinics, then from clinics to the scientific experiments and scientific practices. It is the conclusion of the experimental research and clinical verification(proof), then up to the theory best features and put forward to new discoveries, new knowledge, new theories, all of which are clinical and practicable new theories and can guide the clinical treatments. All of these should move medicine into clinical applications to instruct the clinical theory work so that the patients get benefits.

The contents in these series are the experimental research summary, sorting, and collection into the volumes from more than half century of my practice experience and around 20 years of experimental researches; these scientific research harvest and scientific technological innovation series are all information of myself which contents are international innovation and original innovation. Some of them are advanced in international and independent innovation, all of which are the independent knowledge property.

These contents match the transferring medicine contents. Our scientific research in the 28 peroid are from clinical-----experimentals-----clinical -----experimental---to clinical, then come back clinical to solve the practicable clincial question. and our research models completely match this new medical and scientific models.

The content of transferring medicine: This transferring medicine develop very fast in international which promote that the patients should be center to find out and proved the questios and deeply research the basic research, then apply these basic research harvest into the clinics so that the general medical care level will increase and the patients will get the benefits.The former administrator in healthy department analyze these transferring medicine: First, transferring medicine is a subject which two directory passage; frome clinical to lab and from lab to clinics to deeply understand the disease of the mechanism of ocurrence and progress development prevention health to find out the new strategies of prevention and treatment.

Second, transferring the research scientific results into the practicable intervention method and technology and project(programs) so that they can be widely used.

The whole health organization point out: 21 century medicine should not continue the main research field on the diseases, but on the human health. Academician Chen Lian point out: healthy business model should be transferred into focusing on prevention from the treatment of large later stages of the diseases and move forward the gates of the diseases and control the diseases and to strengthen the prevention medicine research should be important projects for the global medicine models.

The transferring medicine in our country research and the modernization and internationalization of traditional medicine and traditional medications should be one of the important points of our transferring medicine research.

Acknowledgements

This book is for all of people who concern human being health. We are deep grateful to all of people who like our new ways to improve our human being health.

My daughter Lily Xu gives me many smart and creative ideas while we were finishing this book.

I would like to express our sincere gratitude to the following:

1). All of Authorhouse staffs

2). Dr. Xu Ze's family and Dr. Xu Jie's family

3). Mrs. Bo Wu's family and Mrs. Tao Wu's family: especially their daughters Chongshu Luo and Xunyue Wang

4). Medchi CEO: Gene Ransom III gives us great help

Bin Wu, M.D., Ph.D.

Part I Formed XZ-C immunomodulatory anticancer therapy theoretical system

Table of Contents

Foreword

Why do I get the title "Embark on a new way to overcome cancer"? The origin of the title is due to the guidelines and revelations from several experts, scholars, seniors and teacher letters:

Wu Min academician mentioned on July 2, 2001: "The overall impression is that the model from the clinical to the experiment and from experiments to clinical is good, taking the road of combining Chinese and Western is very correct, and sincerely wish you continue to move forward and walk out of a new way to overcome cancer."

On February 22, 2006 Tang Zhao academician mentioned: "...... Chinese medicine and biological therapy are the most promising two anti-metastasis ways, particularly in traditional Chinese medicine, I hope you get out of the characteristic antimetastatic road."

On March 22, 2006 Liuyun Yi academician said: "...... I agreed to your questions and ideas of overcoming cancer in the book very much ...... hope you make a breakthrough in Chinese medicine contribution so that the majority of patients get benefit and so that Chinese medicine develops further and our medical career can reach world levels."

January 9, 2006 Wu Xian academician mentioned: "...... tumor is hard bone to hoe, but it should continue to bite down, but fortunately we are very happy to support, only if effective, whether it is in the treatment of tumors and body, or reduce the radiation and chemical reaction" and on April 10, 2012 the letter mentioned:. "...... I think you walked out a very unique street, traditional Chinese medicine to apply formulations, methods taking medications, pharmaceutical composition, innovations of XZ-C series of drugs, developed your own patents, which should continue down this road."

We thank them for their guidance and help for our research work, scientific thinking, research objectives, research route, research guidelines, research methods. Our research work has been to follow the guidance in the direction of their efforts. In here I give my great gratitude to Wu Min, Tang Zhao, Wu Jiang Zhong, Liuyun Yi and other academicians.

Our 28 years (1985 - present) cancer research work in animal studies, clinical basic research, clinical validation has made a series of scientific and technological innovation, scientific research. After 20 years of hard work, XZ-C Immune Regulation anti-cancer therapy has formed and a new way to overcome cancer has taken out.

20 years of experimental and clinical research in this series has been enthusiastically supported and cordially guided by international renowned foreign scientists and medical dean of general surgery Qiu FaZhu academician. In 1990 when I presented "eight five" key scientific and technological project (further explore the anti-cancer herbal liver cancer, gastrointestinal cancer, cancer, experimental and clinical studies of anti-metastatic precancerous lesions on) application to China Science and Technology department, Academician Qi gave instructions on expert advice: "Study how to prevent cancer metastasis and metastasis is currently a very important topic, the experimental study to investigate prevention methods in clinical practice is feasible, is beneficial to the people's work." Under the influence and guidance of my teacher Qiu Fazhu's rigorous scientific study style, we completed the initial project work above, hereby express my gratitude.

Scientific literature must have nutritional feeding. In 1986 when we have just established a legitimate animal model experimental surgical laboratory to manufacture cancer metastasis experimental research, we read Professor Gao Jin's book "invasion and metastasis - basic research and clinical", read Tang Zhao academician monograph "HCC metastasis, basic and clinical recurrence," which theories of two books make us suddenly understanding, also encouraged and facilitated our experimental work and clinical verification from the other sides. Professor Tang Zhaoyou in his monograph that read: "The next important goal of primary liver cancer study - Prevention of recurrence and metastasis," and said: "The transfer of further recurrence has become a bottleneck to improve the survival rate of liver cancer, is the most important fight against cancer One of the difficulties." This theoretical literature has given us to update thinking, innovative wisdom and courage, but also strengthened the confidence and determination of our experimental group work. In here I gave Tang Zhao academician and Professor Gao Jin my extend gratitude.

For seven years, we used more than 6000 tumor-bearing animal models one after another to explore a fundamental problem. Selecting 200 kinds of Chinese herbal flavor carried by tumor-bearing animal model experiments in vivo anti-tumor screening were completed by my graduates such as Dr. Zhu Siping master, Dr. Zou

Shaomin, Dr. Li Zhengxun Master, Master Dr.Liu Liling, etc., who conducted and completed a lot of painstaking experimental work. Hard work! day and night! they made a contribution to prevent the development of cancer tumor experiments. Here are my sincere thanks.

1. Cancer Therapy concepts

Summary:

1) Traditional concept is that cancer cells keep dividing and proliferation and its treatment goal must be to kill cancer cells so that traditional concept of cancer therapeutics is based on killing cancer cells. In order to achieve cure, it must be to kill the last cancer cell so that people used to expand operations, intensive chemotherapy and radical radiotherapy, but the results are not satisfactory.

2) New model of cancer therapy is that: cure should be regulated, not by killing. The last step of cure of cancer cells should be to mobilize action to control the reproduction of the host, rather than the elimination of the last of the cancer cells.

1. Traditional concept of therapeutic cancer

Traditional therapeutic concepts believe that cancer is that cancer cells keep dividing and proliferating and the treatment goal must be to kill cancer cells. Therefore, the traditional goal of three treatments are based on killing cancer cells.

The principle of current cancer therapeutics is based on the following precondition: in order to achieve the goal of heal, it is necessary to kill or eliminate the last cancer cells. As a result, people adopt the expanded operation and strengthen chemotherapy and radical radiotherapy. However, the curative effects are not so satisfying. At the beginning of 1960s, the extent of surgical operation on tumor tended toward expansion and a series of super-radical operations had been developed. Subsequently, it has been proven by the practice for years that the expansion of extent of surgical removal of the cancer cells, such as breast cancer, lung cancer, liver cancer and pancreatic cancer, has not improved the cancer-free survival time and total survival time. In 1980s, the one receiving intensive chemotherapy and radical radiotherapy could not achieve the improvement of survival quality or elongation of survival time. Since the hematopiesis function and immunologic function of the bone marrow are seriously restricted, some complications endangering the life are coming out. Therefore, it is necessary to establish a new mode to probe into the cancer, strive for opening a new way and renew the concept from the clinical and experimental data.

To sum up, the concept of traditional cancer therapeutics holds the tumor is based on the maniac division and proliferation of the cells, so the cancer cells are the arch criminal, as a result, the target of the treatment goal of the traditional cancer therapeutics is the cancer cell, namely killing-off of the cancer cells.

2. A new concept in cancer therapy

Cure should be through regulation, not by killing

The assumptive new mode of cancer therapeutics includes some new examples and its predominant idea holds that cancer is a kind of disease, the regulation and signal transmission among the cells are disrupted instead of loss and the carcinogenesis is a continuous entity with possibility of reversion.

The understanding of the cancer by the new mode is based on information transfer and regulation and control. It is convinced that the canceration is a process of evolvement step by step, however, it holds that they may be potentially reversed. The new model of cancer believed: heal should be adopted through regulation and non-destruction.

It is indicated by the clinical and experimental experience that the tumor keeps a certain response relation with the host. When the tumor results from the unbalance of regulation and control instead of the autonomy of the tumor, some clinical phenomena can be easily understood. Clinically, it is known by us that the cancer cells can make adaptative response to the environment of the host at high level. The long-term application of immunosuppressant may induce the tumor, when the immunosuppressant is suspended, the tumor can be entirely released. Although the factors inducing the tumor have not been proven, the reaction of host determines the final results. The kidney transplantation tumor with metastasis to the lung will be entirely released after suspension of the antirejection therapy. It looks as if the pregnancy improves the relation between the tumor and the host. Now people have focused on killing the tumor, developed so many therapeutic methods and developed many anti-cancer cytotoxic drugs in the past half a century, however, they cannot prevent the attack and metastasis of tumor.

Viewed from the data, the cytotoxic drugs as the assistant of radiotherapy after operation also cannot prevent the reoccurrence and metastasis of the cancer because most of them severely inhibit the immunity even the non-immunological part of the host reaction. When people increase the concentration and dosage of the chemotherapeutic drugs to make them more aggressive to the cancer cells (such as intensified radiotherapy), we right lead the mechanism of long-term survival or healing to the more dangerous way, even bring about the artificial or iatrogenic immunologic function breakdown.

Viewed from molecular biology, the cancer results from the change in DNA structure. It is the unbalanced differentiation of the cells caused by the genetic information that introduces the normal nucleic acid to the cancer cells via the genetic engineering, inducing the tumor cells to differentiate to the normal cells. Shanghai Tumor Research Institute had extracted RNA from the normal hepatic cells, then incubated and cultivated it together with the liver cancer cells to correct the abnormal genetic activities of the liver cancer cells through the regulation and control reaction of normal liver RNA so as to make it reversed to the normal cells. The scientists now are looking for the bioactive substances related to the genetic information, for example, the normal mRNA can induce the cancer cells to reverse to the normal cells.

The precondition of adopting the cytotoxic drugs to treat the tumor is the understanding that the it is not only possible but also necessary to kill the last cancer cell until it is proven by the clinic application and the lab that the tumor has been entirely eliminated, as is the prerequisite of healing the patient suffering from the tumor. However, according to our experience over 20 years, this argumentation is contradictory. Some clinical cases show that killing can shrink or subside the tumor, however, it cannot directly heal the tumor. Although the dosage of cytotoxic drug is increased and most of the cancer cells are subsided, the survival rate of the patient is not improved. Soon after, it will reoccur and the tumor will be enlarged.

All the obviously healed patients do not seem to adopt the mode of killing the cancer cells. For example, the treatment of tumor with platinum-based drug seems to be related to the induced cell differentiation. The action of interferon and interleukin to the sensitive cells is realized by the regulation and control mechanism. As to the levamisole as the adjuvant for carcinoma of large intestine, it is deemed that its effects are from the change in host reaction.

We had tried out best to kill the cancer cells to treat the cancer before, however, no great achievements had been made. Later, enlarged radical operation, intensified chemotherapy and radical radiotherapy were adopted. However, the results were not ideal and they could not improve the survival quality of the patient suffering from cancer and the survival time of the patient suffering from cancer after operation.

In the recent 50 years, the treatment of cancer by traditional Chinese medicine has made great achievements. A large number of data indicate that the cancer cells can coexist with the host and they may not always damage the host. In the recent 16 years, among 12000 patients suffering from metaphase and advanced cancer treated by Shuguang Tumor Research Institute and Wuchang Shuguang Tumor Special Clinic, some reoccurrence and metastasis patients, such as the patients with anastomotic stoma reoccurrence cancer and gastric carcinoma that cannot be ablated or treated through radiotherapy and chemotherapy, after taking Z-C medicine for a long time over 3-5 years, the conditions are controlled and stabilized, they can survive with tumor (coexist with the tumor) and take care of themselves, the survival quality is good and the survival quality is obviously prolonged.

It is deemed by us that undoubtedly we should kill the foreigners invading the body, however, as to the cancer cells, we shall make a differential treatment just because they are only the variant tissues in the normal body of the host, here we reaffirm that the cancer shall be treated through regulating the control over them by the mechanism instead of the necessary and impossible killing-off of all cancer cells.

Since we have a new cognition of the cancer concept, then, the concept of cancer therapeutics shall renew the thought, the understanding and the concepts and innovate the therapeutic theory and technology.

In view of the experience and lessons of the author over half a century, now we should research the urgent problems in the current cancer study, seek for the breakthrough for clinical research from the weak link of the modern medicine and find the breakthrough of prevention and control from the invasion, reoccurrence and metastasis, look for the anti-reoccurrence and anti-metastasis drugs from the chemical drugs and the natural herbs and deepen the new understanding of the cancer concept at the molecular level, genetic level, integrated treatment level and targeted treatment.

2. Cancer etiology and pathogenesis

Thymic atrophy, immune dysfunction may be one of the etiology and pathogenesis of cancer

This lab has made a series of experimental study on animal to probe into the pathogenic factors and pathophysiology of cancer. Through analyzing and reflecting the results of experimental study, we obtain new findings, new thinking and new enlightenments: one of the pathogenic factors may be thymus atrophy, damaged thymus function and inferior immunologic function. Therefore, Professor Xu Ze initiated that one of the pathogenic factors may be thymus atrophy, damaged function of central immune organ, inferior immunologic function, inferior immunological surveillance and immunologic escape.

1. Cancer etiology, pathogenesis and pathophysiology of experimental research discoveries

Nearly 16 years the author conducted a series of animal studies to search for the etiology, pathogenesis and pathophysiology of cancer, to explore mechanism of cancer invasion, recurrence, metastasis, and to find effective measures to control.

Experimental Surgery is extremely important in the development of medical science and is a key to open the box medicine. Many diseases control methods are achieved after many experiments the stability of the results of animal studies only after clinical application. So, I established Experimental Surgery Laboratory conducting experiments in cancer research, cancer cell transplant purposes, establishing tumor animal model, carrying out the following series of experiments in cancer research: ① to explore the experimental study of cancer etiology, pathogenesis and pathophysiology; ② To explore mechanisms and laws of cancer recurrence, metastasis; ③ investigate the relationship between the tumor and immune and immune organs and between immune organs and tumor; ④ To investigate method of curbing tumor progression, progressive atrophy of immune organs and of immune reconstitution; ⑤ looking for effective measures of regulating cancer invasion, recurrence and metastasis.

From cancer experimental research the author and his colleagues conducted a full four-year experimental cancer research in order to explore the cancer etiology, pathogenesis, invasion, metastasis mechanism to find the regulation, intervention invasion, recurrence, metastasis and effective measures.

Experiment 1: this lab excises thymus (TH) and establishes the cancer-bearing animal model.It is proven by the study conclusions: the occurrence and development of the cancer has remarkably affirmative relation with the thymus of the immune organ of the host and its functions.

Experiment 2: Does the inferior immune lead to the cancer or the cancer lead to the inferior immune at all? Our experimental results: the inferior immune leads to the occurrence and development of the cancer, without the descent of immunologic function, it is not easy to realize the successful inoculation. It is suggested by the experimental results: improving and maintaining the good immunologic function and protecting the good thymus of the central immune organ are the important measures for preventing the occurrence of cancer.

Experiment 3: in studying the relation between the metastasis of cancer and the immune, this lab establishes animal models for liver metastatic carcinoma, which are divided into two groups including Group A applied with immune depressant and Group B not applied with immune depressant. Results: the metastatic lesions in the liver in Group A are obviously more than the ones in Group B. It is suggested by the experimental results: metastasis is related to the immune and inferior immunologic function or application of immune depressant may promote the tumor metastasis.

Experiment 4: When making experiments to probe into the effects of tumor on immune organ, this lab finds that the thymus meets with progressive atrophy with the advance of the cancer. The thymus of the host meets with the acute progressive atrophy after the cancer cells are inoculated, the cell proliferation is prevented and the volume is obviously shrunk. It is suggested by the experimental results: the tumor may inhibit the thymus, resulting in the atrophy of the immune organ.

Experiment 5: we also find through experiment that if some experimental mice are not successfully inoculated or the tumor is very small, the thymus is not obviously shrunk. In order to understand the relation between the tumor and the atrophy of the thymus, we excise the transplanted solid tumor of one group of mice when it grows up to the size of a thumb. After one month, through anatomy, we find the thymus does not meet with progressive atrophy again. Therefore, it is inferred by us that maybe the solid tumor produces one kind of unknown factor to inhibit the thymus, which shall be further studied through experiment.

Experiment 6: it is proven by the above-mentioned experimental results: the advance of the tumor makes the thymus meet with progressive atrophy, then, can we take some measures to prevent the atrophy of the thymus of the host? Therefore, we further perfect the design to seek for the method or drug to prevent the atrophy of the thymus of the cancer-bearing mice through the experimental study on animal. So we make the experimental study to recover the function of the immune organ through cell transplantation of the immune organ. We discuss the atrophy of the thymus of the immune organ in preventing the advance of tumor, seek for the method to recover the functions of the thymus and reconstruct the immune, carry out the cell transplantation of foetal liver, spleen and thymus with the mice and establish the immunologic function through adoptive immunity. It is shown by the results: through the joint transplantation of three groups of cells, namely S, T and L, the entire extinction rate of the tumor in the long term is 46.67% and the one with the entire extinction of the tumor get a long survival life.

Experiment 7: in the experiment to probe into the effects of tumor on the immune organ such as spleen, we find: the spleen can inhibit the growth of the tumor in the early stage of the tumor, however, in the late stage, the spleen meets with the progressive atrophy. It is suggested by the study results: the effects of spleen on the growth of the tumor are embodied into bi-direction, in the early stage, it can inhibit the tumor to a certain extent, however, in the late stage, it fails to inhibit the tumor. The cell transplantation of the spleen can enhance the role of inhibiting the tumor.

Experiment 8: it is suggested by the results of the follow-up survey: control over the metastasis is the key to cancer treatment. Now it is well known that the cancer cell metastasis has multiple steps and links. In order to try to interrupt one link so as to prevent the metastasis, we consider the formation of the regenerative blood vessel of tumor is one of the links in which the metastatic cancer cells can nidate, root and grow into the cancer node or not. In 1986, this lab was making the microcirculation study and we observed the formation of the blood capillary of transplanted tumor node of cancer-bearing mice and its flow rate and flow with the micro-circle microscope; then we tried to seek for the drugs for prevention of the formation of the tumor blood vessel from the natural herbs, observed the formation process of the regenerative blood vessel with Olympus micro-circle microscope photograph system and counted the flow rate and flow of the arteriole and venule, found Common Threewingnut Root acetic ether extract (TG) from the traditional Chinese herbs and carried out the blood vessel inhibition test. It was found from the results: in the first day of inoculation there was no regenerative blood vessel and in the second day it was found that the fine micro regenerative blood vessel grew up. TG can reduce the density of the regenerative blood capillary of the tumor.

Experiment 9: we also found from a large batch of tumor-bearing animal models in the lab that the more the hypodermically inoculated solid tumor of some cancer-bearing experimental mice, the more different the cancer cells of the central tissue of the transplanted solid tumor from the peripheral cancer cells. The center of the node is mostly aseptically necrosed or liquefied its periphery is still surrounded with active cancer cells. Therefore, in the clinical treatment, we adopted the measures to treat the aseptic necroses.

2. Discussion methods of preventing cancer progression and thymic atrophy and of rebuilding the immune function

One of the etiology and pathogenesis of tips from the experimental study is that cancer may be thymus atrophy, thymocyte proliferation is blocked, the thymus dysfunction, immune dysfunction, resulting in immune escape of malignant cells.

Now that along with the progress of the tumor, thymus atrophy occurs, then how to prevent thymus from shrinking? Through animal studies we looked for the way or drugs to prevent mice thymus atrophy and eventually adopted immune organs cell transplantation to restore the immune organs, and achieved exciting results.

In 1986, I got enlightened from the discussion in the satellite meeting of one international micro-circulation academic conference to seek for the micro-circulation drug from the natural herbs and then transplanted the adoptive immune from the biological cells to reconstruct the immune and then sought for a kind of drug from the natural herbs of traditional Chinese herbs that can activate the cytokine, enhance the immunological surveillance, inhibit the tumor and prevent the atrophy of the thymus. All drugs must be subject to the animal experiment and clinical verification, as a result, we made the cancer-bearing animal model and made the in vivo tumor-inhibiting screening experiment on the cancer-bearing animal with over 200 kinds of natural traditional Chinese herbs one by one. Results: the anti-cancer immune-regulating TCM with relatively good tumor-inhibiting rate had been screened. From experimental screening to clinical observation and verification and then to further screening and concentration from the angle of immunopharmacology of TCM, we prepared XZ-C1-10 medicine, which can promote the thymus hyperplasia, prevent the thymus atrophy, improve the immune, protect the bone marrow and promote the function of lymphocyte T and cytokine, with relatively high tumor-inhibiting rate. XZ-C1-10 medicine only inhibits and kills the cancer cells, does not affect the normal cells and can be used for oral administration for a long time. Since cancer is a kind of chronic disease, the division, proliferation and clone of the cancer cells is a long, sustainable and progressive process, so it's better to select the orally administered traditional Chinese herbs with long-term curative effects, without toxin and with slow release. The treatment of cancer with traditional Chinese herbs is carried out after the pathogenic factors are judged on the human body. It shall kill the cancer cells as well as improve the immunologic functions of the organism as well so as to strengthen the anti-cancer capability of the organism, as a result, some refractory cancer with wide metastasis can be controlled, the life of the patient is prolonged, the pain of the patient is reduced, which opens up a new way to further probe into the treatment of the cancer.

Therefore, based on the enlightenment from the study results of a series of animal study regarding pathogenic factors and pathophysiology of the cancer by this lab, we put forward: that thymus resection leads immunologic deficiency, then leads descent of immunological surveillance ad immunologic escape may be one of the pathogenic factors of the cancer and one key of the pathogenesis. It is the new progress of tumor theory in 21st century, offering direction and basis to the cancer therapeutics in 21st century and offering theoretical basis and experimental basis of the immune regulation and control targeted therapy of the cancer. The new finding, enlightenment and thinking is the original innovation and it has not been mentioned in the textbooks and literatures at home and abroad.

One of the pathogenic factors mentioned above by us may be the thymus atrophy and the inferior immunologic function. In case that this new theory and hypothesis is argued and recognized, it will lead to a series of reform and innovation of cancer therapeutics, for example, the reform and innovation of the cognition of cancer therapeutic concept, the reform and innovation of cognition of cancer treatment objective or target; the one of cancer diagnostic procedure and curative effect judgment standard, the one of cancer treatment way and treatment mode and the one of research and development of anti-metastasis drug.

3. Theoretical and experimental evidence of cancer treatment

XZ-C immunomodulatory therapy of protecting thymus and increasing the immune function

Since our study found that the results of laboratory experiments were that thymus was progressive atrophy, and central immune organs were dysfunction, immune function decreased and immune surveillance was low in cancer-bearing mice so the treatment principle must be to prevent thymus atrophy, to promote thymic hyperplasia, to protect bone marrow function, to improve immune surveillance and to control malignant cells immune escape.

Based on the above revelation about cancer etiology, pathogenesis of experimental results, a new theory of XZ-C immunomodulatory therapy and new methods are put forward. The author confirms that treatment principle of protecting thymus and increasing immune function are reasonable and the efficacy is satisfactory after 16 years of cancer clinical verification in more than 12,000 advanced cancer patients.

XZ-C (XU ZE China) immunomodulatory therapy is first proposed by Professor Xu Ze in 2006 in his monograph "New concepts and new methods of treating cancer metastasis," which he believes under normal circumstances, the body's defense was in a dynamic equilibrium between host and cancer; cancer occurs while this dynamic balance was lost. If the state has been adjusted to offset the normal level, it can control cancer growth and make it subside.

As we all know, the incidence of cancer development and prognosis depends on the comparison of two factors, namely, the biological characteristics of cancer cells and the defense capability of cancer cells in host organism itself, such as the balance between the cancer and host which can be controlled. If both are imbalance, the cancer will develop.

Under normal circumstances, the host organism itself against cancer cells have a certain capacity of constraints; but in cancer these constraints are subject to different levels of defense suppression and damage so as to lead to the loss of the immune surveillance of cancer cells, immune escape occurred and to further develop cancer cells and metastasis.

1. Animal experiments revelation

It is found by this lab that the cancer-bearing rats are confronted with the progressive atrophia and damage to the central immune organ, which shall be protected to protect the thymus so as to improve the immunity.

Based on the above-mentioned enlightenment from the results of experimental study on the pathogenic factor and pathogenesis of carcinomatosis by this lab, the new theory and new ways of XZ-C targeted therapeutics of immunity regulation and control initiated by Professor Xu Ze have the theoretical and experimental basis because the findings from the experimental study by this lab indicate that the cancer-bearing rats are confronted with progressive atrophia, damage to the central immune organ, descent of immunologic function and inferior immunological surveillance, so its curative principles shall be based on prevention of progressive athophia, promotion of thymus hyperplasia, improvement of immunity, protection of hematopiesis function of bone marrow, improvement of immunological surveillance and control over the immunologic escape of the canceration cells.

As is now well known, the immune organs include the central immune organs and peripheral immune organ, the former includes the thymus and the bone marrow and the latter includes the spleen and the lymph node. It is validated by the literature and the work in this lab that when the cancer comes, the tumor will produce a factor inhibiting the immune organ, which is temporarily called thymus-inhibiting factor by us and inhibits the thumus, causing the thymus to be progressively atrophic and inhibiting the functions of the central immune organ, in this way, the immunologic function descends and the immunological surveillance of the tumor is lost or weakened, resulting in the further progress of the tumor.

Therefore, the therapeutic theory of the curative principles of thymus protection for immunity improvement and bone marrow protection for hematogenesis initiated by us is reasonable and scientific and has the theoretical and experimental basis. The clinical verification and observation of over 12000 patients suffering from metaphase and advanced cancer in Shuguang Tumor Special Clinic over 16 years, has indicated that the curative principle of thymus protection for immunity improvement and bone marrow protection for hematogenesis initiated, clinically verified, observed by us over 16 years through clinical application is correct and reasonable and the curative effects are satisfying and worth of the patients' confidence.

XZ-C therapeutics of immunity regulation and control was initiated by Professor Xu Ze in 2006 in his monograph New Concept and New Way of Treatment of Cancer

Metastasis. He holds that the cancer and the defense of the organism are in the dynamic balance in the normal conditions and the occurrence and development of the carcinomatosis is caused by the disturbance of the dynamic balance. If the disturbed state can be artificially regulated to the normal state, it can control the growth of cancer and subside the cancer.

As is now well known, occurrence, progress and development and treatment prognosis of the cancer are determined by the contrast of two factors: biological characteristics of the cancer cells and the inhibition and defensive capability of the host organism to the cancer cells, if both of them are in balance, the cancer can be controlled; otherwise, the cancer will advance.

Under the normal conditions, the host organism has a certain capability in inhibiting the cancer cells, however, the inhibition and defensive capabilities are suppressed and damaged to different extent, resulting in the loss of the immunological surveillance and the immunologic escape of the cancer cells, leading to development and metastasis of the cancer cells.

2. The human body has a complete set of anti-cancer immune system and it shall be protected, regulated and activated.

In probing into the curative principle of cancer, we should research which anti-cancer immunological cell line, which anti-cancer cell sub-line, which anti-cancer gene system and which humoral immunity system exists in the human body so as to strengthen the anti-cancerometastasis.

1. Which anti-cancer immunological cells in the human body may be activated and strengthened so as to realize the anti-cancerometastasis? The immunological cells engaged in anti-cancer in the human body include:

(1) Cytotoxic lymphocyte (CTL): it plays a primary role in anti-tumor immunity, CTL in the human body includes CD_3 and CD_8, and CTL has a high content in peripheral blood and spleen and a certain content in thoracic duct, thymus and bone marrow. Under a certain condition, it can produce IL-2, IL-4 and IFN to activate other anti-cancer immunological cells and lethal macrophages, NK cells and lethal B cells to jointly exert the anti-tumor role.

(2) Natural killer cell (NK cell) with the anti-tumor role: NK cells are a group of broad spectrum anti-cancer cells. They do not rely on the antibody or the thymus to kill the

activity and their main role is to surveil and remove the canceration cells in the human body. It is found by the clinical observance that the ones with activity insufficiency of NK have obviously increased incidence rate of malignant tumor. NK cells are an important part in the organism with anti-cancer immunological surveillance function in the early stage.

(3) LAK cells: LAK cells are the most important cancer cells in the modern biological therapeutics and peripheral mononuclear cells in the human body can remarkably kill so many kinds of tumor cells in the human body with the induction of IL-2. LAK cells have a wider anti-cancer spectrum than NK cells while LAK cells can kill the tumor cells that cannot be killed by NK cells.

(4) Macrophage (MO): it plays an important role in anti-tumor immunity in the human body.

2. Which anti-cancer cytokine in the human body may be activated and strengthened so as to realize the anti-cancerometastasis? The anti-cancerometastasis cytokines engaged in anti-cancer in the human body include:

(1) Interferon (IFN): it has the function of anti-cell differentiation and immunoloregulation. It plays a role in anti-proliferation of some tumor cells and its anti-cancer role may be related to the immunoloregulation. It can strengthen the activity of NK cells and MO.

(2) Interleukin-2 (IL-2): this kind of lymphocyte is a kind of T-cell growth factor, with strong function of regulating intrinsic immunity. It can promote the activation of T-cells, NK cells and monocytes as well as the release of INF-a and TNF.

(3) Tumor necrosis factor: its role in cell is the cell toxicant role and it can affect the micrangium of the tumor, resulting in the necrosis of the central portion of the tumor.

In recent years, with the rapid development of molecular biology, molecular immunology, molecular immunological pharmacology and gene engineering, the foundation of molecular level of "anti-cancer organ" and the clinical study are continuously expanded and deepened, its outlook of anti-cancerometastasis is very attracting.

At present, the study on immunotherapy of anti-cancer molecular biology is mainly centralized on "four sub-systems" of "anti-cancer organ", namely "anti-cancer cellular therapy", "anti-cancer cytokine therapy", "anti-cancer gene therapy" and "anti-cancer anti-body therapy".

The basic characteristics of these molecular biological and immunological therapies are as follows: all pharmaceutics of molecular biological and immunological therapies are the inherent substances in the organism and fundamental differences from radiotherapy and chemotherapy are: it has no progressive damage to the normal histiocytes of the organism, especially the cells and the functions of the immune system and the structure and the function of the hemopoietic system of the bone marrow and plays a role in regulation and reinforcement of immunological reaction. As is now well known, radiotherapy and chemotherapy are entirely different from it, the chemotherapy is a kind of non-selective traumatic therapy, killing the cancer cells as well as the normal cells at the same time, which damage the normal histiocytes of the organism, resulting in severe damage to the hemopoietic system and the immunological structure and function, with the severe consequence.

The biotherapy is a kind of therapy stabilizing and balancing the vital mechanism by means of the regulation on biologic reaction. The American scholar Oldham (1984) initiated biological regulation and mediation (BRM) theropy and then initiated the concept of tumor biotherapy based on the therapy.

3. Overview of Study on Similar BRM Anti-cancer Regulation and Control Medicine

Through study on animal experiments by us for 4 years and the clinical verification by the tumor special clinic over 16 years, it is indicated that XZ-C medicine has the roles and curative effects similar to BRM and it is screened from the traditional Chinese herb resources with role similar to BRM.

XZ-C medicine is screened from 200 kinds of traditional Chinese herbs through experiments by Professor Xu Ze (ZU ZE-China, Z-C) in the lab. Firstly, we adopt the culture in vitro of cancer cells and screen 200 kinds of traditional Chinese herbs in vitro one by one, observe the experimental study on the direct damage to the cancer cells in the culture tube by each drug and make the check experiment on tumor-inhibiting rate between the chemotherapy drug CTX and the control group of normal cells in the culture tube. Finally, we select a batch of herbs with a certain tumor-inhibiting rate of proliferation of cancer cells. Then we further establish the tumor-bearing animal model and carry out the experimental study on the 200 kinds of traditional Chinese herbs for the in vivo tumor-inhibiting rate of the tumor-bearing animal model and screen, analyze and evaluate the herbs scientifically, objectively and strictly one by one. It is proven by the results that only 48 kinds of herbs have relatively good tumor-inhibiting rate and another 152 kinds of traditional Chinese herbs are the traditional Chinese herbs commonly used by the herbalist doctors, through experimental screening of tumor-inhibiting rate in vivo by the tumor-bearing experiment, it is proven that they have no anti-cancer role or the tumor-inhibiting rate is very slight.

The screening by this lab is mainly the in vivo tumor-inhibiting experiment of the tumor-bearing animal model. The in vivo chronic experiment on every traditional Chinese herb is observed by one experimental group for 3 months, after screening, 48 kinds of traditional Chinese herbs are selected and then 2 and 3 kinds of dried medicinal herbs are arranged in groups to carry out the tumor-bearing experiments in vivo on the tumor-bearing animal and then it is found by us that the tumor-inhibiting effect of a single dried medicinal herb is not better than the one of the dried medicinal drug compound through tumor-inhibiting experiments. It seems that the single dried medicinal herb only play a role in inhibiting the proliferation of the tumor while the dried medicinal herb compound can inhibit the proliferation of the tumor-bearing rats and play a role in regulating and controlling the organism, enhancing the physical power, improving the immunity, promoting the generation of tumor-inhibiting cytokines, protecting the normal cells and promoting the anti-cancer cytokines as well.

Based on the screening of the single traditional herbs through the in vitro experiments and the tumor-inhibiting experiment screening on the tumor-bearing animal model over 4 years, through experimental optimization and combination and then experiment, this lab finally recombines Z-C$_{1-10}$ compound of anti-cancer, anti-metastasis and anti-reoccurrence through immunity regulation and control and finally it is subject to the clinical verification. Since 1992, we have established the cooperation group to carry out the clinical verification. Up to today from then on, through the clinical verification and observation of over 12000 patients suffering from the cancer in Shuguang Tumor Special Clinic over 16 years, the condition has been stable and improved, the symptom has been improved, the survival quality has been improved and the survival time has been obviously prolonged. So the lesions of many patients suffering from metastasis have been stabilized and have not further spread, as to some patients after operation cannot receive the chemotherapy due to the descent of leucocytes, the metastasis has been controlled after taking the medicine and no metastasis occurs again. Good curative effects have been obtained.

4. Similar BRM Functions and Effects of XZ-C Medicine

Biological response modifier (BRM) is first put forward by Oldham in 1982 to describe BRM. It refers to the ability of regulating the organism's response or reply to surface "attack" by biological response modifier.

The cells and humoral factors of the organism's immunity system are under subtle control, the organism's ability of response or reply will be affected significantly in case of imbalance. Biological response modifier is used to restore the unbalanced organism to normal balance, fulfilling the purpose of preventing diseases.

BRM opened the new field for biological treatment of tumor. At present, BRM is widely recognized in the medical circle as the fourth model of tumor treatment.

BRM is designed to regulate the immunologic function of the organism and restore the function of immune system of the contained organism. Such drug has manifold function mechanisms, but all of them exert regulating functions by activating the organism's immune system.

Biological response modifiers, most of which drive from microorganisms and plants, were previously referred to as immunopotentiator, immunostimulant, immunologic cordial or immunomodulator, now collectively named as biological response modulator or modifier(BRM).

The author screened out XZ-C medicine with good inhibition rate through in vivo experiment on mice inoculated with tumor. It has the functions of improving immunity, protecting centrum immune organ thymus, improve cellular immunity, protecting thymus tissue, protecting hematogenesis of bone marrow, increasing the number of akaryocyte and leukocyte, activate immunologic cytokine, the main pharmacological action of XZ-C improving the immunological surveillance in blood is protecting thymus and improving immunity. 48 types of immunologic drugs with high inhibition rate are screened out by four-year animal experiment, among which 26 types are identified through immune and cytokine level detection as capable of enhancing phagocytic function, or enhancing cellular immunity, or enhancing humoral immunity, or enhancing thymus weight, or promoting proliferation of bone marrow cells, or enhancing T cell function, or enhancing LAK cytoactive; or inhibiting blood platelet coagulation and resisting embolus; or resisting tumor poison and metastasis; or removing free radical. The anticancer mechanism of the above XZ-C medicine is:

Activating the organism's immunocyte system, promoting the enhancement of the host's defense mechanism and effect, achieving the capacity of immune response to cancer.

Activating immune cytokine system of anticancer mechanism of the organism, enhancing the host's immune defense mechanism and improving immunological surveillance of immunocyte of the organism's blood circulation system.

Protecting thymus and improving immunity, protecting bone marrow for hematogenesis, stimulating hematogenesis of bone marrow, promoting recovery of marrow inhibition, increasing leukocyte and akaryocyte.

Mitigating toxicant and side effects of chemotherapy and radiotherapy, enhancing the endurance of the host.

Cancer progress is caused by imbalance between biological characteristics of cancer cells and the organism's pharmaceutical capacity for cancer, XZ-C medicine is used to improve immunity and make them regain balance.

Regulating directly the growth and differentiation of tumor cells.

Increase the volume and weight of thymus, keeping thymus from progressive atrophy, for thymus will go through progressive atrophy when cancer evolves.

Stimulating the host's immune response to anticancer, enhancing the organism's anticancer ability, strengthening the sensitivity of cancer cells to the organism's anticancer mechanism, favorable for killing cancer cells on the way of metastasis.

XZ-C medicine can enable the host to make powerful immune response to cancer cells, achieving the purpose of treating cancer. XZ-C medicine can trigger the following immune responses of the host: enhancing regulation or restoring the host's immune response to tumors; stimulating inherent immunologic functions of the host, activating the host's immune defense system; restoring immunologic functions.

As described above, XZ-C medicine has similar function mechanism to BRM, can have the same treatment effects with BRM in clinic application.

4. Cancer treatment principles

> Theory guides clinic: carry out the treatment in an all-round way aiming at the cancer cells and the host synchronously.

Cancer treatment should change their concepts to establish a comprehensive treatment concept. I believe that cancer treatment should overcome the current one-sided treatment concept targeted only killing cancer cells and change concepts to establish a comprehensive treatment concept. Traditional therapies target alone and only kill cancer cells, but ignore the host itself constrain cancer cells. Therefore, while we advocate the establishment of a comprehensive concept of treatment focus on both tumors and the hosts. It is necessary to establish a new treatment model in order to obtain better therapeutic effect.

After pondering the author presents the impact of cancer occurrence and development of the "Theory of Balance" concept.

If the only goal of cancer treatment to kill cancer cells, but for one aspect, for one-sided treatment, it is impossible to overcome cancer. The goal of treatment should be for both host and cancer cells, both kill cancer cells and protect the host to enhance immune function and to protect thymus, to nurse marrow and blood, and enhance the host ability to anti-cancer, which is the concept of comprehensive treatment, will be possible to overcome cancer.

How to build a comprehensive concept of cancer treatment?

The goal of cancer comprehensive treatment concept is on both tumor and host which the scheme of the clinical treatment of cancer should be on cancer research from both cancer biological characteristics and the response of host organism.

(1) Must pay attention to a set of inherent human anticancer systems which should fully play its role in the immune system, enhancing immune surveillance and preventing escape of malignant cells.

(2) While chemotherapy is used, improving the immune function of the host should be done. To kill cancer cells cannot simply rely on chemotherapy drugs, but must also rely

on the body's cancer-fighting ability to destroy residual cancer cells after chemotherapy because of the limited ability of cytotoxic chemotherapy to kill cancer cells.

1) Time of chemotherapy e is limited and transient effects and time which patients administered chemotherapy to kill cancer cells is only effective about 1-5 days of intravenous injection and its role is to kill cancer cells, which it's just short Time to kill me (1-5 days) and not "once and for all". After 5 days the cancer continues to divide and to proliferate. While chemotherapy ends, efficacy will disappear so it can only relieve short-term improvement in a few weeks, after which you must also rely on the host immune function of cancer-fighting ability.

2) Chemotherapy is "double-edged sword" which is not only to kill cancer cells but also to kill the host bone marrow hematopoietic cells, to decline boost the immune function; therefore, while chemotherapy is used, host immune function must be protected, restored or enhanced.

3) After radiotherapy and chemotherapy cancer cells continue to divide and to proliferate, to clone so that the host need to rely on its own anticancer ability to suppress tumor long-term growth.

Since radiotherapy and chemotherapy all contribute to decreased immune function, therefore, I propose radiotherapy or chemotherapy, should be used with simultaneously immunotherapy, biotherapy, XZ-C immunomodulatory anti-cancer traditional Chinese medicine which is reformed into immunotherapy and chemotherapy and/or immunotherapy and radiotherapy.

(3) Improve the host immune function to inhibit tumor progression. Treatment of cancer in the short term is to rely on chemotherapy drugs to kill cancer cells; in the long term it should rely on the host's immune function, immune surveillance to destroy the remaining cancer cells so that the concept of a comprehensive treatment must enhance host immune function to inhibit tumor progression.

> Professor Xu Ze holds: the treatment of cancer shall get rid of the one-sided treatment outlook of simply killing the cancer cells and we should update the idea, change the concept and establish the treatment outlook in an all-round way. Since the cancer is opposite to the cancer cells and the host, the impaired anti-cancer force of host leads to the occurrence and development of the tumor while the intensive anti-cancer force of the host can control the development of the cancer, just like

the "teeter-totter", as one falls, another rise. Therefore, the treatment of cancer is not only to kill the cancer cells, but also to protect the host and does not harm the host so as to enhance the anti-cancer force of the host and establish the cancer treatment outlook in an all-round way.

I. The objective of traditional therapy is relatively simple, just to kill the cancer cells, which is only one aspect of cancer treatment.

The traditional cancer therapy holds that the cancer is the continual division and proliferation of the cells, so the cancer cells are the arch criminal. Its treatment objective must be to kill the cancer cells.Objective of chemotherapy: to kill the cancer cells, only to kill the cancer cells.

Objective of radiotherapy: to kill the cancer cells, only to kill the cancer cells.

Why the traditional therapy with the objective of simply killing the cancer cells cannot reduce the death rate? Why it cannot prevent recurrence and metastasis? Why it only can play a role in a short-term remission? Why it only can remit the cancer but cannot heat the cancer patients? Is it real that the cancer cannot be cured? Or only simple radiotherapy and chemotherapy cannot cure the cancer? What is the problem in chemotherapy and radiotherapy? What are the defects and the disadvantages? Or is the therapeutic strategy with the objective of simply killing the cancer cells wrong? Are the cancer cells killed in chemotherapy? How many cancer cells are killed? How many cancer cells are remained in the body of the patient? Whether is the chemotherapy drug sensitive or not? Whether does it have drug tolerance? All of these things are remained unknown. Whether it is presented that the traditional therapy does not conform to the actual conditions of the biological characteristics of the cancer cells? It only kills the cancer cells while ignores the host.

II. The objective of traditional therapy ignores the resistance and inhibition of the host itself to the cancer

Actually, the occurrence and development of the tumor, is dependent on the immunologic function of the host and the biological characteristics of the tumor, namely the balance between the biological characteristics of the tumor cancers and the influences of the host on the confinement factors, if both of them are balanced, it is controlled; otherwise, it will be developed.

In the past half a century, the researchers at home and abroad had been focusing on the test on cancer cells to seek the drugs to kill the cancer cells, their ideas were affected by the mode of antibiotics killing the bacteria so as to kill the cancer cells. However, they did not know that they were two entirely different things: the antibiotics only kill the bacteria install of the normal cells and they can be used to make experiments on drug susceptibility while the chemotherapy drug can kill the cancer cells as well as the normal cells, however, it cannot be used to make the experiments on drug susceptibility. **The objective of the traditional therapy only pays attention to radiotherapy and chemotherapy killing cancer cells and ignores the anti-cancer system of the host.** The human body itself has a complete set of anti-cancer cell system while radiotherapy and chemotherapy ignore the anti-cancer cells in the host (NK cell group, K cell group, LAK cell group, macrophage group and TK cell group), the reaction of anti-cancer cell sub-systems IFN, IL-1 and TNF; ignores the reaction of cancer-inhibition gene and cancer-inhibition transfer gene in the host (cancer gene and cancer-inhibition gene as well as cancer transfer gene and cancer-inhibition transfer gene exist in the human body) and ignores the reaction of nervous body fluid system and the incretion system in the host. These organs and their affectois play an important role in adjustment, balance and stabilization of the host organism. These intrinsic anti-cancer factors in the human body shall be protected and activated by all means.

III. Professor Xu Ze proposes the objective or target of cancer treatment should establish the treatment outlook in an all-round way aiming at the cancer cells and the host synchronously.

Since the traditional therapeutic mode with the objective of simply killing the cancer cells has not settle the problem in the past half a century, it is necessary to establish a new treatment mode, update the idea and open a new way.

Through deep consideration and analysis, Professor Xu Ze proposes the concept of "balance theory" affecting recurrence and development of cancer:

Biological characteristics of cancer ⎞ if both of them are balanced, it is controlled;

Restriction capability of host on it ⎠ otherwise, it will be developed

{ Therefore, the objective or target of the cancer treatment must aim at the cancer and the host.

Namely treatment of ① host---immunity---biological factor, cytokine and traditional Chinese medicine for immune regulation and control

target of cancer ② carcinoma---cancer cells---operation, radiotherapy and chemotherapy

Professor Xu Ze holds: if the treatment objective or target only kills the cancer cells, it only focuses on one side, which is unilateral. If the treatment objective or target only focuses on the immune regulation and control, it only stresses on one side, which is unilateral. The above-mentioned treatment outlook is unilateral and is not comprehensive and it is impossible to conquer the cancer. If the treatment objective or target focuses on both the host and the cancer, which can kill the cancer cells, protect the host, strengthen the immunity, protect the chest and the bone marrow, produce the blood and enhance the anti-cancer capability of the host, which is an all-round treatment outlook and it is possible to conquer the cancer.

As to the concept of current traditional therapy, the treatment objective or target only killing the cancer cells is the unilateral treatment outlook, which does not protect the anti-cancer force of the host, but damages the immunity of the host, therefore, it cannot conquer the cancer. It is necessary to establish cancer treatment outlook in an all-round way, that is to say, the objective or target is to focus on both the host and the carcinoma, which not only kills the cancer cells but also strengthen the immunity of the host, conforming to the actual conditions of the biological characteristics of cancer cells, so it is possible to conquer the cancer.

Through reviewing and reflecting the experience and lessons from clinical tumor surgery over 54 years, Professor Xu Ze holds: in order to conquer the cancer, it is necessary to simply kill the cancer cells as well as strengthen the immunity of the host to inhibit the tumor, bring the anti-cancer organ functions of the human body into play and exert their anti-cancer capability to make the anti-cancer resistance of the host stronger, in this way, it can inhibit the tumor for a long time and prevent its development to realize the cancer-bearing survival. Its treatment objective:

1. To control occurrence and development of the tumor, firstly the host shall be taken into consideration, stressing on how to strengthen the anti-cancer capability of the host to inhibit occurrence and development of the tumor.

2. Strengthen the anti-cancer force of the host to inhibit the development of the tumor so as to realize the cancer-bearing survival and prolong the survival period.

3. Try to make the anti-cancer force of the host stronger to inhibit the development of the tumor for a long time to make it stable and dormant, in this way, it will not be developed, resulting in the long-term cancer-bearing survival and becoming a chronic disease.

IV. How to establish the cancer treatment outlook in an all-round way? Stressing on killing the cancer cells as well as strengthening the anti-cancer immunity of the host

The objective or target of cancer treatment outlook in an all-round way aims at both the tumor and the host and research the clinical treatment scheme of cancer from the biological characteristics of the cancer cells and the reaction of the host organism. And then, how to realize the objective?

1. It must be made clear that the human body has a complete set of anti-cancer organ, so it is necessary to bring the reaction of the immune system into play, enhance the immune surveillance and prevent the escape of canceration cells. In fact, the radiotherapy and the chemotherapy cannot kill off all of the cancer cells, the remained cancer cells will be continually divided, proliferated and cloned in geometrical progression, such as one into two, two into four, in this way, it leads to recurrence and metastasis.

2. Radiotherapy and chemotherapy must pay attention to improvement of the immunologic functions of the host synchronously. In order to kill the cancer cells, it cannot simply rely on the chemotherapy drug, it is necessary to rely on the anti-cancer capability of the organism to eliminate the remained cancer cells, why? Because the cytotoxic drug for chemotherapy has limited capability to kill the cancer cells, in addition, the drug effect only lasts a short period.

(1) The chemotherapy reaction time is limited and momentary and the chemotherapy drug cannot kill off the cancer cells once and for ever, it only has the drug effect on killing the cancer cells in the days of intravenous injection for chemotherapy, after chemotherapy, the drug effect disappears and it has no reaction again and it only has the drug effect within 2-3 months even though the chemotherapy is made 4 times even 6 times, after that, it must rely on the anti-cancer capability of the immunologic functions of the host.

(2) The capability of chemotherapy to killing the cancer cells is limited, it cannot kill off all of the cancer cells as per the first order kinetics, it only can kill a part and another part remains again. For example, the patient suffering from acute lymphoblastic leukemia has over 10^{12} cancer cells before administration of chemotherapy drug, after treatment, there are about 10^7 cancer cells surviving, even though the dose is increased, the lethality will not be increased, subsequently, it must rely on the anti-cancer capability of the immunologic functions of the host to eliminate the remained cancer cells.

(3) The chemotherapy is a two-sided sword, which kills the cancer cells as well as the hematopoietic cells and immunological cells of the bone marrow, promoting the decrease of the immunologic function, therefore, it is necessary for the chemotherapy to recover or strength the immunologic functions of the host.

(4) After radiotherapy and chemotherapy, the remained stem cells of tumor are still continually divided, proliferated and cloned, so it is still necessary to improve the anti-cancer capability of the host to suppress the development of tumor for a long term.

Therefore, Professor Xu Ze proposes the current radiotherapy or chemotherapy should be combined with immunological therapy, biological therapy and XZ-C anti-cancer medicine for immune regulation synchronously. It is necessary to reform it to immune + chemotherapy and immune + radiotherapy.

3. How to improve the immunologic functions of the host to suppress the development of tumor for a long time. Viewed from a short term, the radiotherapy kills the cancer cells with chemotherapy drugs, viewed from a long term, it shall rely on the immunologic functions and the immune surveillance of the host to eliminate the remained cancer cells. So the treatment outlook in an all-round way must stress on protecting the chest and improving the immunity to improve the immunologic functions of the host so as to suppress the development of the tumor.

The cancer is a kind of general disease, so it is necessary to research the cancer and consider the clinical treatment scheme from the biological characteristics and behaviors of the cancer. The immune system is specially suitable for eliminated the remained cancer cells, especially the cells in resting stage of the stem cells of the tumor which are difficult to be eliminated by radiotherapy or chemotherapy, which is helpful to prolong the cancer-free survival time. Radiotherapy and chemotherapy only can kill a part of the cancer cells instead of all cancer cells, the rest 10^7 cancer cells are slowly eliminated by the immunological cells of the host organism, so it is difficult to conquer the cancer by radiotherapy and chemotherapy.

Immunological therapy of tumor is an important part of biological treatment of the tumor and it is the key of the treatment outlook in an all-round way. Biological treatment of tumor is based on biological response modifier (BRM), namely BRM theory created by Oldham in 1982. Based on this, Oldham put forward four modality of cancer treatment of tumor treatment in 1984, namely the biological treatment. According to BRM theory, in normal conditions, the tumor and the defense of the organism are in dynamic balance, the occurrence, invasion and metastasis of the tumor are entirely caused by the maladjustment of the dynamic balance. If the maladjusted state can be artificially adjusted to the normal level, it can control the growth of the tumor and make the tumor extinct.

The biological treatment is to adjust the biological response through supplementing, inducing or activating the intrinsic biological active cells (or) factors with cell toxic cytoactive in BRM system in the body in vitro. The biological treatment is different from the three largest traditional therapies, including operation, radiotherapy and chemotherapy, the radiotherapy and the chemoyherapy targets directly attacking the tumor.

The biological treatment of the tumor mainly includes: (1) adoptive infusion of immunologic living cells; (2) application of lymphokine/cytokine; (3) specific active immunity, including tumor vaccine and monovalent vaccine.

The cells and the humoral factors of the organism reaction system are in delicate regulation and control, when they are unbalanced, the reaction or response capability of the organism will be remarkably affected, the adoption of biological reaction moderator is to recover the unbalanced organism state to the normal state so as to realize the objective of preventing the tumor.

The biological reaction moderator is to moderate the immunologic function of the organism, recover the suppressed functions of the immune system of the organism. The reaction mechanism of the drugs is to activate the immune system of the organism to bring its regulation function into play, most of them are from microorganism and the plants.

V. Immune regulation and control therapy is the key of the all-round cancer treatment

It has been proven by 4-year's experimental study and 16-year's clinical verification that XZ-C medicine has the similar reaction and curative effect to BRM and it is the one with the similar reaction to BRM screened from the resources of Chinese traditional herb.

XZ-C medicine is screened through experiment by Professor Xu Ze in China (XU ZE-China, XZ-C) in the lab from 200 kinds of Chinese herbal medicines. Firstly we adopt the culture in vitro of cancer cells, screen 200 kinds of Chinese herbal medicines one by one in vitro, observe the direct damage to cancer cells by the medicines in the culture tube through experimental study and make the check experiment of tumor-suppression rate with the normal cells cultured with chemotherapy drug CTX and in the test tube as the control group. Finally, we select a batch of drugs with the rate of tumor-suppression of the proliferation of cancer cells. Then we further create the tumor-bearing animal model and make the experimental study on 200 kinds of Chinese herbal medicines for in vivo tumor-suppression rate and then screen, analyze and evaluate them one by one scientifically and objectively. It is proven by the experimental results that only 48 kinds of medicines have relatively good tumor-suppression rate while another 152 kinds of Chinese herbal medicines are the common anti-cancer Chinese traditional medicines used by the herbalist doctors, through experimental screening for tumor-suppression rate in the tumor-bearing experimental tumor, which are proven no anti-cancer reaction or little tumor-suppression rate.

XZ-C medicine with relatively better tumor-suppression rate screened through the tumor-bearing rats in the lab by us can improve the immunity, protect the thymus of the central immune organ, improve the cellular immunity, protect the function of the thymus, improve the immunity, protect the hematopiesis function of the bone marrow, increase the erythrocytes and white blood cells, activate the immunocyte factors and improve the immune surveillance in the blood. The main pharmacological action of XZ-C medicine is anti-cancer and improvement of immunity. This group screens 48 kinds of medicines with relatively high tumor-suppression rate through 4-year's animal experiment and then it detects 26 kinds of medicines through immune and cytokine level detection, that can enhance the phagocytic function, or cellular immunity; or humoral immunity; or increase the weight of the thymus; or promote the proliferation of bone marrow cells; or enhance T cellular functions; or increase LAK cytoactive; or increase the active level of the interferon IFN; or increase the active level of TNF; or increase the stimulating factors of CSF colony or inhibit the thromboxane of the blood platelets.

Application principles of XZ-C medicine. BRM and XZ-C medicine with similar reaction to BRM can strengthen immunological reaction of the organism, strengthen the immune surveillance reaction of the organism and they have relatively good effects when the cells meet with catastrophe or the tumor is very small. Through surgical operation or radiotherapy or medication, it will realize the best curative effect when the tumor is minimized.

As to the patient losing the opportunity of operation, with bad body condition, not withstanding radiotherapy and chemotherapy, the immunological therapy has a certain curative effect and reduces the symptom and prolongs the survival time.

After radical excision of the tumor, in order to reduce the recurrence and metastasis, XZ-C medicine can be administered for treatment; when large tumor is excised with operation, in order to eliminate the remained cancer cells and the ones that may be spread remotely, XZ-C medicine can also be administered.

If the tumor cannot be excised, the chemotherapy or the radiotherapy can be made firstly to kill a large number of tumor cells, after the tumor load in the body is reduced, XZ-C medicine can be administered for treatment.

In a word, the host is opposite to the host and the contradiction exists all along the whole process of occurrence and development of the tumor. When the functions of the immune system of the organism are complete, the organism can restrain and eliminate the tumor through cellular immunity and humoral immunity reaction. On the other hand, the growing tumor has so many effects on the immune system of the organism, inhibiting the immunologic functions of the organism and promoting the development of the tumor.

So the cancer treatment scheme must aim at the host and the tumor synchronously. The theory shall be used to guide the clinic; at the same time, the all-round anti-cancer treatment shall be made aiming at the cancer cells and the anti-force forces of the host and the treatment outlook in an all-round way shall be established. The regulation and control shall be used to cure the patients instead of simple killing.

5. Cancer treatment modalities

The new mode combinations multidisciplinary treatment of cancer

Cancer treatment requires a scientifically designed treatment programs, the occurrence of cancer is a disease lose the ability to hang between the immune and tumor development in the balance, loss of immune surveillance, the further development of the tumor, treatment is necessary to restore the balance between stability.

Cancer Treatment requires a "multidisciplinary treatment program". This program is an organic integrated treatment must comply with the actual situation of the patient's condition.

Combinations multidisciplinary treatment must have a reasonable theoretical basis, it must be comprehensive therapy concept, a host of tumor progress and new knowledge transfer has important theoretical value and clinical significance. During cancer invasion and metastasis, two aspects from the tumor and host should be considered, which is theoretical basis for discipline and methods.

Based on the above analysis, diagnosis, treatment, research and drug formulation Hang cancer and anti-metastatic strategies should be considered from two angles to the tumor and the host. This is probably only fundamentally change the current the principle of one-sided treatment programs to kill cancer cells, thereby establishing a comprehensive treatment concept that should be followed.

How to combine multidisciplinary treatment? At first, we should transform the idea and update the approach, establish treatment outlook in an all-round way, arrange intervention, regulation, control and treatment measures in the whole course of disease, i.e. the whole process of cancer occurrence, development, recurrence and metastasis. Now we comprehensively divide the responsibilities of the main treatment methods of all disciplines commonly used at present and coordinate them organically as overall therapy and short-term therapy:

① Overall therapy. In radical surgery the main tumor has been removed and lymph node was dissected, then carried throughout the long course of treatment or biological therapy, immunotherapy, cytokines, gene therapy, XZ-Cimmunomodulatory anti-cancer traditional Chinese medicine, combining Chinese and Western medicine treatment of immune regulation in order to enhance the whole process of anticancer immunity, regulation or control of recurrence and metastasis in the host. It can be used in the whole cancer therapy.

② short-term treatment. Radiotherapy and chemotherapy, only intermittent treatment, or are used short-term to kill the cancer cells, rather than not Full course or long course of treatment, can not "once and for all", because of medication bombs that kill the cancer cells for 3-5 days, followed by no action to kill cancer cells, after a short remission, cancer cells continue to divide, proliferate recurrence, metastasis, because cancer cells can kill 4 cycles or six weeks the public for a long time may develop resistance.

Over the entire treatment and short-course treatment strategy are aimed at the tumor and host two angles to consider, which may fundamentally change only kill cancer cells from the current one-sided treatment concept.

Short-term therapy only in cancer patients in the whole course of a short stage, it should be for the adjuvant treatment (or vice-axis), because it unilaterally against cancer, not long-term, not excessive.

Traditional radiotherapy and chemotherapy for cancer but this factor is limited, one-sided, not comprehensive, and therefore difficult to overcome cancer. Because cancer is a result of the regulation process imbalance, we must address both host and tumor factors, response of the host to determine the final outcome. Cure should by regulation rather than a single killer.

Full treatment from cancer development, recurrence, metastasis, overall disease progression whole process is aimed at the tumor and host two factors to radical surgery foci entity, biological therapy, immunotherapy, gene therapy, cell factor treatment, XZ-C immune regulation medicine and other treatment to improve the host organism anticancer force, this scientific organic integrated comprehensive treatment, is reasonable, in line with cancer pathogenesis, pathophysiology of science, in line with the biological characteristics of cancer cells and biological behavior, therefore, may overcome cancer.

Therefore, the full course of treatment should be used as a cancer treatment spindle, which is the ultimate solution. The short-term treatment should be as countershaft cancer treatment, only palliative, only compatible with the full course of treatment.

Professor Xu Ze holds the combination of multi-disciplinary comprehensive treatment must have reasonable theoretical basis, and the new recognition that the host affects tumor progress and metastasis is of important theoretical value and clinic guiding significance. Two factors including tumor and host shall be considered in formulating anti-carcinoma and anti-metastasis strategies and making comprehensive treatment. Organic integration of discipline, method, technology and medicine with reasonable theoretical basis must be the treatment outlook in an all-round way.

At the beginning of 21st century, carcinoma treatment has entered into the era of multi-disciplinary comprehensive treatment.

Current situation of comprehensive treatment: it takes three traditional therapies as the main body. In most cases, the way of comprehensive application depends on the clinical department for initial diagnosis. Most patients are initially diagnosed in chemotherapy department, in which case they will be subject to chemotherapy firstly and then radiotherapy. If the patients are initially diagnosed in radiotherapy department, then they will be subject to radiotherapy followed by chemotherapy. If the patients are initially diagnosed in surgery department, they will be subject to operation with the presence of operation indications, followed by chemotherapy or radiotherapy, and will be subject to radiotherapy or chemotherapy with the absence of operation indications. The result of such comprehensive treatment is that many patients still fail to prevent recurrence and metastasis, and some even promote the failure of immunologic function.

Biotherapy, immunotherapy, differentiation-inducing therapy, cytokine therapy and immunologic regulation and control therapy of Chinese medicine combined with western medicine have not been incorporated into the treatment scheme of most tumor therapist.

I. The Reason why we put forward the new treatment mode of scientific organic integration

The study on carcinoma therapeutics must be based on tumor biology, both of which must be consistent with each other. Unit now, in the early years of 21st century, the tumor biology has developed into the level of molecular biology, cytokine and gene while the theoretical basis of the traditional cancer therapeutics has been still remaining the cellular level over 50 years which is based on the unceasing proliferation aiming at killing off carcinoma cells. Traditional radiotherapy and chemotherapy aims at killing cancer cells, so cytotoxic drug is used, but the effect is poor which requires increasing the dosage and adding several medicines for combination. In the recent decade, the trend of research on antitumor drugs and status of clinical application indicate the clinical application of traditional anticancer drugs was subject to more limitations due to great side effects, low targeting, the patients' tolerance to drugs, etc.

It can be deemed that the research on anticancer drugs has entered a new stage, facing updating of theories, technologies and ideas. The traditional idea and working method merely aiming at simply eliminating cancer cells by cytotoxic drug as the theoretical basis is under attack.

Since 1980s, with the rapid development of medical molecular, molecular immunology, immunopharmacology, TCM immunopharmacology and cytokine, new bio-therapeutics has emerged, driving the advancement of cancer therapeutics. Biotherapy, immunologic therapy, differentiation inducer, biological reaction regulator, immunological regulation and control TCM at molecular level combined with western medicine are coming out in succession. New tumor vaccine development and gene therapy in recent years presents a more fascinating prospect.

The author holds that cancer therapy needs a scientifically designed treatment plan. In case of cancer, further development of tumor is contributed to imbalance between anticancer immunocompetence and tumor development of the organism and the absence of immune surveillance. Hence, both of them must be recovered to balance and stability through therapy.

II. How to carry out organic, integrated and multi-disciplinary treatment scheme

1. **Professor Xu Ze proposes that carcinoma treatment needs a scientifically designed "organic, integrated and multi-disciplinary treatment scheme". And the scientifically designed organic integration must be consistent with the actual conditions of the patient:**

   (1) Biological characteristics and behaviors of cancer cells, which means that the malignant cells in the organism will be continually progressively divided, proliferated and cloned once becoming cancer cells, from one to two, two

to four......throughout the whole course of cancer occurrence, evolvement, metastasis and recurrence. Hence, treatment measures must stress on control and treatment in the whole course, rather than a certain stage of the course of disease.

(2) Immunologic state of the host. Cancer is in continual evolvement. Cancer cells are featured in uncontrolled infinite proliferation; their canceration results from imbalance in control. A response relationship must be kept between tumor and host, and the response of the host determines the final results.

(3) According to the biological behaviors of cancer cells, multiple-step and multi-link of cancer cell metastasis and its "eight steps", "three stages" and "two points and one line", intervene and intercept cancer cells on the way to metastasis and adopt a new, scientific, organically integrated treatment mode in an all-round way.

2. **The combination of comprehensive multi-disciplinary treatment must have reasonable theoretical basis, that is to say, an all-round treatment outlook and the new recognition of host affecting tumor progress and metastasis must be of great theoretical value and clinical guiding significance.** In working out the strategies of anticancer attack and metastasis and selecting comprehensive treatment, we should consider adopting which discipline, method, technology and medicine to realize the organic integration with reasonable theoretical basis in light of tumor and host.

What is the primary determining factor during occurrence, development and metastasis of cancer? Is it tumor or host? Is it immunological anticancer competence of the host organism or attack and metastasis competence of cancer cells? In the past half century, the research has focused on cancer cell itself, all countries aim at the way of killing the cancer cells. Therefore, traditional treatment is killing cancer cells, which is the single objective. Despite some remarkable progresses, they all fail to solve the problem radically, just addressing secondary symptoms rather than primary ones.

In recent years, more attention is shifted to host factor. Our lab has spent four years in experimental study on tumor origin, pathogenesis, pathologic physiology and cancer attack and metastasis mechanism to explore anticancer immunocompetence and tumor interaction and to seek the control effects on cancer cell attack and metastasis. Through four-year clinic experiment and basic research in our lab, it is found that thymus removal can produce tumor-bearing animal model; with the progress of transplanted tumor, thymus will go through progressive atrophy, which can be prevented by tumor removal; injecting immunologic inhibitor facilitates production of mice tumor-bearing animal model; injecting immunologic inhibitor into tumor-bearing animal mode will increase lung metastasis and liver metastasis lesion; through careful analysis and further consideration, it is found that the relationship between host and tumor and vice versa is the regulation function of the mutual influence between host microenvironment and tumor cells to tumor-bearing animal model. The interaction between cancer cells and host microenvironment finally determines whether and when metastasis lesion can be formed. These indicate the interaction between host microenvironment and tumor cells. **Hence, Professor Xu Ze proposes the "balance" theory which holds that cancer will evolve if the relation between the biological characteristics of cancer cells and the immunological anticancer competence of the host organism is unbalanced; it will be under control and stabilized if the balance is recovered. Thus the treatment must be targeted at two aspects, namely host and tumor, so as to recover them to a balanced and stable state.**

Through experimental exploration of the interaction, interrelationship between host and tumor coupled with clinic practice experience and lessons, we analyze whether cancer cells or host determines the occurrence, development and metastasis and recurrence of cancer. What is behind the death of cancer? Why cancer tumor causes death? **Our current understanding is that the death of tumor patients is mainly contributed to metastasis and recurrence, but how recurrence and metastasis leads to death? According to our preliminary analysis, consideration and understanding, it is contributed to complication and immunologic failure.** So the final result shall be considered as both tumor itself and host.

According to analysis and understanding in our lab, poor immunological function of host organism $\xrightarrow{\text{plus some factor causing cell mutation}}$ malignant mutation of cells most of them are phagocytized by immunologic cells of the organism the rest malignant cells will be continually divided, proliferated and cloned

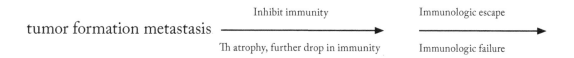

tumor formation metastasis $\xrightarrow{\text{Inhibit immunity}}$ $\xrightarrow{\text{Immunologic escape}}$

Th atrophy, further drop in immunity   Immunologic failure

widespread metastasis.

Professor Xu Ze holds: based on the findings of experimental study in our lab and the data of clinic verification and clinic observation, it is the interaction between cancer cells and host microenvironment and anticancer immunological competence that finally determines cancer progress and that whether and when the metastasis lesion can be formed. The revelation of this regulatory mechanism of interaction

is of great theoretical value and clinical significance. As regards formulation of anticancer metastasis strategies and development of new medicines, we should consider tumor and host factors, which provide theoretical basis for seeking effective intervention methods and developing new medicines. XZ-C medicine developed by us for immunological enhancement through thymus protection and hematopoiesis through spinal marrow protection takes strengthening host factor as the theoretical and experimental basis.

Based on the above analysis, the strategies of diagnosis, treatment, medicine development, anticancer control, antimetastasis should be considered from the perspectives of tumor and host. This may be deemed as the principle of radically changing the current partial treatment scheme with the single aim of killing cancer cells and establishing the treatment outlook in an all-round way previously described.

III. Professor Xu Ze proposes the specific scheme for new combination mode of comprehensive multi-disciplinary treatment Advocated

How to combine multi-disciplinary for comprehensive treatment?

At first, we should transform the idea and update the approach, establish treatment outlook in an all-round way, arrange intervention, regulation, control and treatment measures in the whole course of disease, i.e. the whole process of cancer occurrence, development, recurrence and metastasis. Now we comprehensively divide the responsibilities of the main treatment methods of all disciplines commonly used at present and coordinate them organically as per overall therapy or short-term therapy.

1. Overall therapy: mainly based on radical operation treatment, tumor removal and lymph node elimination are followed by biotherapy, immunotherapy, cytokine therapy, differentiation inducement, gene, immunotherapy with Chinese medicines combined with western medicine, XZ-C medicine in a long term or the whole course, to strengthen anticancer immunocompetence of the host, regulate or control recurrence and metastasis. They can be used in the whole course of cancer disease.

2. Short-term therapy: mainly based on radiotherapy and chemotherapy as the primary form, which is in phases or intermittent, or killing cancer cells suddenly in a short course, but not and cannot cover the overall course or a long course. In this case, the duration of cancer cell elimination can be only four cycles or six cycles, longer duration will produce drug resistance.

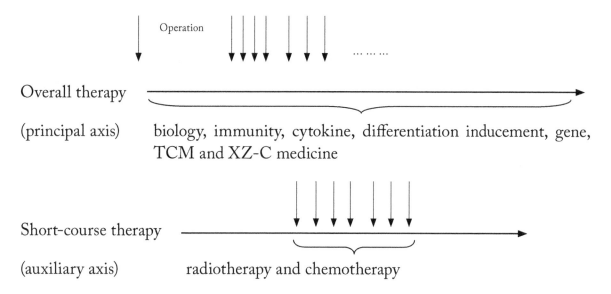

Figure schematic diagram of the combination mode of multi-disciplinary comprehensive treatment

(1) When working out the strategies of the above overall therapy and short-course therapy, we should take tumor and host into account, which may thoroughly change the partial treatment merely killing cancer cells at present. Currently, radiotherapy and chemotherapy only aim at cancer cells, which are partial and incomplete, and fail to consider treatment approaches in light of tumor and host as described above. Apart from this, radiotherapy and chemotherapy will also injure and kill hematopoietic cells and immunological cells of the bone marrow of the host, undermining the immunological function of the host and damaging the host.

(2) Short-course therapy just covers a short stage in the whole course of disease for cancer patients, so it should be deemed as an adjuvant therapy (or referred to as auxiliary axis), for it merely aims at a single aspect of cancer cells.

① Biological characteristics of cancer cells. Cancer stems from malignant mutation of a single cell, the cancer cells are progressively divided and proliferated, from one to two, from two to four…… Cancer is a development process rather than a form or entity. Therefore, the therapy to kill off cancer cells cannot eliminate all cancer cells. As long as several cancer cells remain, they can be continually divided, proliferated and recurred. Moreover, chemotherapy cannot injure tumor stem cells, which are bound to constant division, proliferation, resulting in cancer cells. Hence, the treatment method solely relying on killing cancer cells fails to comply with biological characteristics and biological behavior of cancer cells.

② The effective time of cytotoxic drug is limited. It is only effective during the period of application, and ineffective beyond the period, so it cannot be done once and for all. Its effective time is limited, so the remaining 10^{6-7} cancer cells still need to be eliminated by immunological competence of the host. Moreover, tumor stem cells will continue to form cancer cells. Therefore, radiotherapy and chemotherapy can only relieve the condition for several months but cannot heal it.

③ Chemotherapy killing cancer cells is only the first order kinetics, its lethality is limited and it can only kill 10^{6-7} cancer cells.

④ Chemotherapy drug is a double-edged sword. Apart from killing cancer cells, it can also kill normal cells, hematopoietic cells and immunological cells of the bone marrow of the host, causing drop in immunological function of the host.

Traditional chemotherapy and radiotherapy are only targeted at the factor of cancer cell tumor, which is limited, partial and incomplete, thus it is difficult to conquer the cancer. Because canceration process is the result of regulation imbalance, it must be targeted at host and tumor, and the reaction of the host decides the final result. It should be cured by regulation instead of injury alone.

(3) Overall therapy. It covers the whole course of cancer disease from cancer occurrence, development, recurrence, metastasis, progress, targeted at these two factors, i.e. tumor and host. It applies radical operation to remove cancer lesion entity, and applies biotherapy, immunotherapy, gene treating cytokine, immunological regulation TCM and so on to the host, so as to improve anticancer competence of the organism. Such scientific and organic integration is targeted at two aspects, i.e. cancer cells and host. It is an all-round treatment outlook, which is comprehensive, reasonable and scientific, complies with pathogenesis, pathological physiology, biological characteristics and biological behaviors of cancer cells, and is likely to conquer cancer. Therefore, overall therapy should be the principal axis of cancer treatment, with operation treatment as the main form, biotherapy, immunotherapy, gene therapy, and differentiation inducement therapy, TCM immunological regulation therapy, improving immunity by chest protection and hematogenesis by bone marrow protection distributed and applied in the whole course of cancer treatment.

It is a scientific, reasonable and all-round treatment outlook and a radical method.

Short-course therapy should be auxiliary axis of cancer treatment, with chemotherapy and radiotherapy as the main form. It is only designed to kill off cancer cells and should be combined with overall therapy.

The new treatment mode of scientific and organic integration must have a reasonable theoretical basis, with the theory guiding clinic practice.

Xu Ze holds: the new mode of multi-disciplinary comprehensive treatment described above has a reasonable theoretical basis, comply with the realities of the patient's condition and is rational and scientific.

1. The experience and lessons of clinic treatment practice demonstrate killing cancer cells cannot control cancer or overcome cancer. It is partial and incomplete to merely target at one aspect of cancer cell.

2. The objective or target of cancer treatment should be both host and tumor. As regards which is the main side and who decides the final destiny of the cancer patient, both tumor itself and host should be considered.

3. We must update the approach and transform the idea, fist establish a treatment outlook in an all-round way, scientifically arrange intervention, regulation and treatment measures with the whole course of cancer occurrence, development, recurrence and metastasis.

4. We should work out design and arrangement of "principal axis" and "auxiliary axis" new treatment mode, which is appropriate and scientific, with theoretical basis and in line with the realities of the patient.

5. We must orient human firstly, manage to eliminate toxicant and side effects of radiotherapy and chemotherapy as possible, increase patient safety, study the toxicity and safety of each medicine and technology, which must have appropriate theoretical basis guiding clinic practice.

In short: cancer treatment, whether in early, middle or late stage, requires multi-disciplinary comprehensive treatment and appropriate theoretical basis guiding clinic practice.

Operation is a method of local treatment. Tumor surgeons hold that cancer first occurs in local part, and then attacks the surrounding tissues, shifts to other places through lymphatic vessels and blood vessels. Therefore, they often focus on local part in treatment, i.e. control local growth and diffusion, and especially carry out operation to eliminate lymph nodes shifting through lymph. Although operative treatment has seen constant improvement over the years, its long-term effects fail to be increased significantly. Recurrence and metastasis after operation pose a grave threat to prognosis of the patient, which has attracted great concern of the medical circle, but effective good practice remains absent.

Radiotherapy is also local treatment. Its effect local tumor is to kill off cells with the index of unit dosage. The effects of chemotherapy are greatly affected by cell oxygenation, type of the tumor, cell repair and other factors, and it cannot resist metastasis and recurrence.

Biological characteristics of cancer are attack, recurrence and metastasis, which are vital reasons for failure of operative and chemotherapy treatment.

In recent years, some argues cancer deals with the whole body, so whole body treatment should take chemotherapy as the primary form. Unfortunately, although new medicines come out continually over the past decade, treatment schemes and methods update constantly, the effects of chemotherapy are unsatisfactory. As cell toxicant drug is unselective, it can kill off both cancer cells and normal cells of the host, especially tend to injure immunocytes, with serious toxicant and side effects, inhibiting hematopiesis function of spinal marrow and reduce immunity. Therefore, the writer holds that traditional chemotherapy does not completely comply with the real situation of biological behavior of cancer as we recognized today, for example, attack behavior, metastasis of cancer cells deals with multiple links and steps. Currently, people have realized that antitumor medicine does not necessarily resist metastasis and recurrence.

The biotherapy of tumor newly emerging in 1980s, such as immunotherapy, cytokine therapy, differentiation inducement therapy and gene tumor vaccine therapy, has proved some therapies can regulate the immunity of the patients, but has not proved which immunological preparation or method can induce tumor extinction.

In the last two decades, there are many reports on cancer treatment by tradition Chinese medicine. Its prospect is of concern. Especially with further research on medicine and immunology, it has been recognized that confusion of immunological system is closely related with occurrence and development of tumor. Traditional Chinese medicine has its own characteristics and advantages in treating tumor by regulating immunological function of the organism. Immunological regulation of traditional Chinese medicines and the development of Chinese medicine immunomodulator will be concerned and favored across the world. If combined with operation, radiotherapy and chemotherapy, SZ-C medicine can give full play to its immunological regulation function during treatment, obviously prolong survival time and improve survival quality, displaying characteristics and advantages of traditional Chinese medicine. Its disadvantage lies in that it cannot cause evident change on tumor itself.

Since the methods above are different in action mechanism and effects of cancer treatment, and have their own disadvantages, thus it is necessary to evaluate the advantages and disadvantages of the therapies, "gains" and "losses" of the patients, for example, what are the advantages and disadvantages of adopting this therapy, what will the patients gain or lose? We can draw from the advantages of each therapy to offset their disadvantages, combine the therapies in an organic and appropriate way, forming a comprehensive plan of cancer treatment. Only in this way can we significantly reduce toxic and side effects of the medicine, improve survival quality of the patients and prolong overall survival time. Over the past 16 years, Shuguang Tumor Clinic has applied the comprehensive treatment mainly involving operation +XZ-C medicine to more than 12000 cancer patients at middle and late stage. Most of them have achieved the effects of improving survival quality, stabilizing disease lesion, controlling metastasis, existence with tumor and significantly prolonging life.

6. Cancer metastasis treatment principles

The key of Cancer research is anti-metastasis; the basic principle of cancer therapy is anti-metastatic; the main features of the new concept of cancer treatment is namely to control transfer

It has been seen from the clinical medical practice in about 100 years that the three traditional therapeutics including operation, radiotherapy and chemotherapy have made relatively good curative effects in treating the malignant tumor and so many patients have obtained CR/PR curative effects throaty radiotherapy and chemotherapy and the tumor has been obviously shrunk. However, it is a pity that the tumor meets with reoccurrence, enlargement and metastasis later. Although radiotherapy or chemotherapy is made again, the curative effects on most patients are extremely bad and they die of metastasis and reoccurrence.

The author summarizes the experience and lessons positive and negative from the clinical practice cases over 54 years, forms the following new understanding, puts forward the new theoretical concept and launches the new therapeutic strategies through combining the long-term experimental study with the clinical practice.

I. The key to overcome the cancer is Anti-cancerometastasis

Anti-cancerometastasis is the key to overcome the cancer because the metastasis is the first cause of the death caused by cancer.

In the past one century from 20th century, the goal of tackling the key problem is to kill the cancer cells aiming at the primary carcinoma lesion and metastatic carcinoma lesion. Although the efforts have been made for a century, the cancer mortality has been always taking the first place. The main reason why the mortality is so high is the metastasis. Obviously, the previous traditional therapeutics cannot reduce the stubbornly high mortality. The first cause of its failure is that the goal cannot target the metastasis and control the metastasis.

At the beginning of 21st century, the uppermost problem of cancer treatment is still how to prevent the metastasis. In case that the metastasis after radical operation of cancer cannot be successfully prevented, the cancer treatment cannot get a great-leap-forward development.

Now we deeply realize that the key problem to be tackled is to prevent the metastasis at present. The core of cancer treatment is to prevent the metastasis. Therefore, one of the goals of cancer treatment in 21st century is anti-metastasis.

The above-mentioned problems impel us to update the thoughts and change the ideas to open a new road to find the new therapeutics for preventing metastasis and overcome the cancer while improving the curative effects of the traditional therapeutics as per the traditional ideas. Therefore, we raise: analyzing and understanding the immune state of the host and the multiple steps and links of cancerometastasis based on the biological characteristics of the cancer and the biological behaviors of the cancerometastasis to find a new treatment mode for anti-cancerometastasis.

The academician of Liver Cancer Research Institute of Fudan University, Tang Zhaoxian, raised in *On Clinical Research on Carcerometastasis* on Nov. 9, 2007: "if the cancerometastasis is not studied, the improvement of curative effects is a soap bubble".

Great attention has been paid to the tumor metastasis since 1990s in the world. Metastasis Research Society was established, Clinical and Experimental Metastasis was issued. Cancerometastasis Research Society was established in Tokyo, Japan.

The study on metastasis in China starts relatively late, Professor Gao Jin published *Cancer Invasion and Metastasis------Fundamental Research and Clinic* based on a large quantity of rich experimental data in 1996, which was the first monograph on cancerometastasis and was excellent in both the pictures and their accompanying essay. In 2003, the academician Tang Zhaoxian published his monograph Foundation and Clinic of Metastasis and Reoccurrence of Liver Cancer and he raised in the monograph: "the next important goal of study on primary liver cancer is to prevent and control reoccurrence and metastasis", in addition, he said: "metastasis and reoccurrence have become one bottle-neck of further improving the survival rate of liver cancer and one of the most important difficulties in overcoming the cancer". These monoprahies accelerate the attention to and study on the metastasis by the scholars in China. In 2006, Professor Xu Ze published New Concept and New Way of Treatment of Cancer Metastasis and put forward some theoretical innovations, which was granted with "Three-One-Hundred Original Book" by General Administration of Press and Publication of the People's Republic of China.

2. The basic principle is anti-metastatic cancer therapy

(1 The unique behaviors of invasion and metastasis aiming at the biological behaviors of the cancer cells Metastasis is a malignant behavior. It is well known that the fundamental difference between the benign tumor and the malignant tumor is that the former meets with metastasis while the latter does not meet with the metastasis. If we can take measures to prevent the metastasis of the cancer cells, is the malignant tumor becoming the benign tumor? 85%~95% of the patients die of the metastasis of the cancer. In case of no metastasis, most of the patients will not die. In case that the metastasis does not happen or it is controlled, the cancer is not so terrible. Therefore, the principle of treatment of cancer is to prevent the metastasis, design the therapeutic scheme and intervention scheme of anti-metastasis, research and develop the anti-metastasis drug, try to obstruct and intercept the cancer cells in metastasis and cut off or block one or more links of metastasis so as to control the metastasis..

(2) How to prevent metastasis. The biological characteristics and behaviors of the cancer cells are invasion and metastasis. The reason why the cancer is malignant is mainly the wide harm of invasion and metastasis to the human body. Over a century, the goals of the three traditional therapies have been always aiming at the primary lesion cancer and metastatic carcinoma lesion and ablating the primary carcinoma lesion by operation or treat the metastatic carcinoma lesion with radiotherapy and other local treatment. It is commonly held that the primary carcinoma lesion and the metastatic carcinoma lesion can be seen or touched and they are local, so they can be treated with operation or radiotherapy. Reviewing and reflecting the clinical practice for 54 years, I had made so many radical operation on chest and abdomen based on the above-mentioned understanding, however, after the follow-up survey of 3000 patients after operation made by me in 1985, I was discerning and apprehending quickly and completely that how to prevent the reoccurrence and metastasis after operation is the core to determine the long-term curative effects of the cancer. The primary carcinoma lesion or the metastatic carcinoma lesion may be represented locally while the remote metastasis is systemic.

Since 1970s, in view of the high reoccurrence and metastasis rate of the cancer after operation, in order to control the reoccurrence after operation, the assistant chemotherapy after operation has been adopted, even the chemotherapy before operation (for example, on breast cancer) has been made, however, the results have not been so satisfactory and the assistant chemotherapy after operation on the patients cannot prevent the reoccurrence and metastasis. As to some cases, the chemotherapy is intensified, resulting in adynamia of immunologic function. All these issued shall be seriously and calmly thought, reviewed, analyzed and reflected by the clinicians so as to find how to prevent the reoccurrence and metastasis to treat the cancer.

In the recent 20 years, the understanding of the molecular metastasis mechanism of cancer has made great progress, however, there have been no actually effective measures for preventing the metastasis of the cancer cells at home and abroad. Although some new anti-cancer drugs have come out in recent years, the curative effects cannot be improved to our satisfaction. The reason why some cancer cells cannot be radically cured by the exploration in the middle and late stage is that the lymph node meets with the remote metastasis. It is important and key to inhibit the cancerometastasis so as to reduce the death rate of cancer and improve the curative effects.

The goal of tackling the key problem is relatively simple, just to kill the cancer cells, which does not entirely conform to the actual condition of the biological characteristics of the cancer at present, for example, the invasion behaviors of the cancer cells, metastasis link and multi-step, molecular biological mechanism of metastasis, immunoreactivity of the organism and inducement of reoccurrence and reoccurrence after incubation for several months even several years. Now it is known by the people at present that the anti-cancer drug does not always prevent the metastasis or kill the cancer cells.

Therefore, it is held by the author that now it is key to prevent the metastasis so as to overcome the cancer and it is core to study how to prevent the metastasis so as to cure the cancer.

3. The main features of the new concept of cancer treatment, namely the transfer of control

Killing cancer cells in human body should resort to two kinds of force: one is foreign force from operation, radiation therapy and chemotherapy, the other is intrinsic force from patient's autoimmunity. Although medicament, operation and therapeutic techniques are important to patient's therapy, intrinsic immunity of human body is more important. Many problems must depend on patient's self force, such as nutrition problem, it is hard to attain the object if the patient organism can't absorb and utilize despite given sufficient nutriment. Take healing of incision as another example, it must rely on patient's intrinsic healing function and exogenous factor can only influence or accelerate its healing.

Intrinsic immunity of human body can kill cancer cells. Literature material shows that a tiny tumor (1-8g) can release several millions or hundreds of thousands of cancer cells to blood within 24h, but most (99.99%) of them will be killed by human body immune system can kill cancer, only less than 0.1% can survive and grow to metastatic carcinoma. The data from our own laboratory show that Kunming mouse can kill 99% of cancer cells by its autoimmunity within 24h when injected 10^5 S_{180} malignant cells to caudal vein. More cancer cells will be killed if the mouse takes $XZ\text{-}C_1$ and $XZ\text{-}C_4$ immunization regulation and control traditional Chinese medicine. Anti-cancer Metastasis Lab of Wuhan Shuguang Tumor Special Clinic has implied $XZ\text{-}C_1$ and $XZ\text{-}C_4$ to patients regularly in recent 10 years, it is shown by clinical data statistics that certain amount of cancer cells in metastasis can indeed be killed.

Human body has certain anti-cancer ability and there is a complete anti-cancer mechanism and system in host body with the anticancer effect of anticancer cell cluster (NL cell cluster, K cell cluster, LAK cell cluster, macrophage cluster and TK cell cluster), the anticancer effect of anticancer cytokine system, FN, IL-2, TNF and LT, and the effect of anti-oncogene and inhibiting cancer metastasis gene, therefore, it must be protected, activated and brought into play.

The generation and development of cancer is close related to immunologic hypofunction of the body. The carcinoma can directly infringe immune organ to worsen or inhibit immunologic function and can release immunosuppressive factor to bring down the immunity of host or to induce the intracorporeal suppressor cell to increase. The Thymus of host has been inhibited in case of cancer and chemotherapy inhibits bone marrow, just like one disaster after another. Traditional therapy neglects the intrinsic anticancer ability of human body and the anticancer force of anticancer cell, anticancer cytokine, antioncogene and anti-metastasis gene in anticancer system, in this way, the whole central immune organ shall be damaged and can not be effectively protected, which is why the curative effect of traditional therapy can't be improved.

Consequently, the author suggests attaching great importance to exerting and relying on the intrinsic force of anticancer system of the host.

Main characteristics of Xu Ze's cancer therapeutics: control over metastasis, protection of immunity of the patient instead of simply killing the cancer cells.

7. New Concept of treatment of cancer metastasis

Treatment of the cancer group on the metastasis way

Cancer in the body exists in the form of a major conventional cancer therapeutics think there are two forms; the new concept of cancer treatment think that there are three forms; there is the third form of cancer in the body of research and understanding of the process; the goal of cancer treatment should be the third existing form.

After 50 years of clinical experience in surgical oncology practice and 10 years of laboratory research I carried out careful sorting and summarizing and formed an unique new understanding and new concept of cancer metastasis and proposed new methods and new technology of anti-metastatic cancer therapy.

Its main contents include: ① cancer in the body exists in three forms; ② the whole process of two points and One Line of Carcinoma Development ③ cancer metastasis" eight steps and a three-stage "theory; ④ the third field of human anti-cancer metastasis treatment (5) metastasis treatment "trilogy"; ⑥ independently developed XZ-C immunomodulatory anticancer Chinese medication.

The following series of new understanding, new theories, new concepts have not yet been mentioned so far in the literature and textbooks. After lessons of half century practice and 10 years of experimental research, analysis, reflection and wake up, it converses to real theory which founded new concepts and has become distinctive anti-metastatic cancer in therapy theoretical system and have independent innovation and creative and original intellectual property rights.

1. Traditional cancer therapeutics that there are two forms

There are two forms of cancer existing in human body: one is the primary lesion of primary tumor and another is the metastatic node or metastases.

The goal or target of treatment of traditional cancer therapeutics aims at these two existing forms, namely the primary tumor or metastatic tumor just because no matter the primary tumor or metastatic tumor is composed of cancer cell while the goal of treatment is to kill the cancer cell.

The main reason for the failure of conventional therapy is recurrence and metastasis.

2. XU ZE New Concept of Cancer Treatment Holding Three Forms Exist

The author first published an new theory which the third form of cancer group which exists in our body is the cancer cells on the route of metastasis. The author holds that the cancer existing in the human body has three forms: the first one is the primary lesion of primary tumor; the second one is metastatic node or metastatic tumid lymph node; the third one is the cancer cell and cancer cell group and micro-metastasis in metastasis routing which the main reason for the failure of conventional therapy is recurrence and metastasis.

The third manifestation is the thousands of cancer cells or cancer mill groups or slight cancer embolus in metastasis routing, which cannot be seen or touched. These potential, hidden and roving metastatic cancer cells, which cannot be examined through endoscope, ultrasonic, CT and MRI and so on, is the largest threat to the life of the patient suffering from cancer.

In operation, the third group of cancer cell and micro-metastasis in metastasis routig which cannot be seen by eyes, for example, in radical operation for carcinoma of stomach, the phyma of stomach cancer and metastatic tumid lymph nodes can be seen by us, however, whether the cancer cell exists in the vein of stomach wall or portal vein blood stream cannot be seen? And how many cancer cells exist? And where the cancer cells in the vein blood stream go? Whether the cancer cell groups touched and extruded into the vein flood stream arrive at the stomach vein or the portal vein even the portal vein branch in the anus? It is impossible to not touch the cancer tumor in operations research and abscision of tumor of stomach cancer and cleaning down of lymph node, since the operation by hand necessarily makes a large number of cancer cells extruded and exfoliated, flowing into the blood circulation through out-neoplasm vein and rushing into the blood stream of portal vein, however, which cannot be seen by the operation doctor. These cancer cells rushing into the blood stream of portal vein will flow into the portal vein system.. Generally, the various immunological cells in the portal vein will carry out the immune surveillance over the cancer cells in the blood circulation of the portal vein and will phagocytize them. However, in a short time, the immunological cells in the portal vein system cannot phagocytize these cancer cells rushing abruptly. After a period of time, some cancer cells escape the immune surveillance, the cancer cells surviving after impact of blood stream may implant in the sinus hepaticus, the blood vessel produces and forms the intrahepatic metastasis.

The phenomenon as well as a fact has not been thought and discovered that is a dynamic manifestation of the cancer cell existing in the human body. The anti-cancer metastasis and recurrence lab of this experimental surgical research institution, through analysis and research of the metastasis rule of over 10000 clinic patients suffering from cancer, has been aware of this phenomenon and find it, that is to say that the essence of the metastasis is the cancer cells in the metastasis routing and the goal of anti metastasis and the target of treatment should aim at the cancer cells in metastasis routing, namely the third manifestation of cancer existing in human body; in the past, since the people had not been aware of this point, they only cured the primary lesion and metastasis and tried to shorten or eliminate it, but not knew that the shrinkage of the tumor did not mean that it did not metastasis. The traditional therapy of treatment fails in reoccurrence and metastasis in a long term.

3. Cancer in the body of a third form of research and understanding of the process

(1) Where are metastasis cancer cells?

Since it is cognized by us that the key to cure the cancer is to anti-metastasis, how to realize the anti-metastasis? And how to cognize the detailed process, step and mechanism of the metastasis of cancer cells? How these cancer cells move? What is their movement rule? Where is the weak link of the cancer cell in metastasis routing? Which link(s) should be stricken or blockaded? The goal of striking the cancer metastasis must be objectified.

(2) Experimental study tracked the fate and the role of the way in the metastasis cancer cells

In order to settle the above-mentioned problems, the experimental surgical anti-metastasis and recurrence lab was established by us to carry out the fundamental research of experimental tumor, implant the cancer cells, establish the animal model of tumor and develop a series of experimental tumor research: probing into the mechanism and rule of cancer invasion and metastasis; probing into the relationship between the tumor and immunity and the immune organ as well as the one between the immune organ and the tumor; finding the effective measures to regulate and control the invasion and metastasis of cancer. This lab has spent 3 years in the experimental research on the animal model of cancer metastasis and the experimental observation for observing and tracing the fortune and rule of the cancer cells in the metastasis routing.

In animal experiments cancer cells could not be found in mice blood 48h after 10^5 cancer cells were injected. **These injected cancer cells are eliminated completely?**

Through analysis and presumption, it is possible that some cells transfused into the circulation system are killed because they do not adapt the environment or they are damaged due to the impact of the rapid blood stream or are obstructed by the impediment micro-circulation, however, most of the cancer cells entering the blood circulation, are mainly the immunizing ability of the mouse, which are killed by a large number of immunological cells in the blood circulation of the mouse. Therefore, in the treatment of anti-metastasis, the treatment of cancer cells and cancer cell groups in the metastasis routing must protect the immunizing ability of the host body and it is necessary to try to mobilize, recover and activate its immunologic function of the immune system, instead of striking, damaging and reducing or avoiding striking, damaging and reducing the immunizing ability and functions of immune system of the host body as much as possible. How to try to protect, mobilize and activate the immune functions of the host to deal with the cancer cells in metastasis routing is an important anti-metastasis strategy.

(3) The way in which the transfer of cancer cells present in the form

Some new approaches through the animal experiment and some experimental achievements are obtained. However, it is difficult to verify many experimental results just because that the clinical verification must last 3~5 years before the long-term curative effect can be evaluated. Usually, good effect is obtained in the experimental research, however, it is difficult to observe the remarkable clinical effect just because that the subject investigated in the lab is the mouse while the clinical object is the patient, the experimental results are not always be applied to clinic and it must be subject to the clinical verification and observation for 3~5 years even 8~10 years before the long-term reoccurrence and metastasis of cancer can be understood.

Why the patients meet with the occurrence even wide metastasis and spreading where-after or before long even after the primary lesion or metastasis of these patients are appropriately even satisfactorily cured? Where these metastasis and reoccurrence cancer cells exist in which form? What causes the difference in metastasis time from several months to several years? We remain perplexed despite much thought. Where are these cancer cells hidden in the human body? Why are they so pertinacious? The popular explanation of the patients' families is that "the cancer is alive and it can move". The author realized and found that the forms of the cancer cell in human body were not only the primary lesion and metastasis; the third manifestation, namely the cancer cell and cancer cell group exist in the metastasis routing. The third manifestation has been not mentioned in the literatures and teaching books up to today. Just because that the people have not cognized it, resulting in ignore of the special manifestation of the cancer cell in the metastasis routing.

(4) How cancer cells can survive during the metastasis way

Many patients are subject to the comprehensive treatment such as radiotherapy and chemotherapy over the primary lesion or metastasis tumor by means of various traditional therapeutic methods, the cancer cell meets with metastasis chronically and duratively, thus where these cancer cells exist or hide? Through research, it is deemed by us that these cancer cells has slow or quick metastasis speed in the metastasis routing; under a certain conditions, they may meet with dormancy and rest in GO stage; sometimes, the cancer cells are active, entering the cell cycle. The so-called "condition" may be relevant to the factors such as the cancerous protuberance and local micro-environment of the host; it also be related to the cyto-dynamics of the cancer cells. In facts, these thousands of cancer cells in metastasis routing are most dangerous. They are the hidden enemy; the cancer cells with metastasis potential surviving in the metastasis routing will slowly and gradually form the new metastasis. They are in the active and slow attack. However, the presently traditional therapeutic method is to wait for the new metastasis and then cure it.

The reason why the cancer cells survive in the metastasis routing is because that it can escape the immune surveillance of the immunological cell in the blood circulation. If the cell toxicant chemotherapy is used to cure the metastasis, it is possible to kill many immunological cells, resulting in further weakening the immune surveillance of the immunological cells in the blood circulation of the patient and surviving of more cancer cells in the metastasis routing due to escaping the immune surveillance, forming more new metastasis.

4. Target for cancer therapy should be the three existing forms

Cancer treatment goal or "target" should be one of the goals against cancer in the body exists in three forms, namely treatment for primary lesions; second goal of treatment for tumor foci; third goal of treatment for the transfer of cancer cells en route group.

(I) The key to anti-cancer metastasis is to aim on cancer cells on the metastasis routing

Presented at the human n the third manifestation is being transferred during the multi-step, multi-factor fine the way cancer cells, cancer cells and micro-thrombus metastasis group because this issue has not yet been recognized and did not cause enough attention, but did not specifically discuss how their diagnosis, treatment methods and countermeasures. In fact, the key to anti-cancer metastasis was to surround and annihilate the cancer cells, blocking or interference and, cutting off the transfer of new treatment modalities way.

(2) The way for the transfer of cancer cells, the cancer treatment may cause change and renewal.

The new doctrine or a new theoretical understanding, upon demonstration confirmed, may cause a chain reaction like tumor treatment changes and updates, such as changes in cancer treatment in understanding the concept and updated target for cancer therapy or "target" change and renewal of understanding, to change and update on cancer diagnosis method of looking for anti-cancer, anti-metastasis caused major changes and updates on the research and development of new drugs for cancer treatment modalities and major changes in treatment methods and updates as well as cancer metastasis, recurrence study, pathological cells from the cell level to change and update oncology molecular biology, gene expression at the molecular level oncology.

(3) The way for the transfer of cancer cells, will bring new hope for the fight against cancer

① conventional cancer therapeutics think there are two forms: The first manifestation is the primary cancer,; the second is the manifestation of tumor foci. This traditional therapeutic concept, followed the more than 100 years, the treatment goal or "target" is for the two forms - the primary tumor or metastatic foci. Isolated treat these two "target" on the dynamic relationship between the two, a causal relationship, affiliation is not taking into account. As primary foci is how to form a tumor foci, and how to stop its transfer. Therefore, the traditional concept of cancer therapeutics is incomplete, imperfect, flawed, because it ignores the way cancer metastasis, and cancer metastasis is the most important biological characteristics and biological behavior. There is no way for the transfer of cancer cells is blocking, you can not control the transfer of cancer cells, it is difficult to obtain cancer treatment all the more possible.

② The author provides new concept of cancer which there are three forms: The first manifestation is the primary foci; the second is the manifestation of tumor foci; third manifestation is being transferred on the way cancer cells, cancer cells Group and micro thrombus metastasis. This new concept is more complete and more comprehensive, it illustrates the dynamic relationship between the three, garden fruit relationships and dependencies is a complete new concept of cancer therapeutics, fully explain the whole process of cancer development and how control the whole process of transfer of cancer metastasis, this new doctrine proposed to combat cancer brought new hope.

(4) Press the metastasis pathway, the design of new anti-metastatic therapy mode annihilate interdiction

summary, cancer treatment includes not only surgery for resection of the primary tumor and the implementation of the first two forms, surgery or radiotherapy or chemotherapy for the treatment of metastatic immunity stoves, should also include a third form of treatment for the goal or target, that is shifting the way for red cell carcinoma group, conducted surround and annihilate interdiction, enhance host immune surveillance, interference prevents cancer metastasis. By transfer pathways of cancer cells, multi-step transfer of line, multi-factor, multi-link molecular transfer mechanisms, design of new anti-metastatic treatment modalities, for cancer intervention and interdiction of new treatments.

Metastasis cancer group on the routing or micrometastases, although no clinical manifestations, but it does exist, only to enter the molecular biological level, the gene level, molecular level of immunity in order to find and recognize, overexpression of various tumor markers such as now already that could be undertaken, molecular immunology and genetically modified micro-metastasis detection. Individual cancer cells (ITC) in the blood, bone marrow presence detection can be obtained at the molecular level, the level of detection of new molecular targets, indicators of immune molecules, cytokines, tumor markers, will continue to emerge, we believe that in the near future we will reach the pre-and early diagnosis of cancer micrometastases.

8. How to stop cancer cells metastasis? Cancer metastasis treatment trilogy

To understand cancer cell metastasis steps so that the treatment goal will be more specific; More specifically, trying to break each step; three measures ("trilogy") of anti-cancer metastasis treatment

1. Try to Do Well in Each Step

As to how to make clearer the extremely complicated dynamic and continuous biological process of carcinoma metastasis with multi-step and multi-element, through repeated thinking and carefully analysis, we summed up and put forward Eight Steps of Metastasis of Cancer Cells in the aforesaid. Based on Eight Steps, we tried to make clearer and more particular of the concept of extremely complicated dynamic and continuous biological process of carcinoma metastasis with multi-step and multi-element with respect to understanding. In order to take scientific measures to obstruct and intercept each metastasis step and destroy it one by one, it is necessary to make clear the concept of each step in the metastasis process. Only when the target of each step is made clear, can the prevention and cure countermeasures be carried out, researched and probed into.

In the above, we have mentioned "Three Stages" of carcinoma metastasis and illuminated it in details. The reason why "Three Stage" is put forward is that one of the keys to therapy of cancer is to anti metastasis, however, at present, the understanding of the concept of metastasis is still ambiguous and it is not clear and particular. People only understand the severity of the harm of the metastasis to the patients, however, it lacks of effective prevention and therapeutic countermeasures with clear concept and detailed profile. In order to take scientific measures to obstruct and intercept each metastasis step, based on the Eight Steps, Three Stages and the molecular mechanism of carcinoma metastasis, we try to establish the preventive and therapeutic countermeasures for each stage and called it Xu Ze Three Steps of Therapy of Carcinoma Metastasis.

2. Trying to Get a Good Idea about the Object

The basic process of carcinoma metastasis is: the cancer cell falling from the primary tumor---degrading the basement membrance---migrating into blood capillary and small vein---survived cancer cell adhering to endothelial cell of blood capillary or basement membrance under the exposed endothelium---passing through wall---growing up in the remote target organ and forming the metastatic carcinoma, which is an extremely complicated, dynamic and continuous biological process, composed of several relatively independent but interlocked steps. In each step, a series of molecular biological events will happen between cancer cells, and between the cancer cells and the host cells, finishing the whole metastatic process and finally forming the metastatic carcinoma.

That is to say, it is necessary for the cancer cells to be subject to and finish the whole metastatic process before forming the metastatic carcinoma. any failure of each step will result in the stop of the whole metastatic process, which presents that if we take measures to destroy the metastatic steps one by one and carry out the strategy and tactics of obstruction and interception of the cancer cells in the routing of the metastasis, it is certainly possible to break or intercept the metastatic routing and intercept and kill the cancer cells in the routing of metastasis.

Xu Ze New Concept and Mode of Therapy of Carcinoma and Carcinoma Metastasis are to try to intercept one or several steps or links of the above-mentioned metastatic process so as to control the metastasis.

In order to realize the above-mentioned objectives, what measures shall be taken by us for anti metastasis? With which theory? Which technology and which drug? In which step or in which stage and link to intercept the cancer cells in the routing of the metastasis?

3. Three Steps of Therapy of Carcinoma Metastasis

1. First step of anti carcinomatous metastasis: in this stage, the metastatic process of cancer cells is as follows: cancer cells falling from the primary carcinoma---adhering to the stroma outside the cells---degrading ECM to open up a road for cancer cells---carrying out cell movement via the adherence of degraded stroma or the degraded stroma for adherence---then arriving at the external wall---degrading basement membrane of blood vessel---doing Amoeba movement, firstly stretching out the pseudopodium---then passing through the wall.

Prevention and cure countermeasures: this stage is the intervention and repression countermeasure before the cancer cell falls from the primary carcinoma and enters the blood vessel. In this stage, the therapeutic "targets" are mainly anti-adherence, anti-degradation, anti-movement and anti cancer cell attack. The therapeutic goal is to prevent the cancer cells from entering the blood vessel so as to realize the goal of "turning the enemy back at the border".

2. Second step of anti carcinomatous metastasis: in this stage, the metastasis process of cancer cell: it will pass through the wall and enter the blood circulation. The cancer cell will be interweaved in various blood cell components including blood plasma and blood or will be adhered to cancer cell group together with homo-cancer cell, or will be adhered to slight cancer embolus together with the alloplasm such as blood platelet and white blood cell and float in venous system → turn back to the right ventricle → circulate → enter pulmonary vein → turn back to left ventricle together with the venous blood, some cancer cells can stay in the pulmonary microcirculation blood vessel (forming the pulmonary metastasis lesion), some will enter the pulmonary vein → turn back to the left ventricle via the pulmonary microcirculation. The cancer cell, interweaved in the blood, enters the aorta and then jets into the small artery of the parenchymatous viscera and then enters the microcirculation of each organ (especially the parenchymatous organ, such as liver, kidney, brain and porotic substance of bone through the impact force and vertex flow and pump flow of the heart valve blood. Most of the cancer cells in the circulation will be damaged and killed by the immunological cells in the circulation or the strong blood impact force and shearing force, the tiny minority of the survived cancer cells form the micro-cancer embolus, adhering to the endothelial cell of the micrangium, degrading the basement membrance and passing through the blood vessel.

In this stage, the cancer cell will contact various immunological cells in floating in the blood circulation and cannot survive possibly due to being captured and phagocytized by various immunological cells in the blood. Few survived cancer cells will be adhered to the endothelial cell of the blood vessel due to escaping from the monitoring of the immunity in the blood circulation.

Prevention and cure countermeasures: in this stage, the "target" of therapy of carcinoma metastasis is to protect and enhance the immunologic function of various immunological cells in the blood circulation, activate the immunological cytokine and resist adherence (homogenous adherence of cancer cells and cancer cells, alloplasmatic adherence of cancer cells with blood platelet and so on), resist movement, resist aggregation of blood platelet, resist high coagulation and resist cancer embolus.

Therapeutic goal: activating the immunological cell, protecting function of thymus organization, improving immunity, protecting the bone marrow and producing the blood and promoting the cancer cells floating in the blood circulation to be captured, phagocytized, surrounded and annihilated and intercepted by the immunological cell group.

The second step is the main battlefield to kill off the cancer cells floating in the blood circulation as well as the main countermeasures to interfere and repress the carcinoma metastasis.

3. Third Step of anti carcinomatous metastasis: the metastasis process of the cancer cell in this stage: the cancer cell escapes the monitoring of the immunological cell in blood circulation and the annihilation of the immunological cell, passes through the wall and anchors itself in the organs with agreeable local microenvironment for settlement, in this way, the new blood capillary of tumor forms and then it gradually forms the metastatic carcinoma.

Prevention and cure countermeasures: the interference and repression countermeasures, mainly aiming at improving the histogenic immunity of the local microenvironment and regulating the local microenvironment to make it adverse to the survival and nidation and repress the angiogenesis factor and the new angiogenesis.

To sum up, space allocation of Xu Ze Three Steps of Therapy of Carcinoma Metastasis is in the blood circulation and the time allocation is in three different stages. It attaches importance to improvement of the host immunity. It can be summed up and concluded as Table 1.

Table 1 Xu Ze Three Steps of Therapy of Carcinoma Metastasis

Metastasis stage of cancer cell	Metastasis process	Prevention and cure countermeasures
The stage before the cancer cell intrudes the circulation First step of anti metastasis	Separating the cancer cell from the primary cancer→degrading ECM→adherence and de-adherence→ movement→before entering the blood vessel.	• anti-adherence • anti-degradation • anti-movement • anti stroma metal protease

Transportation stage of cancer cell in blood circulation Second step of anti-metastasis	The cancer cell group and micro cancer embolus float in the blood circulation and are damaged due to being phagocytized and captured by the immunological cell and be subject to the shearing force of the blood.	• enhancing and activating various immunological cells in circulation, improving the immunologic function as the main battlefield of killing off the cancer cells in the routing of the metastasis • anti-adherence • anti-aggregation of blood platelet • anti cancer embolus • TG
The stage in which Cancer cell escapes the blood circulation and anchors "target" organ Third step of anti metastasis	After cancer cell escapes from the blood vessel, it anchors the organ for nidation, forms the new blood vessel and forms the metastatic lesion.	• Inhibiting angiogenesis factor • Inhibiting angiogenesis • Improving immunological regulation • Improving the immunity of local microenvironment.

9. Cancer treatment methods and drugs

Outline

XZ-C immunomodulatory anticancer medicine are from traditional Chinese herbal medicines which are selected 48 kinds of anti-tumor Chinese herbal medicine with better inhibitory rate. After made up into the composition of the compound, and then tested by inhibiting cancer-bearing mice tumor experiments in cancer-bearing mice experiments, the compound inhibitory rate inhibition rate is much greater than single herbs. XZ-C1, XZ-C4 God grass, agrimony, Shu Yang Quan etc 28 Chinese herbal medicines, of which XZ-C1-A, XZ-C1-B 100% inhibit cancer, 100 percent don't kill normal cells, with righting improvment of the role of the body's immune function. From our experiments XZ-C pharmacodynamics, study results show: they has a good inhibitory rate on Ehrlich ascites carcinoma, S182, H22 hepatocellular carcinoma; there are obvious synergy and toxicity attenuation; experiments also demonstrated that the immune XZ-C the regulation of traditional Chinese medicine have significantly improved immune function.

After the acute toxicity test in mice, no obvious toxicity, no significant side effects for long-term oral clinical taking (2--6 years). XZ-C can significantly reduce the toxicity while oral immune regulation medicine during chemotherapy. Intermittent oral XZ-C drugs make leukocytosis, hemoglobin increased while Chemotherapy. Advanced cancer patients, mostly weakness, fatigue, loss of appetite, after taking XZ-C immunomodulatory anticancer medicine 4-8-12 weeks, more significantly improved appetite, sleep, relieve pain, gradually recuperate.

Experiments have been carried out in the research and clinical validation work

Experimental studies

Our laboratory conducted the following new cancer screening experiment study from traditional Chinese medicine, anti-metastatic drugs:

I. In vitro screening test: the use of cancer cells in vitro was observed for cancer drugs directly damage cancer cells. Cultured cancer cells in a test tube, were placed raw meal drug products (500ug / ml) to observe whether there is inhibition and inhibition rate of cancer cells.

2. In vivo antitumor screening test: manufacture cancer-bearing animal model for the screening of Chinese herbs for cancer-bearing animal experiments suppressor rate, batch experiments with 240 mice were divided into eight experimental groups, each group 30, para. 7 group was the control group, Group 8 with 5-Fu or CTX as the control group. The whole group of mice were inoculated with EAC or S180 or H22 cancer cells inoculated 24h, the crude product by oral feeding crude drug powder, long-term feeding the herbs screened each mouse was observed survival inhibition rate was calculated.

Our experimental study for four consecutive years, with more than 1000 per year tumor-bearing animal models, four years made a total of two tumor-bearing animal models, mice each were carried out after the death of the liver, spleen, lung, thymus, 'kidney pathological anatomy, in the 20000 times slices.

3. Results: In our laboratory animal experiments after screening 200 kinds of Chinese herbal medicine, the selected 48 kinds indeed carry, even excellent inhibition of cancer cells, the inhibition rate of more than 75-90%. The group of animal experiments made screening test 152 had no significant anti-cancer effect.

Clinical Vertification:

On the basis of successful experiments on animals to clinical validation

1. Methods: built oncology clinics and combination Research Group of anti-cancer, anti-metastasis and anti-recurrence, keeping the medical records, built perfect follow-up and observation system to observe the long-term efficacy and clinical validation. From experimental study to clinical verification means the clinical application on the basis of successful experimental study. Then new problems are found during the clinical application, which need fundamental experimental studies. Afterwards new experimental results are applied to clinical verification. Experiments → clinic → experiments once more → clinic once more, recurrent ascent continuously; through eight-year clinical practical experiences, knowledge also continues to improve. Summation, analysis, reflection and evaluation ascend to theory, putting forward new knowledge, new concept, new thought, new strategy and new therapeutic route and scheme.

Clinical criteria are: good quality of life, longer survival.

Results: XZ-C immunomodulatory anticancer Chinese medicines have significant treatment effect after applying through a lot in advanced cancer patients treated with observation,

2. Clinical information

(1) Hubei Branch of China Anti-cancer Research Cooperation of Chinese Traditional Medicine and Western Medicine, Anti Carcinoma Metastasis and Recurrence Research Office and Shuguang Tumor Specialized Outpatient Department had treated 4, 698 carcinoma patients in Stage III and IV or in metastasis and recurrence with Z-C medicine combined with western medicine from 1994 to Nov. 2002, among which there were 3, 051 men patients and 1,647 women patients. The youngest one was 11 years old and the oldest one was 86 years old, the high invasion age was 40~69 years. All groups of the patients were entirely subject to the diagnosis of pathological histology or definitive diagnosis with ultrasonic B, CT and MRI iconography. According to the staging standard of UICC, all the cases were entirely the patients in medium and advanced stage over Stage III. In this group, there were 1,021 hepatic carcinoma patients, among which there were 694 primary lesion hepatic carcinoma patients and 327 metastatic hepatic carcinoma patients; there were 752 patients suffering from carcinoma of lung, among which there were 699 patients suffering from the primary carcinoma of lung and 53 patients suffering from the metastatic carcinoma of lung; there were 668 gastric carcinoma patients, 624 patients suffering from esophagus cardia carcinoma, 328 patients suffering from rectum carcinoma of anal canal, 442 patients suffering from carcinoma of colon, 368 patients suffering from breast carcinoma, 74 patients suffering from adenocarcinoma of pancreas, 30 patients suffering from carcinoma of bile duct, 43 patients suffering from retroperitoneal tumor, 38 patients suffering from oophoroma, 9 patients suffering from cervical carcinoma, 11 patients suffering from cerebroma, 34 patients suffering from thyroid carcinoma, 38 patients suffering from nasopharyngeal carcinoma, 9 patients suffering from melanoma, 27 patients suffering from kidney carcinoma, 48 patients suffering from carcinoma of urinary bladder, 13 patients suffering from leukemia, 47 patients suffering from metastasis of supraclavicular lymph nodes, 35 patients suffering various fleshy tumors and 39 patients suffering from other malignancies.

3. Medicine and medication: the treatment aims to protect thymus and increase immune system, protect bone marrow so that improve the immune surveillance and to control cancer cells escape. From traditional Chinese medicine the treatment aims are to support healthy energy to eliminate evils, soften and resolve the hard mass and supplement qi and blood. $XZ-C_1$, $XZ-C_2$, $XZ-C_3$, $XZ-C_4$, $XZ-C_5$, $XZ-C_6$, $XZ-C_7$, $XZ-C_8$, ... $XZ-C_{10}$, according to different kinds of cancers, disease conditions, metastasis situations and according to disease syndrome, choose the above medications. According to the analysis and differentiation of the diseases, anti-cancer powder shall be taken orally and the anti-cancer apocatastasis paste shall be applied externally for the solid tumor or the metastatic tumor. In case of being in pain, anti-cancer aponic paste shall be applied externally. Icterus removal soup or dropsy removal soup shall be taken orally for the patients suffering from icterrus and the ascites.

4. Curative results: The symptom was improved, the quality of life was improved, the survival time was prolonged

(1) Among the 4,277 carcinoma patients in medium and advanced stage who took Z-C medicine with the return visit over 3 months, the case history had the specific observation record of the curative effect, see Table 1. It improved the quality of life of the patients in an all-round way, see Table 2.

Table 1 General information about 4,277 patients suffering from recurrence and metastasis

		Hepatic carcinoma	Carcinoma of lung	Gastric carcinoma	Esophagus cardia carcinoma	Rectum carcinoma of anal canal	Carcinoma of colon	Breast carcinoma	adenocarcinoma of pancreas
No. of cases		1 021	752	668	624	328	442	368	74
Male: female		4:1	4.4:1	2.25:1	3.1:1	1:1	2.1:1	Female	3.2:1
Focus	Primary	694 (68.6%)	699 (93.9%)						
	Metastasis	327 (31.2%)	53 (6.1%)						
Usual metastasis part in this group		Metastatic lung (2) From the stomach (31.2%)	Metastasis of supraclavicular lymph nodes (11.6%)	Metastatic lever (23.8%) Lung metastasis (3%)	Upper metastasis of compact bone (13.1%)	Reoccurrence rate (14.8%)	Metastatic lever (16.0%)	Metastasis of supraclavicular lymph nodes (17.5%)	Metastatic lever (11.7%)
		From esophagus cardia (19.5%) From recta (31.2%)	Brain metastasis (3.1%) Bone metastasis (4.6%)	Metastasis of peritoneum (29.1%) Upper metastasis of compact bone (6.1%)	Metastatic lever (8.3%)	Metastatic lever (7.0%)	Metastasis of peritoneum (6.0%)	Metastasis of axillary lymph nodes (15.0%) Bone metastasis (5.0%)	Rear metastasis of peritoneum (39.1%)
Age	high invasion (year) %	30~39 (76.2)	50~69 (71.6)	40~49 (73.4)	40~69 (80.4)	40~49 (75.2)	30~69 (88.0)	40~59 (65.9)	40~59 (70.0)
	Oldest (year) %	11	20	17	30	27	27	29	34
	Youngest (year) %	86	80	77	77	78	76	80	68

Table 2 Observation of curative effect on 4 277 patients: fully improving the quality of life of the carcinoma patients in medium and advanced stage

Improvement	Vigor	Appetite	Reinforcement of physical force	Improvement in generalized case	Increase of body weight	Improvement of sleep	The restriction of improvement activity and capability released activity	self servicing, normal walking	Resumption of work, Engaged in light work
No. of cases	4071	3986	2450	479	2938	1005	1038	3220	479
(%)	95.2	93.2	57.3	11.2	68.7	23.5	24.3	75.3	11.2

In this group, all of them were the patients in medium and advanced stage. After taking the medicine, their symptoms were improved to different extents with the effective rate of 93.2%. With respect to the improvement of the quality of life (as per Karnofsky Performance Status), it rose to 80 scores on average after administration from 50 on average before administration; the patients in this group met with the different metastasis and dysfunction of the organs about Stage III. It was reported by the previous statistic information that the mesoposition survival time of this kind of patients was about 6 months. The longest time among this group of the cases reached up to 11 years; another patient suffering from hepatic carcinoma had taken Z-C medicine for ten years and a half; two patients suffering from hepatic carcinoma met with frequency encountered carcinomatous lesion in the left and right liver and it entirely subsided through secondary CT reexamination after the patient took Z-C medicine for half a year and the state of the disease had been stable over half a year. One patient suffering from double-kidney carcinoma met with the widespread metastasis of abdominal cavity after removal of one kidney, after taking Z-C medicine, he was entirely recovered and began to work again. 3 patients suffering from carcinoma of lung, with the lung not removed through explaraton, had taken Z-C medicine over three years and a half. 2 patients suffering from gastric remnant carcinoma had taken Z-C medicine for 8 years. 3 patients suffering from reoccurrence of rectal carcinoma had taken Z-C medicine for 3 years. 1 patient suffering from metastatic liver and rib of the mastocarcinoma had taken Z-C medicine for 8 years. 1 patient suffering from the recurrent bladder carcinoma after operation of renal carcinoma had not met with the carcinoma for 9 years and a half after taking Z-C medicine. All of these patients were the ones in the medium and advanced stage that could not be operated once more or treated with radiotherapy or chemotherapy. They only took Z-C medicine without other medicines for treatment. Up to today, they are reexamined and get the medicine at the out-patient department every month. Through taking the medicine for a long time, the state of the disease is controlled in the stable state to make the organism and the tumor in balanced state for a relatively long time and get a relatively good survival with tumor, in this way, the symptoms of the patients are improved, the quality of life is improved and the survival time is prolonged.

(2) As to 84 patients suffering from solid tumor and 56 patients suffering from enlargement of upper lymph node of metastatic compact bone, after taking Z-C series medicines orally and applying Z-C3 anti-cancer apocatastasis paste, they met with good curative effects, see table 3.

Table 3 Changes of 84 patients suffering from solid tumor and 56 patients suffering from metastatic mode after applying Z-C paste externally

	Solid tumor				Enlargement of upper lymph node of metastatic compact bone			
	Disappearance	Shrinkage 1/2	Softening	No change	Disappearance	Shrinkage 1/2	Softening	No change
No. of cases (%)	12	28	32	12	12	22	14	8
	14.2	33.3	38.0	14.2	21.4	39.2	25.0	14.2
Total effective rate (%)	85.7				85.7			

(3) 298 patients suffering from carcinoma pain obtained the obvious pain alleviation effects after taking Z-C medicine orally and applying Z-C anti-cancer apocatastasis paste externally, see Table 1-4.

Clinical menifetation	Pain			
	Light alleviation	Obvious alleviation	Disappearance	Avoidance
No of cases	52	139	93	14
(%)	17.3	46.8	31.2	4.7
Total effective rate (%)	95.3			

5. Exclusive research and development of products: XZ-C immunomodulatory anticancer medicine products (Profile)

Independently developed XZ-C (XU ZE China) series of anti-cancer immune regulation medicine preparation, from experimental research to clinical validation, in animal experiments on the basis of success in clinical practice, clinical experience over the years a large number of clinical cases verification, a significant effect. The results are self-invention, the Department of independent innovation and intellectual property rights.

Looking from traditional Chinese medicine, and screening anti-cancer, anti-metastatic investigational new drug:

The purpose is to screen out non-resistance, non-toxic side effects, a high selectivity, long-term oral anti-cancer, anti-metastatic and anti-recurrent cancer drug. It is well known now for the world's anti-cancer agent does inhibit proliferation of cancer cells, but it only kill cancer cells but also kill normal cells, especially the bone marrow of immune cells, a host of serious damage, because of chemotherapy cytotoxic and non-selectivity. And traditional chemotherapy can suppress the immune function and inhibit bone marrow function. Traditional intravenous chemotherapy treatment is interrupted, the cancer cells cannot be treated during the gap period which cancer cells continued proliferation and division. Although chemotherapy drugs can inhibit the proliferation of cancer cells, but because of its toxic side effects when cancer has not yet been eliminated, administration had to stop. After treatment, cancer cell proliferation up again, and began to have resistance. When resistance, this dose would not work so as to increase the amount executioner. However, if the dose is increased, it may endanger the lives of patients. If the chemotherapy drug resistance has been given, then the cancer is not only ineffective; Contrary to killing only patient's normal cells so cancer cells resistance to cancer drugs and toxics of cancer drugs on the host side effects is a long vexing problem. And we are looking for new drugs, the purpose is to avoid these drawbacks.

According to the theory of cell cycle, anticancer agents must be able to continue long applications so that cancer foci can bath in anti-cancer agents long lasting time, and is available without stopping to prevent their cell division and to prevent recurrence and metastasis. Must be long years, have been conducting long-term, it is best to long-term oral drugs to control existing foci and prevent nascent cancer cells to form. Due to large toxicity the currently used anticancer medication cannot long continuous use, but only short cycle applications. Existing anticancer medication has suppressed immune function, bone marrow suppression, suppression thymus, bone marrow suppression side effects. The formation and development of cancer is due to the patient's immune system to reduce lost immune surveillance, therefore, all anticancer medications should be increased immunization, protection immune organs, immune suppression and should not use drugs.

To this end, we conducted the following experiment laboratory screening of new anti-cancer research from the traditional Chinese medicine, anti-metastatic drugs:

(A) The method of cancer cells in vitro, the experimental study of Chinese herbal medicine suppressor screening rates:

In vitro screening tests: The cancer cells in vitro was observed for sore drugs directly damage cells.

Screening in vitro culture of cancer cells in vitro tests respectively allowing raw and crude drugs of crude product (500ug / ml) to be used and to observe whether there is inhibition of cancer cells, we believe that 200 kinds of traditional Chinese medicine herbs have anticancer function performed one by one in vitro screening tests. And under the same conditions with a normal fiber cell culture to test the toxicity of these cells, and then compared.

(B) Building cancer-bearing animal model for the screening of Chinese herbs for cancer-bearing animal experimental tumor suppressor rate

Suppressor in vivo screening test, each batch experiments with mice 240, divided into 8 groups, each group 30, the first group was the control group 7, group 8 with 5-Fu or CTX control group, the whole group of small mice was inoculated with EA C or S 180 or H22 cancer cells. After inoculation 24h, each rat oral feeding crude product of crude drug powder, long-term feeding the screened the herbs, observed survival, toxicity, computing prolong survival rate calculated suppression sores.

So, we conducted experimental study for four consecutive years, and has conducted a 3-year incidence of tumor-bearing mice and transfer mechanism, the experimental study of the mechanism of relapse, and experimental studies to explore how cancer causing death of the host each year with more than 1,000 tumor-bearing animals model, made a total of nearly four years, 6000 tumor-bearing animal models, mice each were carried out after the death of the liver, spleen, lung, thymus, kidney pathological anatomy, a total of 20,000 times slice to explore to find out whether There may be slight carcinogenic pathogens, with microcirculation microscope 100 tumor-bearing mice were tumor microvessels bell establish and microcirculation.

Through experimental study we first found in China a medicine to inhibit tumor angiogenesis TG had a significant effect, more than 80 cases have been used in clinical treatment of patients Hang metastasis being observed.

Results: In our laboratory animal experiments screened 200 kinds of Chinese herbs and screened48 kinds of certain and excellent herbs with inhibition of cancer cell proliferation, inhibition rate of more than 75 to 90%. But there are some of commonly used Chinese medicine which consider to have the anticancer roles, after animal in vitro and in vivo inhibition rate anti-cancer screening, showed really no effect, or little effect which 152 kinds of medications having no anti-cancer effect had removed from the phase-out of animal experiments.

Screening out of this real 48 kinds of traditional Chinese medications with having good tumor suppression rates, and then optimized the combination and repeated tumor suppression rate experiments in vivo, and finally developed immunomodulatory anticancer Chinese medication XU ZE China1-10 with Chinese own characteristics China (ZC $_{1-10}$).

$Z-C_1$ could inhibit cancer cells, but does not affect normal cells; $Z-C_4$ specially can increase thymus function, can promote proliferation, increased immunity; $Z-C_1$ can protect bone marrow function and to product more blood.

Clinical validation: Based on the success of animal experiments, clinical validation was conducted. Namely the establishment of oncology clinics and Western medicine combined with anti-cancer, anti-metastasis, recurrence Research Group, retained patient medical records, to establish a regular follow-up observation system to observe the long-term effect · face from experimental research to clinical evidence, the discovery of new clinical validation process issue, went back to the laboratory for basical research, then the results of a new experiment for clinical validation. Thus, a clinical experiment again and again clinical experiment, all experimental studies must be clinically proven in a large number of patients observed 3--5 years, or even clinical observation of 8 to 10 years, according to evidence-based medicine, and can have long-term follow-up assessment information, verified indeed have a good long-term efficacy, the efficacy of the standard is: a good quality of life, longer survival. XZ-C sectional immune regulation anti-cancer medicine made after a lot of applications in advanced cancer patients verification, and achieved remarkable results.. XZ-C sectional immune regulation anti-cancer medicine can improve the quality of life of patients with advanced cancer, enhance immune function, increase the body's anticancer abilities, increased appetite and significantly prolong survival.

(C) XZ-C immunomodulatory anticancer Chinese medication Mechanism of Action

With the deepening of traditional Chinese medicine research, it is known to produce a lot of traditional Chinese medicine and biological activity of cytokines and other immune molecules having a regulatory role, this time to clarify XZ-C from the molecular level immunomodulatory anticancer Chinese medication immunological mechanisms very important.

1. XZ-C immunomodulatory anticancer Chinese medication can protect immune organs, increasing the weight of the spleen and chest pay attention.

2. XZ-C immunomodulatory anticancer Chinese medication for hematopoietic function of bone marrow cell proliferation and significant role in promoting.

3. XZ-C immunomodulatory anticancer Chinese medication on T cell immune function enhancement effect on T cells significantly promote proliferation.

4. XZ-C immunomodulatory anticancer Chinese medication for human IL-2 production has significantly enhanced role.

5. XZ-C immunomodulatory anticancer Chinese medication activation of NK cell activity and enhance the role, NK cells with a broad spectrum of anticancer effect, can anti-xenograft tumor cells.

6. XZ-C immunomodulatory anticancer Chinese medication for LAK cell activity can enhance the effect, LAK cells are capable of killing of NK cell sensitive and non-sensitive solid tumor cells, with broad-spectrum anti-tumor effect.

7. XZ-C immunomodulatory anticancer Chinese medication to induce interferon and pro-inducing effect, IFN has a broad-spectrum anti-tumor effect Wo immunomodulatory effects, IFN can inhibit tumor cell proliferation, IFN can activate the skin to kill cancer cells and OIL cells.

8. XZ-C immunomodulatory anticancer Chinese medication for colony stimulating factor can promote credit enhancement, CSF not only involved in hematopoietic cell proliferation, differentiation, and in a host of anti-tumor immunity plays an important role

9. XZ-C immunomodulatory anticancer Chinese medication can promote tumor necrosis factor (TNF) role, TNF is a class can directly cause tumor cell death factor, its main biological role is to kill or inhibit tumor cells.

D. Bilogical response modification(BRM), traditional chinese anticancer medicine similar to BRM and tumor treatment

1. Biological reaction modification (BRM) explores the new field of the tumor biological therapy. Currently BRM as the fourth methods of the tumor treatment gets widely attention in the world.

Oldham in 1982 built BRM theory. Based this in 1984 he advanced the fourth modality of cancer treatment-----biological therapy again. According to this, in the normal condition, there is the dynamic equilibrium between the tumor and the body. The development of the tumors, and even invasion and metastasis, completely is caused by the loss of this equilibrium. If this unbland situation is adjusted to the normal level, the tumor growth can be controlled and will disappear.

The anticancer mechanism of BRM in details as the following:

1) Improve the host defence abilities or decrease the immune inhabitation of the tumors to the host to reach the immune response to the tumors.

2) Look for the biological active things in natural or gene combination to enhance the host defense abilities.

3) Reduce the host response induced by the tumor cells

4) Promote the tumors to division and mature to become the normal cells

5) Reduce the side effects of the chemotherapy and redio therapy and enhance

The host toleration.

2. XZ-C immune regulation anticancer medicine have the functions and curative effects similar to BRM

After four years experimental research and 16 years clinical research which are the drugs similar to BRM selected from traditional Chinese medicine.

XZ-C is the drugs that XU ZE in China professor selected from two hundreds of the anticancer herbs after the experiments. At first the culturing tumor were done. The in vitro was done One by one to select and abserve the direct damage to tumor cells in the culture setting and the control groups of the rate of the anticancer are the chemotherapyxxxx and the normal culture tube cells. The results are to select the a series of the medicine of the anti-cancer proliferation, then made the animal modes which 200 drugs were used on one by one. These experiments of the analysis and evaluation are steps by steps, scientific, practical and strict, etc. The results proved that48 of them have the excellent tumor inhibition effects, however the rest 152 of the tumors anticancer medicine are all common old anticancer medicine which proved no anticancer or less inhibition of the tumors in the animal models during these medicine selection experiments.

The medicine which the author selected on the tumor animal models and had excellent anticancer rat XZ-C can improve immune function, protection of the central immune organs such as thymus and, improving the cell-mediated immune functions, protecting the thymus function, protect the bone morrow function, increase the red blood cells and white blood cells number, active the immune factors, improve the immune surveilence in the blood ect.

XZ-C the main anticancer pharmacology function si anticancer and increase of the immune function. The above XZ-C has the following function as:

1). Activing the host immune system to promote the host immune function to reach the immune respond to the tumors.

2). Activing the host immune factors of the anticancer systems to strengthen the host immune function and improve the immunce surviellence of the host immune systems.

3). Protecting the thymus and bone marrow, improve the immune system, and stimulate the bone marrow function to reduce the inhibition of the bone marrow and increase the white blood cell and red blood cells etc.

4). Reduction of the side effects of the chemotherapy and radioactive therapy to increase the tolerance of the hosts.

5). Increaseing thymus weight and stop the shrinkle of thymus because when the tumor develop thymus goes on shrinkles.

As the above statement, the basic mechanism of XZ-C is similar to BRM and the clinical application is similar to those of the BRM.

(A) XZ-C1 "Smart grams cancer"

The main components are eight Chinese herbs.

Anticancer pharmacology

1. Detoxification, increasing blood circulation, righting, dispelling evil without injury, strong inhibition of cancer cells and inhibition of cancer cell metastasis without inhibition of normal cells.

2. In anti-cancer in vivo tests in mice, they have inhibitory activity in the mice Ehrlich ascites tumor cells which there had been significant differences in the control group.

3. Can prolong survival of mice bearing cancer, increased the survival rate of 26.92%.

4. The main prescription drugs Z-C1-A and Z-C1-B has a stable and significant anticancer effects, 100% inhibition of cancer cells, cancer cell mitotic reduced

and degenerated and necrosed seriously and epithelial cells or fibroblasts is no impact in the administration group. XZ-C1-D extract have inhibitory activity on human cervical cancer cells, on mouse sarcoma s180 inhibition rate was 98.9%, several other ingredients also have a strong anticancer effect.

5. Z-C1 Herbs inhibition effect on Mice bearing H22 hepatoma tumor: z-c1 drug inhibition rate was 40 percent in the second week, the first four weeks was 45%, the first six weeks of 58%; in the control group CTX medication first two weeks inhibition rate was 45%, the first four weeks inhibition rate was 45%, 49% for the first six weeks.

6. Z-C1 medicine influence on survival in mice bearing H22: life-prolonging rate was 85% in z-c1 group; life extension was 9.8% in CTX control group; in Z-C1 group Thymus did not shrink; however thymus shrank in Control group.

Clinical application

1. Indications: esophageal cancer, stomach cancer, colorectal cancer, lung cancer, breast cancer, liver pain, bile duct cancer, pancreatic cancer, thyroid cancer, nasopharyngeal cancer, brain tumors, renal cancer, bladder cancer, ovarian cancer, cervical cancer, various sarcoma and a variety of metastasis, recurrent cancer.

2. Usage: after taking z- c1 continuously 1 - 3 months, the patients felt better. This medication can be taken for long-term and can be taken one dose every other day after three years; can be taken two doses weekly after 5 years to retain immune function and cytokine long-term stable at a certain level.

Toxicity Test

ZX-C1 can be used for long-term. The acute toxicity test showed that when adult mice was fed a dose 104 times (10g / Kg body weight), respectively, in 24, 48, 72, 96 hours of observation, 30 purebred mice didn't die. The median lethal dose (LD5O) didn't have any number so that it is a rather safe prescriptions.

In the oncology clinic it has been used for many years and some patients have taken more than three to five years and more than 8 to 10 years in order to maintain immunity and to stop recurrence. It can be taken for long-term and it is quite safe oral cancer.

(B) XZ-C2

Ingredients: 9 kinds of anticancer herbs

Anticancer pharmacology

1. Animal experiments show that it can prolong L7212 mouse (mouse leukemia) survival, well-behaved compared to the control group, there were statistically significant.

2. Can improve inhibition rate in the L7212 in mice

3. Z-C1-A and Z-C2-B on mouse sarcoma (s180) has a strong inhibitory effect.

Application

Indications: leukemia, upper gastrointestinal cancer, tongue, larynx, nasopharynx cancer, cervical cancer, bone metastasis, esophagus cancer or gastric ulcer anastomotic recurrence narrow (no longer surgery). It has general effect on Acute leukemia lymph and has obvious efficiency of each of the other type of leukemia. It has a more significant effect on Bone metastasis

Usage: one capsule Qid generally or two capsules tid

Leukemia 3 capsules tid after meal and seven days for a course.

(C) XZ-C3 topical pain Patch

Prescription Content: kaempferol, turmeric, etc. 14 flavors

Anticancer pharmacology

1. Detoxification, anti-inflammatory pain, qi Sanjie pain;

2. Increasing the blood circulation, reducing swelling and pain, played a total of detoxification, swelling and analgesic effect, while the most prominent role in cancer treatment is to stop pain.

3. For point application, applicator than simply pain, can better play the efficacy and achieve rapid pain relief purposes.

Clinical application

Indications: liver cancer, lung cancer pain, back pain from pancreatic cancer, bone pain, neck and supraclavicular lymph nodes metastasis.

Usage: A total of research and go take honey, mix, stir into a paste backup, lung disease spreads in milk root point (nipple straight down 5, 6 ribs), liver cancer spreads on the door hole (milk midline 6-7 rib room), treated and covered with gauze and tape securely, severe pain 6h for a second, lesser pain, 12h replacement of 1: continuous use to relieve pain or disappeared.

Experience: Treatment of 84 cases of liver cancer, lung cancer pain patients, have analgesic effect, general medicine three times, will receive different levels of pain relief, 3 to 7 days after a significant analgesic effect, some basical pain.

(D) ZX-C4 anticancer medication of protecting thymus and increasing immune function (5g / bag)

Ingredients: including 12 valuable herbs

Anticancer pharmacology

1. To promote lymphocyte transformation, enhancing immune function, increased white blood cells, inhibit cancer cell, Warming blood.

2. Ehrlich ascites tumor cells transplanted into the abdominal cavity of mice, one day after transplantation and 7 Days 2 times for chemotherapy drugs in mice, while serving z -c4 (2g / kg) per day is significantly enhanced the effectiveness of chemotherapy drugs effect.

3. To suppress leukopenia and weight loss induced by chemotherapy medicinal MMC MMC

4. While serving Z-C4, it was found to inhibit cancer cells in terms of improving the effect of intravenously injected anticancer chemotherapy drugs than simply using more than three times in cancer-bearing mice.

5. Chemotherapy drugs for cancer-bearing mice can damage special thymus, spleen and other immune organs, but after adding the service z-C4, thymus, spleen and other organs completely don't shrink, showed z-C4 have effects on the immune organ protective nature function.

6. ZX-C4 extract in Ehrlich ascites disease mouse prolonged the mice life span of up to 167.1%, the average survival time of mice in the control group 15.2 days, and z-c4 administration group is 25.4 days, while reticuloendothelial system function in mice showed significantly higher.

7. Z-C4 allows the chemotherapy drugs cisplatin quickly to mitigate its effects, can enhance the effectiveness of cisplatin. z-C4 can be 100% inhibition of cisplatin toxicity chloroplatinic day conventional dose amount that is human can be. z-c4 not resist cisplatin Chen Hang crazy. z-C4 can protect the kidney, the renal damage cis-platinum chlorine hardly occurs. Z-C4 has highly promising anticancer drug.

8. Z-C4 patients after cancer surgery have a significant effect, gastrointestinal, liver, pancreas and other ulcer disease after radical: all manifestations of physical decline, decreased immunity, fatigue, burnout, loss of appetite and anemia, after 1 a 2 weeks from the beginning can be oral or tube feeding, oral Z-C4 granules, 7.5 g daily, before meals three times a blunt, 12 weeks, during which can be chemotherapy or immune therapy.

9. Z-C4 medicine antitumor effect in mice bearing hepatoma H22: z-c4 first two weeks of medication inhibition rate was 55%, the first four weeks inhibition rate was 68%, the first six weeks inhibition rate was 70% the control group, CTX (cyclophosphamide Yu amine) Week 2 inhibitory drugs was 45%: the first four weeks inhibition rate of 49%.

10. z-C4 medicine for liver cancer H22 bearing mice survival, z-C4 group extend survival rate 200%, CTX group life span was 9.8%.

11. Z-C4 can significantly improve immune function, can increase white blood cells and red blood cells, liver and kidney function had no effect on the liver, kidney slices without damage. CTX cause leukopenia, reduced immune function, kidney sections have kidney damage.

12. Z-C4 treated group Thymus do not shrink and slightly hypertrophy, CTX thymus control group significantly shrink. Z-C4 on mouse sarcoma (S180) has a strong inhibitory effect.

Clinical Application:

Indications: various types of cancer, sarcoma, a variety of advanced cancer, metastasis, recurrence of cancer, radiotherapy, chemotherapy, post-operative patients. It can be applied all kinds of cancer, especially dizziness, weakness, fatigue, lazy words, less gas, spontaneous sweating, heart palpitations, insomnia, blood deficiency were more applicable.

Z-C4 medicine was used before surgery and after starting the medication and medication every four weeks to do a clinical and laboratory tests, for 20 weeks. Test items: conscious and objective symptoms, body weight, total protein and albumin, total cholesterol, dielectric, ALT AST blood and platelets, lymphocytes, T cells and B cells, r globulin, urinary protein.

Treatment Results: ① increase in the number of lymphocytes, inhibit the role of leukopenia; ② no impact on liver function; ③ protect the kidney function, kidney damage is not so; ④ can significantly reduce the chemotherapy and radiotherapy-induced rash, stomatitis etc; ⑤ postoperative, after chemotherapy, effective physical recovery after radiotherapy, can increase appetite, improve the general malaise and weight gain.

ZX-C4 reduce side effects of radiotherapy and chemotherapy and improve the overall state of the patient after surgery. It is a very valuable rehabilitation medication.

Experience: Modern medicine for the treatment of advanced cancer presents a variety of methods, but there are still some problems, it is still not convinced that the combined use of chemotherapy for advanced disease if certain effective drugs. Even if effective, but it also brings serious side effects, may be considered modern medical treatment for cancer is to kill cancer cells, is offensive, while the Chinese places to enhance the body's own functions to draw even tone pull eliminate cancer. To this end, it should find a way to reduce or eliminate symptoms, improve or treat the disease with few side effects, the treatment can prolong life, and Z-C4 being has the features and advantages.

Through experiments ZX-C4 has the role of enhanced anticancer effect; promote B cell mitosis role; the catch into the effects of radiation damage hematopoietic system recovery; the promotion of the role of phagocytic cells; thymus increased protective immunity, protection of bone marrow Blood role.

Toxicity Test

Z-C4 can be used long-term. Acute toxicity experiments showed that the median lethal dose (LD50) can not do, is safe and herbs, has been used in the specialist clinic for many years, some patients long-term use three to five years, or even take 8-10 years to maintain immunity, prevent cancer recurrence and metastasis. This anticancer and antimetasatasis medication can be taken by oral for long-term oral and is quite safe.

(5) The following XZ-C various immunomodulatory anticancer medicine series and the experimental and clinical contents are too many and too long so that here only gave names and profiles were omitted.

1. XZ-C5: for liver cancer
2. XZ-C6: for bladder cancer
3. XZ-C7: for Lung cancer
4. XZ-C 8: protect bone marrow and increase blood, attenuated toxics of radiotherapy and chemotherapy
5. XZ-C9: pancreas cancer, prostate cancer.
6. XZ-C10: for brain tumor

All of above of a variety of cancer anticancer, antimetastasis, recurrent research Chinese medicine are based on the experimental study and applied by specialist in outpatient clinics more than 20 years and achieved good results.

Our research Chinese medications for cancer complications in out-patient center of cancer treatment:

1. Anticancer eliminate water soup for pleural effusion and ascites
2. Drop yellow soup for liver cirrhosis and jaundice
3. Anticancer soup after surgery for postoperative recovery
4. Starvation soup for cancer loss of appetite
5. Through Quiet soup for anastomotic stenosis
6. Adhesiolysis soup for adhesions after surgery for cancer

Above all research product formulations. Observation by cancer specialist clinic over the years this big boy patient, have achieved good results, reduce patient suffering, improve the survival quality first, extended survival.

10. Immune pharmacology of XZ-C Immune regulation anti-cancer medications

Compared traditional Chinese immunization pharmacology with western immunity pharmacology which they have their own characteristics and advantages. Traditional Chinese medicine through clinical experience accumulated a large of medications which have role in regulating the immune function, especially beneficial traditional Chinese medicines generally having dynamic regulation of the immune benefits.

Whether single herb or drug prescription will have a variety of active ingredients, and unlike Western medicine (synthetic drugs) is a matter of a single structure. Traditional medications are multifaceted roles. In addition to the regulation of immune function, traditional medications have certain roles on each function of the whole systems.

XZ-C traditional Chinese medicine immunomodulator have a major role in regulate cell-mediated immunity (Cellular imnunity) including cytokines or lymphokines, traditional Chinese medicine has the main role in the stem cells immune such as the thymus, gonads and lymphatic systems and T, B cells and various cells factors.

There have been a few ancient medicine concepts through righteousness and no evil, which constitute an integral part of traditional Chinese medicine and its essence of this theory is a few two-dimensional three functional balance, enhance resistance to disease. In fact, its main role is to enhance immune function. Immunity pharmacology is an emerging interdisciplinary, a bridge contact between pharmacology and immunology. XZC immunomodulatory agents have obvious immune function.

XZ-C immune regulation medication XZ-C$_{1-10}$ anti-cancer metastasis and recurrence clinical observation Adaptation

1. Distant metastases: such as liver metastases, lung metastases, bone metastases, brain metastases, abdominal lymph node metastasis, mediastinal metastasis, malignant pleural effusion, malignant ascites.
2. After chemotherapy and radiology therapy.
3. The patients who cannot tolerate the radiology and chemotheray such as the elderly or other diseases.
4. The surgery can not remove the cancer or can not tolerate surgery.

11. Formed theoretical system of XZ-C anticancer treatment

After 20 years of self-reliance, hard work, Professor Xu Ze completed national science and technology commission of the application of "eight five" basic and clinical research and technological topics. Series of nearly one hundred scientific research papers summarized the information and several books were published. This book collected and summarized his formed theoretical system of XZ-C cancer Therapy which the theoretical basis and experimental evidence and clinical observation verification were undergoing for cancer treatment.

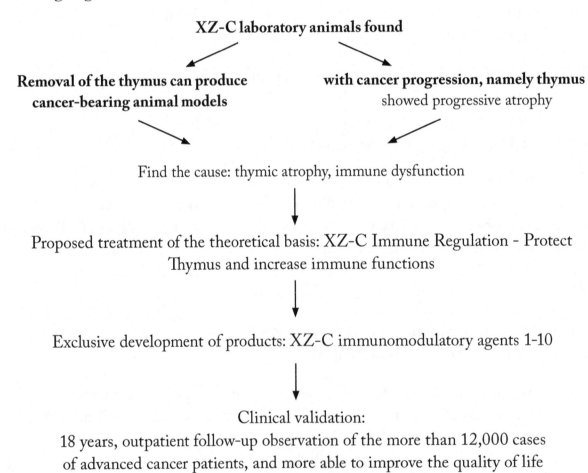

XZ-C laboratory animals found

Removal of the thymus can produce cancer-bearing animal models

with cancer progression, namely thymus showed progressive atrophy

Find the cause: thymic atrophy, immune dysfunction

Proposed treatment of the theoretical basis: XZ-C Immune Regulation - Protect Thymus and increase immune functions

Exclusive development of products: XZ-C immunomodulatory agents 1-10

Clinical validation:
18 years, outpatient follow-up observation of the more than 12,000 cases of advanced cancer patients, and more able to improve the quality of life and prolong survival, satisfactory

Theoretical System XZ-C cancer therapy

12. Our research journey of thinking and scientific thinking

Our 28 years of cancer research work of scientific thinking and scientific journey thinking can be divided into three phases profile:

(A) The first phase of 1985-- 1999

- From the follow-up questions to find and ask a question → → research questions;
- From the review, analysis, reflection to find current problems of traditional cancer therapies and to be further studied and improved;
- Recognize that there is a problem and it should change the thinking, changing concepts;
- Summary information, sorting, collection, published the first monograph "new understanding and a new model for cancer therapy" in January 2001 by Hubei Science and Technology Publishing House.

(B) The second phase after 2001 -

- The "target" and key of cancer research and treatment is anti-metastatic cancer therapy;
- Conducted a series of basic and clinical validation studies of anti-cancer metastasis, recurrence and rised to the theory of innovation, put forward new ideas, new methods of anti-metastasis;
- Summarized information, sorted into collection, published "new concepts and new methods of cancer metastasis treatment" second monograph January 2006 by People's Medical Publishing House, Xinhua Bookstore issued in April 2007 won the People's Republic of China and Publication issued by the department "Three hundred" original book award.

(C) The third phase after 2006 -

A. Study the whole process of development of cancer prevention and treatment;
B. Reform and innovation of cancer research and development;

C. "three early" is the strategies of cancer prevention and treatment

D. I have been 55 years in the tumor surgery, more and more patients, the incidence of cancer is also on the rise, the mortality rate remains high, so I deeply appreciate, not only pay attention to the treatment of cancer, but also to focus on prevention from cancer source. There is a series of related studies, summary data, sorting and collection which was published, the third of my monograph "The new concept and a new approach to cancer treatment," in October 2011 by People's Medical Publishing House, Xinhua Bookstore. Later it was published in English on March 26, 2013 in Washington publication, international distribution.

Part II Basic and Clinical

Table of Contents

Experimental research, pharmacology and molecular medicine immunity level Chinese and Western medicine combined with Cancer Research

A. Step out a XZ-C immune regulation at the molecular level in Chinese and Western medicine Pharmaceutical combination of new roads to overcome cancer

B. Walk out a way of a traditional Chinese medicine immune regulation, regulation of the immune vitality, prevent thymus atrophy, promote thymic hyperplasia, protection of bone marrow function, improve immune surveillance at the molecular level

Foreword

Experimental Surgery is extremely important in the development of medical science and is a key to open the box of medicine. The method of prevention and treatment of many diseases has achieved stability after many times of animal studies, then applied to clinical outcomes in order to promote the development of the medical industry.

In order to development of science and innovation of technology, the laboratory is a key. I deeply appreciate the importance of the lab. I was the first group of university students after the liberation of the college entrance examination. I didn't further degree study, nor went aboard for study, but I made a number of world-class results, The key is that I have a good laboratory. In the 1960s I participated in cardiopulmonary bypass surgery laboratory. In the 80s I built with liver cirrhosis room laboratory. In the 90s I built the Institute of Experimental Surgery in order to conquer cancer as the main direction. In my lab equipment condition is better and there are animals such as mice, rats, guinea pigs, rabbits, dogs, monkeys and other animals, a better operating room sterilization can make various major surgery such as the chest, abdomen operations and postoperative observation successfully, also a variety of designs and conceive of the experimental operation can achieve outcomes or conclusions.

Therefore laboratory conditions are the key which is to build well-equipped laboratories.

University teachers should take dual tasks, first do a good job teaching; the second is the development of science.

University teachers should have a good laboratory for scientific research, follow the scientific concept of development, based on the known science, to explore the unknown science, and the future of science, new disciplines, interdisciplinary, cross-disciplinary, facing the frontiers of science, for innovative, forward, to science hall, brick by Tim Watts.

In summary, the experimental research and basic research are important. The absence of experimental research and breakthrough of basic research is difficult to improve the clinical efficacy and is difficult propose new understanding, new concept, new theoretical insights. The experiment is the key and I have a good laboratory, was director of the Institute of Experimental Surgery and is also director of clinical surgery, experimental research, basic research and clinical validation facilitate balanced.

Basic medical research is very important to the progress of fighting against the disease. The experimental oncology is basic science of cancer prevention research and promotes the deepening development of China's cancer research.

Our experimental Surgery Institute conducted a series of experiments of exploring the mechanism study of cancer occurrence, invasion and recurrence. After a full four-year experimental cancer research, it was found that: thymic atrophy and immune dysfunction may be one of a tumor etiology, pathogenesis. How to prevent thymus atrophy? Regulates immune function? How to boost the immune? How to protect thymus function? The answer is: to overcome cancer should be immune regulation and combine Chinese and Western medicine at the molecular level to walk out a new Chinese style road.

Experimental Study

1. New discovery of anticancer and cancer metastasis research

Revelation of anticancer metastasis research

I am a clinical surgeon, why do I do cancer research? This is due to the petition results of following up a group of cancer patients.

In 1985, I did petition letters for more than 3000 cases of thoracic and abdominal cancer patients which I operated surgery myself.

Results: most patients were relapse and metastasis recurrence or metastasis during postoperative 2--3-year and some even several months or 1 year.

The findings of these results of follow-up: the key to influence long-term outcome of the surgery is recurrence and metastasis.

Therefore, it presents us with an important question which clinicians must pay attention to research recurrence, prevention and treatment measures of metastasis in order to improve long-term outcome after surgery. Therefore, the basis and clinical experimental study of the metastasis needed. Without basic research breakthroughs, it is difficult to improve the clinical efficacy.

So we established the Experimental Surgery Laboratory (later in 1991 established the Hubei Medical College, Institute of Experimental Surgery, research direction for the fight against cancer).

We conducted a study from the following two aspects: one for animal studies; a clinical study. On the basis of successful experiments on animals, then used in clinical, clinical validation. After 28 years of hard work, summer and winter, and conducted a series of experimental studies and clinical validation work, we made a series of scientific and technological innovation achievements in scientific research.

New discovery

(1) From the follow-up found that:

① Recurrence and metastasis is the key to influence long-term outcome of the surgery.

② Clinician must pay attention to and study the prevention measures of the recurrence and metastasis.

(2) It was found from cancer research:

① Removal of the thymus (Thymus, TH) can produce cancer-bearing animal models, injection of immunosuppressive agents can also contribute to the establishment of a cancer-bearing animal models. The study concluded, apparently to prove: the occurrence and development of the cancer has remarkably affirmative relation with the thymus of the immune organ of the host and its functions. If TH was not cut, it is difficult to manufacture animal models. Repeating several experiments, results were confirmed.

② Does the inferior immune lead to the cancer or the cancer lead to the inferior immune at all? Our experimental results: the inferior immune leads to the occurrence and development of the cancer, without the descent of immunologic function, it is not easy to realize the successful inoculation. It is suggested by the experimental results: improving and maintaining the good immunologic function and protecting the good thymus of the central immune organ are the important measures for preventing the occurrence of cancer.

③ in studying the relation between the metastasis of cancer and the immune our lab establishes animal models for liver metastatic carcinoma, which are divided into two groups including Group A applied with immune depressant and Group B not applied with immune depressant. Results: the metastatic lesions in the liver in Group A are obviously more than the ones in Group B. It is suggested by the experimental results: metastasis is related to the immune and inferior immunologic function or application of immune depressant may promote the tumor metastasis.

④ When we investigate for how tumor impacts on immune organ, it was found that with the progress of cancer, thymus is showed a progressive atrophy. The thymus of the host meets with the acute progressive atrophy after the cancer cells are inoculated, the cell proliferation is prevented and the volume is obviously shrunk. It is suggested by the experimental results: the tumor may inhibit the thymus, resulting in the atrophy of the immune organ

⑤ Through experiments, we also found that: that if some experimental mice are not successfully inoculated or the tumor is very small, the thymus is not obviously shrunk. In order to understand the relation between the tumor and the atrophy of the thymus, we excise the transplanted solid tumor of one group of mice when it grows up to the size of a thumb. After one month, through anatomy, we find the thymus does not meet with progressive atrophy again. Therefore, it is inferred by us that maybe the solid tumor produces one kind of unknown factor to inhibit the thymus, which shall be further studied through experiment.

⑥ it is proven by the above-mentioned experimental results: the advance of the tumor makes the thymus meet with progressive atrophy, then, can we take some measures to prevent the atrophy of the thymus of the host? Therefore, we further perfect the design to seek for the method or drug to prevent the atrophy of the thymus of the cancer-bearing mice through the experimental study on animal. So we make the experimental study to recover the function of the immune organ through cell transplantation of the immune organ. We discuss the atrophy of the thymus of the immune organ in preventing the advance of tumor, seek for the method to recover the functions of the thymus and reconstruct the immune, carry out the cell transplantation of foetal liver, spleen and thymus with the mice and establish the immunologic function through adoptive immunity. It is shown by the results: through the joint transplantation of three groups of cells, namely S, T and L (200 experimental mice), the entire extinction rate of the tumor in the long term is 46.67% and the one with the entire extinction of the tumor get a long survival life.

⑦ In the experiment to probe into the effects of tumor on the immune organ such as spleen, we find: the spleen can inhibit the growth of the tumor in the early stage of the tumor, however, in the late stage, the spleen meets with the progressive atrophy. It is suggested by the study results: the effects of spleen on the growth of the tumor are embodied into bi-direction, in the early stage, it can inhibit the tumor to a certain extent, however, in the late stage, it fails to inhibit the tumor. The cell transplantation of the spleen can enhance the role of inhibiting the tumor.

In short, from the above series of experiments it was found that thymus atrophy and immune dysfunction may be one of the etiology and pathogenesis of cancer, should be to study further from thymus function and organizational structure, immune dysfunction and how to boost the immune, immune reconstruction, new methods and new ways how to protect Thymus and increase immune function. The following review the structure and function of the thymus and look for cancer treatment.

2. Experimental observation of tumor effects on thymus

Generally it is believed that the body's immune function status affects the occurrence, development and prognosis of cancer, while cancer of the immune status will dampen demand. Both reinforce each other and complex. When doing the animal experiments on the influences of spleen on the tumorous growth, the author have observed that the immune organs thymus, spleen of the cancer-bearing mice have changed a lot. It seems that this process presents a certain law. In order to study further on the relationship and laws between tumors and spleens or thymus, the following experiments are designed to observe dynamically the changes of conversion rates of thymus, spleen and lymphocyte of cancer-bearing mice in different phases and probe into the relationship between them.

【Materials and Methods】

(1) Experimental animals and grouping 40 Kunming mice were randomly divided into four groups, rats aged 40 ~ 50d, weighing 15 ~ 18g. Male and female, regardless.

I   groups: healthy control group, is not healthy mice inoculated with cancer, were killed after thymus, spleen and peripheral blood experiment observation.

II   group: intraperitoneal inoculation of Ehrlich ascites tumor cells in 0.1×10^7 个, 3d sacrificed after observation.

III group: inoculation of tumor cells (ibid.), The first 7 days sacrificed observation.

IV   groups: the first 14 days of the death of tumor cells inoculation observation.

Take the results from the experiment of the spleen effects on tumor growth in 100 tumor-bearing mice with the autopsy after terminally dead as thymus and spleen change in the advanced tumor stages. The average diameter of thymus in advanced tumor-bearing mice was 1.2 ± 0.3mm and the average weight was 20 ± 5 mg with hard texture. The spleen was withering, average weight was 60 ± 12 mg with hard texture, color gray, significantly reduced the growth center, and fibrosis.

(2) Experimental methods

Each group of mice were sacrificed at the prepared time and reserve the whole blood specimens from each mouse (with heparin) 1ml to do lymphocyte conversion test, and then anatomize them immediately; observe the range of soakage, volume of ascites and the situation of all viscera; emphasize on observing the anatomical shape of thymus, spleens and lymph nodes and take out the thymus and spleen integrally, then measure their volume with a vernier caliper; weigh them respectively using analytical balance and send them to the department of defection.

[Results]

(1) Thymic weights of mice in each group after inoculated with cancer cells in different phases

Analysis of variance of Table 1, Table 2. Table 1, Table 2 with a graph showing the results, to delineate the thymus weight change curve (Figure 1)

Table 1 Comparison of thymic weights of mice in each group (mg)

Group	Group I Control	Group II on the 3rd after inoculated	Group III on the 7rd after inoculated	Group IV on the 14rd after inoculated	Group On the 25th after inoculated	Group On the 30th after inoculated
Xij	72.8	78.2	90.0	40.0	25.13	16.90
	50.0	83.4	66.0	32.2	29.46	17.00
	56.4	89	85.4	39.8	28.90	19.05
	96.4	68	106.5	23.5	26.77	18.16
	77.4	74.8	51.7	38.0	27.00	16.98
	100.7	95.4	77.8	36.0	28.00	20.01
	87.5	115.0	73.0	46.0	26.78	19.23
	76.8	56.4	60.0	20.0	27.69	18.98
	112.7	43.0	49.4	55	31.37	18.54
	51.0			20	28.90	15.15
åX	781.07	703.2	736.3	350.5	280	180
N	10	9	10	10	10	10
CI	78.17	78.13	73.63	35.05	28.00	18.00
SC²	66261.79	58566.66	57033.75	18467.25	7867.44	6518.612

Table 2 Analysis of variance of table 1

Resources of variation	SS	V	MS	F	P
Between groups within groups	12967.10 11777.12	3 35	4322.36 336.48	12.85	<0.01
Total	24744.22				

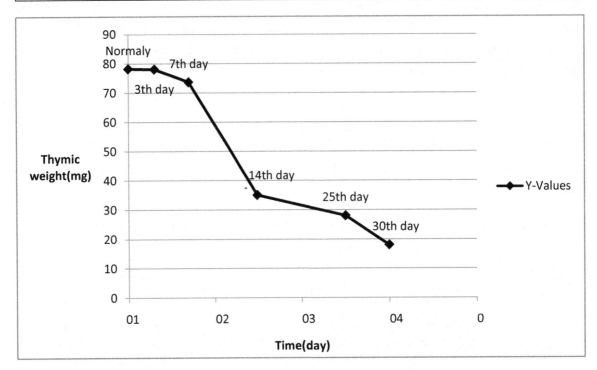

Figure 1 the curve of variation on the thymic weights

It can be noticed that thymus of the cancer-bearing mice present the regular change from table 1, table 2 and figure 1. Within 7 days after inoculation, thymuses have no obvious change observed by eyes; however their weights begin to lose weight. After 7 days, they present acute progressive atrophy; in the later period, the diameter of the thymuses reduce from the normal level 5~8 mm to about 1mm and the weights decrease from 76.1mg to 20mg with the texture becoming hard and the functions declining even lost, which indicates that the cellular immune functions are operated and inhibited increasingly with the development of tumors, and the immune functions are declined to a lower level with tumors growing more and more rapidly.

(2) Pathological changes in thymus

Thymus: Thymus presents progressive atrophy during the whole course of disease; on the 3rd day after inoculated with cancer cells, thymus shrinks slightly and the color is gray; on the 7th day, thymic volume shrinks obviously and the cellular proliferation is stopped with reduced mature cells; during the later period of tumors, thymus shrinks extremely and its volume is as big as a sesame with the diameter of 1 mm and hard texture.

(3) The experimental results showed that after inoculation of the tumors, thymus rapidly shrinkle and continue shrinkle during the whole process so that thymus rapidly lost the anticancer immune response. The experiment showed that thymus change its construction after the inoculation of the tumors and shrinkls during the whole process. In the later stage thymus weight decrease from 78.13+13.2 mg to 20+5mg, the diameter of the volume decrease from 5-8mm to 1mm. The cell proliferation clearly decreased.

Due to the shrinkle of thymus, the cell proliferation inhibited, the mature cell decrease or loss, the index decrease, the metabilish decrease, the cell activities decrease, the decrease of the secretory of thymus hormones, the cell-mediated immune function must be damaged and the defense of the mice decrease, the tumor cells of transplantation grow rapidly. XXX etc reported that along with thymus shrinkle in the mice there is the proliferation of the bone marrow ad the decrease of the xxx cells which was considered there were close relationship between them. Therefore, the inhibition or damage to the host immune system are many aspects, which affects the whole immune system. The experiment of the lymphocyte transformation rates showed that after the inoculation of the tumors, the transformation rates decreased, in the later stage into50%, showing the inhibition of the cell-mediated immune system. The details of how the thymus can be inhibited and shrinkled need to research further.

Thymus also produces a variety of hormones to promote the differentiation of immune lymphoid stem cell maturation. Although thymus is lymphoid organs, but due to the presence of blood thymus barrier, thymus doesn't contact with the antigens directly to play a role in the effect. Therefore there are not tumor-specific antigen stimulation and proliferation of enlargement. The tumors secrete immunosuppressive factors able to act on the thymus, so that thymus is atrophy, dysfunction.

The immune therapy of the tumors is the field which many physicians have great interests.

Since the 1980s, due to the rapid development of immunology and biotechnology which provide an opportunity of tumor immunotherapy, biological response modifiers(BRM) was proposed as fourth treatment in addition to surgery, radiotherapy, chemotherapy which is tumor biological therapy. Using biological modulators to treat cancer may have hoped to promote the development of effective new therapies for immune therapy.

Summary, the host and the tumor are against with each other during the tumor occurrence and development, which exist all the time. In the healthy immune system, our bodyhave ability to limit and to kill the tumor cells. On the other hand, the growth of the tumor produces a lot of influence on the body's immune system which suppresses immune function and promotes tumor development.

3. Shape and position of the thymus

Thymus is cone-shaped and can be divided into left and right leaves which are not symmetrical and is soft, elongated flat strip and is connected by connective tissue. The size of the thymus has a large difference in different age groups. Thymus grows fast in late period of embryonic development and neonatal. The period from birth to 2 years old is the best period of development of the thymus weighing 15 ~ 20g. With age, the thymus continues to develop and to increase, but slow during postnatal development. In puberty it reached to 25 ~ 40g. After puberty, the thymus begins to shrink. Thymus in adult still maintain the original shape, but its structure has changed dramatically such as a significant reduction in lymphocytes and thymus tissue is replaced by fat tissue more.

The adult thymus is behind sternum and on the front of mediastinum. Its rear is with the innominate vein and aortic arch adjacent to both sides of the mediastinal pleura and lung. Thymoma and thymic enlargement can compress the above organs corresponding clinical symptoms.

Children thymus is larger with upper end extending root of the neck and with sometimes up to the lower edge of the thyroid gland. Sometimes the lower end can be inserted into the anterior mediastinum up to the front of pericardial.

4. Thymus structure and function

(1) Coating: thymus tissue surface is coated with a film, a film composed of dense collagen fibers, elastic fiber and matrix and other substance. Coating of the connective tissue fibers extends into the substance of the thymus. The thymus is divided into many lobules. Leaflets around are the cortex and medulla is in the dark side. There is a mesh stent composed of epithelial cells between these two.

(2) Cortex: thymic cortex is located around the portion of the leaflets by dense lymphocytes and epithelial reticular cells. Lymphocytes near cortex is large which is original cell type. Middle lymphocytes were medium-sized, mostly small lymphocyte is in the inner layer. Scattered macrophages is within the cortex. Hematopoietic stem cell proliferation and differentiation of T lymphocytes process is from shallow to deep.

(3) Medulla: thymic medulla is located deep leaflets composed by epithelial reticular cells and a small number of lymphocytes. Thymus bodies are scattering in the medulla. Small bodies are circular or oval made of several layers of epithelial reticular cells and arranged in concentric circles.

Thymus function

Thymus function is more complex. Thymus is lymphoid organs and has endocrine functions. Some authors will list it in the endocrine system. Its main function is to develop and to manufacture T lymphocytes and thymic hormone secretion. T cells within thymus need a suitable internal environment to develop. Thymic epithelial reticular cells can secrete a variety of solidarity hormones: thymosin, thymopoietin, thymulin, thymic humoral factor(THF) and ubiguitin, etc. These hormones and macrophages within thymus together form a nurturing T cell microenvironment. Thymosin and thymopoietin can promote lymphoid stem cell differentiation to T cells, stimulate T cell proliferation and stimulate hypothalamus to secrete ACTH and LH; thymopoietin can induce T cell differentiation; other hormones can promote early T cell division and have to promote synergy of T cell maturation.

Original lymph stem cells don't have immune function; later convert into T cells with immune function, then migrate to peripheral lymphoid organs such as lymphoid tissue, lymph nodes, spleen, etc. by blood circulation to be involved in the immune response after antigen activation. Although thymus atrophy and degradation in adult, there is still the ability to secrete thymic hormones. When the body's lymphoid tissue damage, T cells have a significant reduction. In thymic hormone action lymphoid stem cells in thymus can still be converted to T cells.

T lymphocyte

Two distinct types of thymocytes are produced in the thymus: CD4/CD8. All T cells originate from <u>haematopoietic stem cells</u> in the <u>bone marrow</u>. In the bone marrow haematopoietic stem cells become haematopoietic progenitors; on the way to thymus haematopoietic progenitors are expanded by cell division to generate a large population of immature thymocytes; in the thymus the earlist thymocytes are *double- negative* (CD4⁻CD8⁻) cells, later become *double-positive* thymocytes (CD4⁺CD8⁺); finally mature to *single-positive* (CD4⁺CD8⁻ or CD4⁻CD8⁺) thymocytes. About 98% of <u>thymocytes</u> die during the development processes in the thymus by failing either positive selection or negative selection, whereas 2% matured naïve T cells leave the <u>thymus</u> and begin to spread throughout the body, including the <u>lymph nodes</u>. As the thymus shrinks by about 3% a year throughout middle age, there is a corresponding fall in the thymic production of naive T cells, leaving peripheral T cell expansion to play a greater role in protecting older subjects.

Phenotypic change of T cell differentiation during development.

To induce T cell differentiation and mature in the thymus, the main factors include: ① thymic stromal cells (TSC) interact directly with thymocytes by adhesion molecules on the cell surface; ② thymic stromal cells secrete a variety of cytokines (such as IL-1, IL-6, IL-7) and thymus hormone-induced thymocyte differentiation; ③ thymus cells themselves secrete a variety of cytokines (such as IL-2, IL-4) playing an important role on thymocyte differentiation and maturation itself. In addition, thymic epithelial cells, macrophages and dendritic cells play a decisive role to self-tolerance of thymocytes differentiation, MHC-restricted as well as the formation of T cell subsets.

5. Body's immune function

Especially cellular immunity and T lymphocyte function decreases with age, the structure and function of thymus gradually degenerate in adulthood. Thymus is a central organ of immune system and the base of T lymphocyte differentiation and maturation. Thymic epithelial cells produce and release thymosin which plays an important role in differentiating T lymphocyte precursors into mature T cell immune activity. Thymus is the first organ of the body degradation, and then began a decline after sexual maturity and the ability to produce and secrete thymosin also gradually decreased with age.

Thymus research began in the early 1960s, it was found that closely related to immune function. Miller et al (1960) found that when thymus was removed in animals (neonatal mice), immune function will not develop completely and the number of circulating T cells was significantly reduced. Since 50 years thymus has been recognized as the center of the immune organ and is the first mature organ in the body and the structure and function of the thymus reach a peak while sexual maturity; thereafter with age increase, it is gradually shrinking and degradation and immune function in adult animals is gradually being replaced by the spleen and other lymphoid tissues. The thymus is the core of tissue T lymphocyte development, but it is also the base producing a variety of immune factors (lymphokines, cytokines). Thymosin is the main immune modulators secreting from thymus and now there are a variety of thymosin (peptide) products for the Clinical and Experimental Research. There is a foreign specialized periodicals called "thymus" (thymus) which regularly publishes reports on the thymus research and clinical treatment.

6. Thymus immune function and NIM theory

From the beginning it is believed that it was a single regulatory system independent to other physiological systems. So far it is considered that thymus and the neuroendocrine system are interconnected functional network system. Since the late 1970s Besedovsky (1977) proposed neuroendocrine immune network theory (NIM) which has been recognized as the core guide for thymus and immune function. Thymus and central nervous system and peripheral immune response functions form the system's three-point line connection. Central cerebral cortex, hypothalamus, pituitary is higher regulation center; peripheral lymphoid organs and tissues, cells and cytokines to regulate and implementation units subordinate immune network; intermediate hub is thymus called NIM middle line. NIM path can be divided into three: ① down line that reached down from the central median line to middle line and down line; ② up line from each cytokine feedback information to the central site; ③ middle line access to thymus for the spindle, combined with the spleen and other lymphoid tissue and bone marrow progenitor cell nucleus. Recent studies have shown that the thymus plays an important role in the NIM activities. For example, Fabres (1983) put forward - the concept of "thymic neuroendocrine network", Goldstein AL (1983) that "neuroendocrine - thymus axis" of thought, expression can be described as the thymus special significance in the NIM network.

Thymus starts to degrade after sexual maturity and secreted thymosin and other hormones are also reduced so that T lymphocyte differentiation and immune function decrease. The main reason for human and mammalian aging degeneration has the close relation to atrophy of the thymus.

While Increasing age, thymic atrophy naturally and life is gradually aging, the thymus is an important factor affecting the level of the body's immunity. Experiments show that removal of the thymus in adult rats (2 months) can accelerate its own immune dysfunction and aging. Six months after removal of thymus in rats (2 months) lymphocyte immune activity in spleen decreased, only of 51.6% in the same age without removal of the thymus.

7. Thymus exocrine

Thymic hormone vitality can be detected by available bioassay method. The experiment proved the vitality of the thymus hormone decline with increasing age. With thymic atrophy it decreases. In the animals with removal of the thymus serum cannot be measured. Thymus is the main source of thymic hormone. Thymus hormones are substance secreted by thymocytes regulating immune function.

The thymus is the important organization of body's immune function, secrete and generate thymulin etc, and secrete IL-1 and IL-2 and other interleukins to adjust thymus intrinsic function and viability ingredient; at the same time regulated by the pituitary secretion of prolactin. Now the research about thymus immunomodulator primarily provides evidence indicating that exogenous hormone (such as prolactin, growth hormone, thyroxine, etc.) can rejuvenate the thymus recession and maintain immunomodulatory force. Thymic involution can be reversed which is common developmental prospects of modern immunology and endocrinology.

8. Impact of chemicals on the immune function

Cyclophosphamide (Cy) or hydrocortisone pine (HC) is commonly used in clinical medicine can cause decreased immune function, and other long-term injections can cause the thymus, spleen and lymph node atrophy, and decreased immune function.

In short, Although Cy and HC has a certain inhibition in immune function, after Cy medication is used with 3 W, thymus atrophy; after 6W spleen began to shrink; in 6 ~ 12W proliferation of peripheral blood T lymphocyte decreased significantly.

9. The name and function of the thymus hormone

Since the early 1960s by the famous scientists Good and Miller and others first reported thymus function is "central" organ systemic immune system since the rapid development of cellular immunology. In the early 1970s the hypothesis about the thymus hormone secretion was proposed, several "constructive" but not yet sure of the thymus hormones or hormone-like ingredients have come out, they are extracted from the whole thymus peptides ingredients. Recent studies have shown that thymic epithelial cells (TEC) is to produce thymic hormone component of cells divided into two categories: interleukin-class (Ils) and thymosin class ingredients. Foreign studies have demonstrated that there are four kinds of thymic hormone: (1) thymosin-α; (2) thymulin; (3) thymopoietin; (4) thymichumoral factor (THF). Thymulin is 9 peptide binding component requiring a zinc binding to keep biological activity. Multiple thymus ingredient mostly are extracted from bovine thymus abroad.

10. Immunity Regulation and Immune Enhancers

At present immune enhancers can be divided into several categories by different sources.

The first class of immune enhancers derived from microorganisms

Fungal glucan ingredient containing β-1,3- glucoside chain has demonstrated better clinical effect, they can promote MΦ killing bacteria and tumor cells and induce the release of a single factor (monokine), such as interleukin-1 (IL-1), tumor necrosis factor (TNF), colony stimulating factor (CSF) and the like.

The second largest category of immune enhancer is thymus extract.

Thymus peptides extracted from animal. The world (including our) has a variety of products available which have immunological pharmacological activity, also known as thymic hormone. Thymosin zinc complex (zinc thymulin complex) is the active ingredients secreted by thymic epithelial cells. A variety of other crude thymic extract has clinical effects. Its main role is to enhance T cell activity in vivo, but no effect produce new T cells. In other words, activation of T cells can enhance the body against germs and anti-tumor; and anti-aging vitality animal's immune function subsided. Clinically they are used for the treatment of other chronic infectious diseases and cancer.

The third category of immune agents to promote the development of recombination cytokines since 1980s.

These biologically active factors has achieved significant benefits in clinical treatment, of which the most prominent is rIFN-r, rIFN-α, IL-2 (IL-1 to IL-2), TNF, rCSF (such as GM-CSF). This can be a significant innovations immunity pharmacology or breakthrough, recently appeared monoclonal antibodies (Mabs) and the human gene antibody (H-Ab), these new components can be summarized as recombinant peptide immune substances.

Purification about a variety of immune substances has made significant progress and now we have a variety of effective products available, which indeed has proved clinical usefulness of chemicals is not too much.

11. Research Progress of Chinese herbal pharmacology of anticancer immunity

Anti-cancer research of Wolfberry Polysaccharide, Polyporus Polysaccharide, Poria Polysaccharide, Mushrooms Polysaccharide, Versicolor, Ganoderma Polysaccharide, White fungus Polysaccharide

Anti-tumor mechanism and prospects of polysaccharide drugs and Immune polysaccharide anticancer medicine research progress:

Polysaccharides can improve the body's immune surveillance system, including natural killer cells (NK), macrophages (MΦ), cytotoxic T cell (CTL), T cells, LAK cells, tumor infiltrating lymphocytes (TIL), interleukin (IL) and other cytokines to achieve the purpose of the activity of killing tumor cells.

Although many polysaccharides alone have some anti-tumor effect, two kinds of immune enhancers combining two polysaccharides will be higher effects. Polysaccharides with the use of chemotherapy or radiotherapy may further improve the outcome.

Research and Development Overview

Thomas and Burnet's immune surveillance theory proposed that immune system can eliminate cells with a mutation of tumor cells in vitro in order to maintain a single cell type each cell. The body's immune surveillance system including cellular immune and humoral immune, cellular immune is particularly important to reject tumor cells. Immune cells performing cellular immune function include natural killer cells (NK), macrophages (MΦ), recently proposed LAK cells and tumor infiltrating lymphocytes (TIL), the anti-tumor effect of the latter than the LAK cells is 50 to 100 times, play a stronger role. If these effector cells is inhibited it is difficult to play a role in immune surveillance system. Elston reported that in 19 cases of chorionic cancers with cellular immune response only three cases died; however 24 patients with no immune response or immune response was significantly lower, 13 patients died, indicating that the level of immune function plays an important role in cancer therapy. By enhancing immune function to prevent cancer, it will undoubtedly have a bright future.

In accordance with domestic and foreign research, polysaccharides drugs including LBP, on the one hand it can play antibacterial, antiviral, anti-tumor, anti-aging, anti-side effects of chemotherapy and anti-autoimmune disease function; also have a variety of biological functions such as lowering blood pressure, blood fat, anti-vomiting, and blood sugar. These aspects will also be an important direction for LBP-depth research and application development.

LBP compared with other polysaccharides, consisting of a glycopeptide, the role of strong, small amount, water-soluble, stable and easy oral absorption, it can be considered a highly effective immune T cell adjuvant. But LBP, a crude extract of the plant, has yet to cooperate with the experts to purify and modify LBP including degrading into different molecular weight oligosaccharides and oligosaccharides and polysaccharides, etc. which is expected to further enhance the immune activity of LBP in order to find to a newer immunologically active drugs.

Immune is closely associated with aging. Many scholars further study also found that the aging process causes cellular immune function degradation mainly due to the thymus with age and shrink, and thus it was suggested that the thymus is to control the aging process in the immune function of the biological clock. LBP has the role on Thymus, the main part of the immune senescence. The main results show as follows: ① LBP main role in thymic T cell selection; ② Ding Yan and other reports that LBP can promote an increase in the number of mature T cells in the thymus, but also enhances the "emptying" function, so that the outer periphery of thymocyte proliferation playing thymus central role of immune regulation, and enhance resistance to disease and aging; ③ Our experiments have shown that six months after daily consumption of LBP solution, in LBP group thymic atrophy recovery, increase in weight; in control animals thymus atrophy, but it didn't reach adulthood normal levels. The facts suggest that LBP can reverse thymus degeneration caused by aging. The above can be clearly understood that the relationship between thymus and aging.

12. Characteristics of traditional Chinese medicine immunity pharmacology

Compared with western immunity pharmacology advantages of traditional Chinese medicine immune pharmacology have their own characteristics or advantages, but also have shortcomings. The advantages of Chinese immunology medications roughly as follows:

The first is the long-term clinical application and have accumulated a lot of herbs to regulate the body immune function, especially having generally dynamic regulation of the immune benefits.

Rich source of traditional Chinese! traditional Chinese medicine is effective medicine during long-term clinical application and have significant pharmacological effects after extraction (including immunomodulatory effects). The research process can save people, save time and have high efficiency.

Secondly, whether single herb or medicine prescriptions contain a variety of active ingredients, unlike Western medicine (synthetic drugs) is a single structure. The roles of traditional Chinese medications are many, in addition to the regulation of immune function, have a certain effect on the overall function of the system and various organs. These effects in turn are interconnected and combined.

Chinese medications regulate immune function by generally tonic that is within the normal range of adjustment, with two-way adjustment as the main feature. Tonics can be called immunomodulatory drugs, causing non-specific immune response.

Tonic medication which there is regulation of immune function, shows the correlation between dose and benefits under the general experimental conditions, in particular a normal healthy animal experiments are obvious. When the animal is low in immune vitality(for example, the animals with removal of thymus, the aging animal or chemotherapy drugs cyclophosphamide under suppression and tumor animals), tonics medications improve immune function even more significant.

Immune pharmacology is an interdisciplinary formed by combining immunology and pharmacology. Traditional Chinese medications immunity pharmacology in our immune pharmacology occupies a special importance. TCM immunity pharmacology can be understood as the new field grafting modern immune pharmacology and TCM.

As early as the 1970s, Professor Zhou Jinhuang have been calling for the creation of integrative medicine pharmacology, clearly put forward the theory of Chinese medicine from starting to study and clarify the role of Chinese Herbal Medicine.

TCM theory has its obvious overall concept emphasizing the balance of the body and maintain balance when internal and external environment change. The body appears syndromes while losing balance and coordination.

Modern medicine also places great emphasis on a stable internal environment. The stable adjustment factors for Internal environment is the three systems of nervous, endocrine and immune systems.

As a system these play their independent regulatory role, but it is also interrelated and influence each other so as to achieve a relatively stable internal environment purposes.

"Nervous, endocrine, immune, regulating network" (NIM Network) is the research focus immunity pharmacology.

Through a lot of research work Professor Zhou Jinhuang developed NIM ideas which was conceived with a wide range of practical significance, is in line with scientific laws of life, but also with traditional Chinese medicine as a whole ideology coincides. Extensive, in-depth study of the role of traditional Chinese medicine on NIM network on basic theory can greatly develop Chinese medications and make it to the world more quickly.

13. New discoveries from cancer research experiments:

(1) Removal of the thymus (Thymus, TH) can be manufactured bearing animal model for sure;

(2) These results suggest that: the metastasis is related to immune function; immune deficiency may promote tumor metastasis;

(3) It was found that: the host thymus was acute atrophy after inoculation of cancer cells which cell proliferation is blocked and volume was significantly reduced;

(4) It was found that: When solid tumors grow to large thumb, they were removed. A week later there was no further thymus atrophy;

(5) In our laboratory we were looking for immune reconstitution methods by using mice fetal liver, fetal thymus, fetal spleen cell transplantation to reconstitute while exploring to stop thymus atrophy. The results showed that in S, T, L three groups of cell transplantation, recently complete tumor regression was 40%, long-term tumor regression rate was 46.67%.

From the above experimental findings, thymus atrophy and immune dysfunction may be one factor in cancer incidence and pathogenesis, we should start from the body's immune function, especially cellular immunity, T lymphocyte function and immune function of the thymus to explore and seek immune regulation approach in the molecule levels.

In view of the development of Chinese medicine immunity pharmacology, traditional Chinese medicine theory has its obvious overall concept, emphasizing the balance of the body and maintain balance when changes in internal and external environment, loss of balance, the body appeared syndromes.

Modern medicine also places great emphasis on a stable internal environment. Internal environment stable adjustment factors are three systems: nervous, endocrine and immune systems. "Nervous, endocrine, immune regulatory network" (NIM Network) is the research focus immune pharmacology.

There are a lot of traditional Chinese medications regulating the body's immune function, especially having generally dynamic regulation of the immune benefits. During 28 years we have conducted a series of experimental research to find new drugs from natural medications to find new anti-cancer drugs and anti-cancer metastasis, to prevent thymus atrophy and to increase immune anti-cancer medication; looking only inhibit cancer cells without inhibiting normal drugs; from traditional Chinese medication to look for preventing atrophy of the thymus and adjusting the relationship between the host and tumors, preventing recurrence and metastasis drugs.

Existing anti-cancer drugs inhibit the patient's immune function, suppress bone marrow and thymus and immune surveillance was lost so that cancer further develops. Therefore, we must strengthen the research, all the anti-cancer drug used must be able to increase immune function and protect the immune organ, and should not be immune suppression drugs.

14. Research of Action Mechanism of XZ-C Anticancer Medications

Looking for anti-cancer, anti-metastasis of new drugs in natural medicine (TCM) in the experimental work within our laboratory over a long period, a batch of 200 kinds of traditional considered to be "anti-cancer medicine," were screened in the experiments of tumor inhibition in tumor-bearing animal models, the results found that only 48 kinds do have some even better inhibition of tumor proliferation of cancer cells. Optimized combination, and then in vivo anti-tumor experiments in tumor-bearing animal models such as liver cancer, lung cancer, stomach cancer and others to consist of Z-C1 ~ 10 particles, Z-C1 can inhibit cancer cells, but not normal cells, Z-C4 can protect thymus and improve immune function, Z-C8 can protect marrow liters of blood, ZC immune regulation medication can improve the quality of life of patients with advanced cancer, increase immunity, enhance physical fitness, improve appetite, prolong survival.

With more and deeper researches on traditional Chinese medicine, it has been proved that many kinds of traditional Chinese medicine can regulate and control the production and biological activity of cytokine and other immune molecules, which is meaningful to explain the immunological mechanism of XZ-C traditional Chinese anti-carcinoma medicine for immunologic regulation and control from the level of molecule.

I. Protecting Immune Organs and Increasing the Weight of Thymus and Spleen

That XZ-C traditional Chinese medicine can protect immune organs resulting from the following active principles.

1. XZ-C-T (ASD): Using its 15g/kg and 30g/kg extracting solution (equivalent to 1g original medicine) along with 12.5mg/kg, 25mg/kg ferulic acid suspension to feed the mice for seven days in a raw can increase the weight of thymus and spleen obviously, especially the effects of the group with high dose are more apparent. Intraperitoneal injection of EBM polysaccharide can also alleviate thymus and spleen atrophy obviously caused by perdnisolone.

2. XZ-C-O (PMT): Extract PM-2, feed the mice with 6g/(kg·d) PMT decoction for successive seven days which can increase the weight of thymus and celiac lymph nodes and antagonize the reduction in the weight of immune organs caused by perdnisolone. Drenching the mouse of 15 months old with 6g/kg decoction (with the concentration of 0.5g/ml) for 14 days can increase the weight and volume of thymus, thicken the cortex and raise cellular density apparently. The combined use of PM and astragalus root can promote non-lymphocyte hyperplasia and benefit the micro environment of thymus.

3. XZ-C-W (SCB): SCB polysaccharide can gain weight of thymus and spleen of a normal mouse. Lavage with it enables cyclophosphane to control the gain in the weight of thymus and spleen.

4. XZ-C-M (LLA): Drench a mouse with LLA decoction for seven days resulting in increasing the weight of thymus and spleen.

5. XZ-C-L: For a 15-month old mouse, its thymus degenerates obviously. Astragalus injectio can enlarge the thymus significantly. The cortex under microscope is thickened and the cellular density increase obviously.

II. Effects on Proliferation, Differentiation and Hematopiesis of Marrow Cells

The following active principles of XZ-C traditional Chinese medicine have effects on hematopiesis of marrow cells.

1. XZ-C-Q (LBP) extracts (PM-2):

(1) Effects on the proliferation of hematopoietic stem cell (CFU-S) of a normal mouse: inject PM-2 with the dose of 500mg/(kg·d)×3d or 10mg/(kg·d)×3d LBP into the experimental mice respectively by venoclysis and kill them in the ninth day. It can be found that the number of spleen CFU-S in the group with administration increases obviously. The number of CFU-S in group PM-2 is 21% higher than that of the control group and it is 36% in the group with LBP.

(2) Effects on colony forming unit of granulocytes and macrophages (CFU-GM): the experimental results indicate that LBP with the dose of 5~30mg/(kg·d)×3d can increase the number of CFU-GM and PM-2 can also strengthen the effect of CFU-GM with the effective dose of 12.5~50mg/(kg·d)×3d. In the early stage of cultivation, most

CFU-GMs are units of granulocytes and then units of macrophages increase gradually. In the anaphase units of macrophages take over the dominance.

From the above experiment, it can be found that PM-2 and LBP can promote hematopiesis of normal mice obviously. The experiment proves that during the process of restoring hematopiesis damaged by cyclophosphamide, PM-2 and LBP stimulate the proliferation of granulocytes at first, and then marrow karyocytes multiply; at last these two promote the restoration of peripheral granulocytes.

2. XZ-C-D (TSPG):

Ginsenoside, which is the active principle of ginseng to promote hematopiesis, can bring the recovery of erythrocyte in peripheral blood, haemoglobin and myeloid cell of thighbone in the mice of marrow-inhibited type, increase the index of myeloid cellular division and stimulate the proliferation of myeloid hematopoietic cell in vitro so as to make it into cell cycle with active proliferation (S+G$_2$/M stage). TSPG can promote the proliferation and differentiation of polyenergetic hematopoietic cells and induce the formation of hemopoietic growth factor (HGF).

3. XZ-C-H (RCL):

Steamed Chinese Foxglove can promote the recovery of erythrocyte and haemoglobin for animals with blood deficiency and accelerate the proliferation and differentiation of myeloid hematopoietic cell (CFU-S) with the effect of predominance and hematosis significantly. Peritoneal injection of rehmannia polysaccharides for successive six days can promote the proliferation and differentiation of myeloid hematopoietic cells and progenitor cells as well as increasing the number of leucocytes in peripheral blood.

4. XZ-C-J (ASD):

ASD polysaccharide has no effects on erythrocytes and leucocytes of normal mice, but for those damaged by radiation, injection of ASD polysaccharide can influence the proliferation and differentiation of both polyenergetic hematopoietic stem cells (CPU-S) and hemopoietic progenitor cells. But its decoction has no obvious effects.

5. XZ-C-E (PEW):

Poria cocos (micromolecule chemical compound extracted from Tuckahoe polysaccharide) is the active principle that can strengthen the production of colony stimulating factor (CSF) and improve the level of leucocytes in peripheral blood inside the mouse's body. It can also prevent the decline in leucocytes caused by cyclophosphamide and accelerate the recovery with the effects better than sodium ferulic which is used to increase leucocytes.

6. XZ-C-Y (PAR):

Its polysaccharide can obviously resist the decline in leucocytes caused by cyclophosphamide and increase the number of myeloid cells to promote the proliferation of myeloid induced by CSF as well as the recovery and reconstitution of hematopiesis for the mice irradiated by X ray. It can also increase the number of hematopoietic stem cells and myeloid cells along with leucocytes.

III. Enhancing Immunologic Function of T Cells

The active principles of XZ-C traditional Chinese medicine and their effects are following.

1. XZ-C-L (AMB): It can raise the percentage of lymphocytes in peripheral blood obviously. The LBP in small dose (5~10mg/kg) can cause the proliferation of lymphocytes, indicating that LBP can promote the proliferation of T cells apparently. 50mg/(kg·d)×7d is the best dose in that it will have no effects if lower than the level and it will bring the effects down if higher than the level. Oral administration of LBP can raise the conversion rate of lymphocytes for the sufferers who are weak and with fewer leucocytes.

2. $XZ-C_4$ It can regulate immune system and active T cells of aggregated lymphatic follicles, as well as stimulate the secretion of hemopoietic growth factor in T cells. Among the crude drugs of $XZ-C_4$ the extract from the hot water of atractylodes lancea rhizome can obviously stimulate the cells of aggregated lymphatic follicles, which is regarded as the base of $XZ-C_4$ immunoloregulation.

IV. Activating and Enhancing NK Cell Activity

Natural killer cell, NK cell is another kind of killer cell in lymphocytes for human beings and mice, which needs neither antigenic stimulation, nor the participation of antibodies to kill some cells. It plays an important role in immunity, especially in the function of immune surveillance as NK cell is the first line of defense against tumors and has broad spectrum anti-tumor effects.

NK cell is broad-spectrum and able to kill sygeneous, homogenous and heterogenous tumor cells with special effects on lymjphoma and leucocytes.

NK cell is an important kind of cells for immunoloregulation, which can regulate T cells, B cells and stem cells, etc. It can also regulate immunity by releasing cytokines like IFN-α, IFN-γ, IL-2, TNF, etc.

The active principles in XZ-C traditional Chinese medicine and their effects are following.

1. XZ-C-X (SDS)

Divaricate Saposhniovia Root can strengthen the activity of NK cells of experimental mice. When combined with IL-2, it can make the activity of NK cell higher, indicating that its polysaccharide can give a hand to IL-2 to activate NK cells and improve the activity.

LBP can strengthen T cell mediated immune reaction and the activity of NK cells for normal mice and those dealt by cyclophosphamide. Peritoneal injection of LBP can improve the proliferation of spleen T lymphocytes and strengthen the lethality of CTL increasing the specific lethal rate from 33% to 67%.

2. XZ-C-G (GUF)

Glycyrrhizin can induce the production of IFN in the blood of animals and human beings and strengthen NK cell activity at the same time. Clinical tests made by Abe show that after intravenous injection of 80mg GL, the raise of NK cell activity reaches 75% among 21 sufferers. Peritoneal injection of 0.5mg/kg GL on mice can strengthen the activity of NK cells in liver.

3. XZ-C-L (AMB)

Its bath fluid can promote NK cell activity of mice both in vivo and in vitro, and can also induce IFN-γ to deal with effector cells under the certain concentration of 0.1mg/ml. Cordyceps sinensis extract can strengthen NK cells activity of the mouse both in vivo and in vitro. Fluids with the concentrations of 0.5g/kg, 1g/kg and 5g/kg can strengthen NK cell activity of mice.

(5) Effects on Iterleukin-2 (IL-2)

The active principles in XZ-C anti-carcinoma traditional Chinese medicine and their effects are following.

1. XZ-C-T

EBM polysaccharide can enhance obviously the production of IL-2 for human beings when the concentration is 100ug/ml. At higher concentration (2500ug/ml and 5000ug/ml), it will lead to inhibition. Hypodermic injection of barrenwort polysaccharide for seven days in a row can significantly improve the ability of thymus and spleen of the mouse induced by ConA to produce IL-2.

2. XZ-C-Y

PAR polysaccharide has strong immune activity and is able to promote the production of IL-2. For the mouse bearing S-180 tumor, it can raise the ability of spleen cells to produce IL-2 obviously。

3. XZ-C-D

Ginseng polysaccharide has great promotion on IL-2 induced by peripheral monocytes for both healthy people and sufferers with kidney troubles. The effects are relevant to the dose positively.

(6). Function of inducing interferon and promoting inducement of interferon from XZ-C:

IFN are broad-spectrum in resisting tumors and can regulate immunity. It can also inhibit the proliferation of tumor cells and activate NK cells and CTL to kill tumor cells. Meanwhile, IFN can cooperate with TNF, IL-1 and IL-2 to enforce anti-tumorous ability.

The active principles in XZ-C anti-carcinoma traditional Chinese medicine and their effects are following.

1. XZ-C-Z

250mg/kg or 500mg/kg CVQ polysaccharide can improve significantly the level of IFN-γ produced by mouse spleen cells.

2. XZ-C-D

Ginsenoside (GS) and panaxitriol ginsenoside (PTGS) can induce whole blood cells and monocytes of human beings to produce IFN-α and IFN-γ. It can also recover the low level of IFN-γ and IL-2 to the normal.

The IFN potency of ASH polysaccharide on S-180 cell line of acute lymphoblastic leukemia and S_{7811} cell line of acute myelomonocytic leukemia produced after acanthopanax polysaccharide stimulation is 5~10 times more than that of normal control group.

3. XZ-C-E

Hydroxymethyl Poria cocos mushroom polysaccharide has many kinds of physical activity like immunoloregulation, promoting to induce IPN, resisting virus indirectly and alleviating adverse reaction resulting from radiation. Do IFN inducement dynamic experiment on S-180leukaemia cell line by using 50mg/ml Hydroxymethyl Poria cocos mushroom polysaccharide. The results indicate that its potency to induce interferon at all stages is better than that of normal inducement.

4. XZ-C-G (GL)

It can induce IFN activity. Make peritoneal injection of 330mg/kg GL on mice. IFN activity reaches the peak after 20 hours.

15. Cytokines induced by XZ-C Anticancer Medications

(1) Z-C4 anticancer medication can induce endogenous cytokines

① Experimental study: Z-C4 has a variety of immune-enhancing effect with induced endogenous cytokine closely related.

② Z-C4 inhibit the reduction of leukocyte, neutrophils and thrombocyte.

③ Z-C4 by interleukin -1β (IL-1β) not only has a direct effect, but also enhances the tumor necrosis factor (TNF), interferon (IFN) and other cytokines, which may be an indirect mechanism.

④ Z-C4 can raise Th1 cytokines so that it has effects on anemia and leukopenia after chemotherapy.

⑤ Z-C4 can not only protect the bone marrow, but also play a direct role in cell differentiation by cytokines.

In short, Z-C4 induces tumor cell differentiation and natural death due to autocrine which is a substance secreted itself and in turn acts on its own. Looking to the future, Z-C4 may become induced differentiation therapy for cancer cells.

(2) Z-C4 inhibits cancer progression and metastasis

Invasion and metastasis of cancer cells obtained in the proliferation of malignant nature of the process, this phenomenon is called malignant progression. Advances in cancer research requires good reproducibility animal model. Thus cancer QR-32 model isolated from mouse fibrosarcoma made this good reproducibility. Even though the mice were implanted subcutaneously nor hyperplasia, QR-32 will be completely self-limiting; it does not appear input vein metastatic nodules in the lung. However, if the body of foreign substances as gelatin sponge together with QR-32 subcutaneously was transplanted into mice, in vivo QR-32 becomes proliferative cancer QRSP.

(3) Z-C1 + Z-C4 immune regulation anti-cancer medicine

Z-C1 + Z-C4 immunomodulatory anticancer medicine has the following characteristics

① Overall improvement in the quality of life of patients with advanced cancer.

② Protect the thymus enhance immunity, protect the bone marrow and enhance hematopoietic function, improve immune and regulatory capacity.

③ Enhance physical fitness, reduce pain, improve appetite.

④ Enhance the therapeutic effect and reduce the side effects of chemotherapy.

16. Experimental and clinical efficacy of XZ-C immunomodulatory anticancer medication

(1) Tumor inhibitory effect of anti-cancer medicine Z-C1 ~ 4 on tumor-bearing hepatoma H22 mice

It was found on H22 mice two weeks, four weeks, six weeks after the using the medication, the inhibition increases with prolonged treatment time, on 6 weeks XZ-C4 inhibitory rate reaching 70%, followed by twice repeating the test, results are stable, indicating that the inhibitory effect of Chinese medicine is slow, gradual increase, namely anti-tumor effect and the cumulative medicine dose was positively correlated.

Effect of Anti-cancer medicine XZ-C1 or XZ-C4 on lifetime of H22 liver cancer tumor-bearing mice:

Experimental results show that anticancer medicine XZ-C1, XZ-C4 can significantly prolong the survival time of tumor-bearing mice, especially XZ-C4 significantly prolong the survival of more than 200%, not only that, XZ-C4 also significantly improve the immune function, protect the immune organs, to protect the bone marrow, reducing chemotherapy and radiotherapy drug toxicity, the mice were fed up to 12 service months with no any side effects. The above experimental studies provide a useful basis for clinical applications.

(2) Clinical efficacy On the basis of experiments, since 1994 clinical application on various types of cancers, mostly for stage III, stage IV patients, namely: exploratory surgery unresectable advanced cancer; advanced cancer indications who cannot have surgery; recently or long-term metastasis or recurrence after various cancer surgery; a variety of advanced cancer of the liver metastases, lung metastases, brain metastases and cancer pleural effusion, ascites carcinoma; various cancer surgery can only do gastrointestinal anastomosis or colostomy and can not be resected: not surgery, no radiotherapy and no chemotherapy.

Systematic observation:

After 20 years of clinical application, Z-C1, Z-C4 anticancer medication achieved a significant effect for long-term use and no adverse reactions. Clinical observations demonstrate Z-C1, Z-C4 anticancer medicine can improve the overall quality of life in advanced cancer patients, improve the overall immunity, control cancer cell proliferation, consolidate and enhance the long-term effect. Oral and topical drug to soften XZ-C and to narrow surface of metastatic tumor has a good effect, with intervention or cannula drug pump therapy, can protect the liver, kidney, bone marrow and immune system organs and enhance immunity.

(3) XZ-C analgesic effect of anti-cancer

Pain in advanced cancer patients is more obvious and painful symptoms, usually pain medication for cancer pain without much effect, narcotic analgesics addiction and dependence; ZC anticancer analgesic cream has strong analgesic effect and last longer. In 298 cases it was clinically proved to have significantly effective rate 78.0%, the total efficiency of 95.3%, can be re-used with no significant side effects, non-addictive. Analgesic effect is stable and relieves pain for cancer patients to improve the quality of life.

Through experimental research and clinical validation, our experience is: Chinese medications with Chinese characteristics has its unique advantages in terms of cancer treatment, such as a strong overall concept, highlighting the role of conditioning, side effects are mild, can relieve pain, relieve symptoms, significantly improved quality of life of patients, can mobilize immune function and overall disease resistance, improve treatment.

B. Results

① The tumor-inhibition effect of Z-C Medicine on Rats bearing hepatic carcinoma H_{22}: in the second week after administration of $Z-C_1$, the tumor-inhibition rate was 40% and the one in the fourth week was 45% and 58% in the sixth week. The tumor-inhibition rate after administration of $Z-C_4$ was 55%, 68% in the fourth week and 70% in the sixth week. (P<0.01) the tumor-inhibiting rate after administration of CTX was 45% in the second week, 45% in the fourth week and 49% in the sixth week (See Fig. 1 and 2)

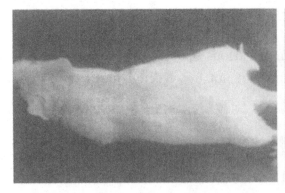 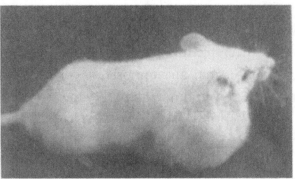

Figure 1 Z-C1, C4 treatment group   Figure 2 Control group
30d after inoculation of hepatoma H22   30d after inoculation of hepatoma H22

(2) The effect of Z-C medicine on the survival time of the rats bearing hepatic carcinoma H_{22}: the average survival time of $Z-C_1$, $Z-C_4$ and CTX was longer than the one of the normal saline control group (P<0.01); Z-C medicine played a role in obviously prolonging the survival time. Through comparison with the control group, the life elongation rate of $Z-C_1$ group was 85%, the one of $Z-C_4$ group was 200% and the one of CTX group was 9.8%. The rats in $Z-C_1$ and CTX in Group B met with death in 75d. 6 rats bearing carcinoma in $Z-C_4$ survived after seven months.

(3) Both $Z-C_1$ and $Z-C_4$ medicine improved the immunologic function and $Z-C_4$ obviously improved the immunologic function, increased the white blood cells and red blood cells, without any effect on the hepatic function and kidney function and without damage to the hepatic and kidney section. CTX decreased the white blood cells and reduced the immunologic function with the renal damage to the kidney section. The thymus in the control group was obviously atrophic (Fig. 1-4) while the one of $Z-C_1$ and $Z-C_2$ therapy group was not atrophic but a little hypertrophic (Fig.1-3).

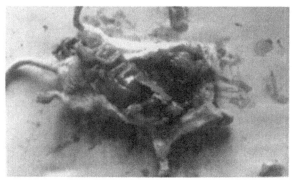 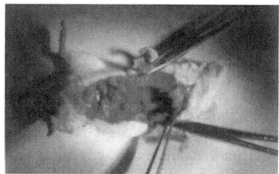

Figure 3 Z-C4 group
30d after inoculation of hepatoma H22
thymus hypertrophy

Figure 4 Control
30d after inoculation of liver cancer H22
marked atrophy of thymus

Pathological section of thymus in the control group: the cortex of the thymus was atrophic, the cells were discrete and the blood vessel met with sludge (Fig. 1-5). The pathological section of the thymus in $Z-C_4$ therapy group displayed that the cortical area of the thymus built up, the lymphocyte was dense, the epithelium reticulocyte increased and the thymus corpuscles increased (Fig. 1-6).

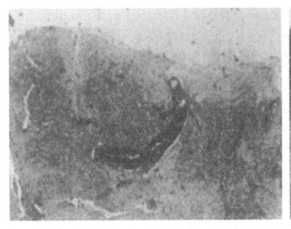 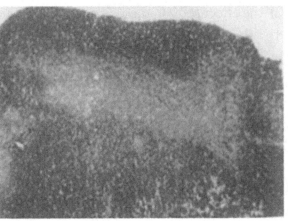

Figure 5 thymic tumor-bearing control group, HE × 100 lymphocytes decreased cortical atrophy, Cortex form a lymphocyte empty band degree

Figure 6 Z-C4 treated thymus HE × 100 thymic cortex and medulla thickening, lymphocyte high, intravascular congestion intensive

C. Clinical Application

1. Clinical information

(1) Hubei Branch of China Anti-cancer Research Cooperation of Chinese Traditional Medicine and Western Medicine, Anti Carcinoma Metastasis and Recurrence Research Office and Shuguang Tumor Specialized Outpatient Department had treated 4, 698 carcinoma patients in Stage III and IV or in metastasis and recurrence with Z-C medicine combined with western medicine from 1994 to Nov. 2002, among which there were 3, 051 men patients and 1,647 women patients. The youngest one was 11 years old and the oldest one was 86 years old, the high invasion age was 40~69 years. All groups of the patients were entirely subject to the diagnosis of pathological histology or definitive diagnosis with ultrasonic B, CT and MRI iconography. According to the staging standard of UICC, all the cases were entirely the patients in medium and advanced stage over Stage III. In this group, there were 1,021 hepatic carcinoma patients, among which there were 694 primary lesion hepatic carcinoma patients and 327 metastatic hepatic carcinoma patients; there were 752 patients suffering from carcinoma of lung, among which there were 699 patients suffering from the primary carcinoma of lung and 53 patients suffering from the metastatic carcinoma of lung; there were 668 gastric carcinoma patients, 624 patients suffering from esophagus cardia carcinoma, 328 patients suffering from rectum carcinoma of anal canal, 442 patients suffering from carcinoma of colon, 368 patients suffering from breast carcinoma, 74 patients suffering from adenocarcinoma of pancreas, 30 patients suffering from carcinoma of bile duct, 43 patients suffering from retroperitoneal tumor, 38 patients

suffering from oophoroma, 9 patients suffering from cervical carcinoma, 11 patients suffering from cerebroma, 34 patients suffering from thyroid carcinoma, 38 patients suffering from nasopharyngeal carcinoma, 9 patients suffering from melanoma, 27 patients suffering from kidney carcinoma, 48 patients suffering from carcinoma of urinary bladder, 13 patients suffering from leukemia, 47 patients suffering from metastasis of supraclavicular lymph nodes, 35 patients suffering various fleshy tumors and 39 patients suffering from other malignancies.

(2) Medicine and medication: the treatment aims to support healthy energy to eliminate evils, soften and resolve the hard mass and supplement qi and blood. $Z\text{-}C_1$ is the compound, 150ml to be taken on the daily basis, $Z\text{-}C_4$ is powder, 10g to be taken on the daily basis. According to the analysis and differentiation of the diseases, anti-cancer powder shall be taken orally and the anti-cancer apocatastasis paste shall be applied externally for the solid tumor or the metastatic tumor. In case of being in pain, anti-cancer aponic paste shall be applied externally. Icterus removal soup or dropsy removal soup shall be taken orally for the patients suffering from icterrus and the ascites.

(3) Therapeutic evaluation: it pays attention to the short-term curative effect and iconography indexes as well as the survival time of long-term curative effect, quality of life and immunologic indexes. Attention shall be paid to the changes in subjective signs in administration of drugs. It will be effective when the subjective signs are improved and last over one month; otherwise, it will be ineffective. As to the quality of life (Karnofsky Performance Status), it will be effective when it is improved and lasts over one month, otherwise, it will be ineffective. As to the evaluation standard of the curative effect of solid tumor, it can be divided into four levels according to the changes in size of tumor: Level I: disappearance of tumor; Level II: tumor reduces 1/2; Level III: softening of tumor; Level IV: no change or enlargement of level tumor.

Effect of treatment

(1) The symptom was improved, the quality of life was improved, the survival time was prolonged: among the 4,277 carcinoma patients in medium and advanced stage who took Z-C medicine with the return visit over 3 months. It improved the quality of life of the patients in an all-round way, see Table 1.

Table 1 Observation of curative effect on 4 277 patients: fully improving the quality of life of the carcinoma patients in medium and advanced stage

Improvement	Vigor	Appetite	Reinforcement of physical force	Improvement in generalized case	Increase of body weight	Improvement of sleep
No. of cases (%)	4071	3986	2450	479	2938	1005
	95.2	93.2	57.3	11.2	68.7	23.5

The restriction of improvement activity and capability released activity	self servicing normal walking	Resumption of work Engaged in light work
1038	3220	479
24.3	75.3	11.2

In this group, all of them were the patients in medium and advanced stage. After taking the medicine, their symptoms were improved to different extents with the effective rate of 93.2%. With respect to the improvement of the quality of life (as per Karnofsky Performance Status), it rose to 80 scores on average after administration from 50 on average before administration; the patients in this group met with the different metastasis and dysfunction of the organs about Stage III. It was reported by the previous statistic information that the mesoposition survival time of this kind of patients was about 6 months. The longest time among this group of the cases reached up to 11 years; another patient suffering from hepatic carcinoma had taken Z-C medicine for ten years and a half; two patients suffering from hepatic carcinoma met with frequency encountered carcinomatous lesion in the left and right liver and it entirely subsided through secondary CT reexamination after the patient took Z-C medicine for half a year and the state of the disease had been stable over half a year. One patient suffering from double-kidney carcinoma met with the widespread metastasis of abdominal cavity after removal of one kidney, after taking Z-C medicine, he was entirely recovered and began to work again. 3 patients suffering from carcinoma of lung, with the lung not removed through explaraton, had taken Z-C medicine over three years and a half. 2 patients suffering from gastric remnant carcinoma had taken Z-C medicine for 8 years. 3 patients suffering from reoccurrence of rectal carcinoma had taken Z-C medicine for 3 years. 1 patient suffering from metastatic liver and rib of the mastocarcinoma had taken Z-C medicine for 8 years. 1 patient suffering from the recurrent bladder carcinoma after operation of renal carcinoma had not met with the carcinoma for 9 years and a half after taking Z-C medicine. All of these patients were the ones in the medium and advanced stage that could not be operated once more or treated with radiotherapy or chemotherapy. They only took Z-C medicine without other medicines for treatment. Up to today, they are reexamined and get the medicine at the out-patient department every month. Through taking the medicine for a long time, the state of the disease is controlled in the stable state to make the organism and the tumor in balanced state for a relatively long time and get a relatively good survival with tumor, in this way, the symptoms of the patients are improved, the quality of life is improved and the survival time is prolonged.

(2) As to 84 patients suffering from solid tumor and 56 patients suffering from enlargement of upper lymph node of metastatic compact bone, after taking Z-C series medicines orally and applying Z-C3 anti-cancer apocatastasis paste, they met with good curative effects, see table2.

Table 2 Changes of 84 patients suffering from solid tumor and 56 patients suffering from metastatic mode after applying Z-C paste externally

84 cases of physical mass and 56 Lymph nodes on the neck tumor after applying Z-C paste externally.

	Solid tumor				Enlargement of upper lymph node of metastatic compact bone			
	Disappearance	Shrinkage 1/2	Softening	No change	Disappearance	Shrinkage 1/2	Softening	No change
No. of cases (%)	12 14.2	28 33.3	32 38.0	12 14.2	12 21.4	22 39.2	14 25.0	8 14.2
Total effective rate (%)	85.7				85.7			

(3) 298 patients suffering from carcinoma pain obtained the obvious pain alleviation effects after taking Z-C medicine orally and applying Z-C anti-cancer apocatastasis paste externally, see Table3.

Clinical Symptoms	Pain			
	Light alleviation	Obvious alleviation	Disappearance	Avoidance
No of cases	52	139	93	14
(%)	17.3	46.8	31.2	4.7
Total effective rate (%)	95.3			

17. XZ-C immunomodulatory anticancer medicine is the outcome of the modernization of traditional Chinese medicine

XZ-C immunomodulatory anti-cancer medications are not the experience side, nor is the name of the old Chinese side, but the combination of Chinese and Western medicine and traditional Chinese medicine with modern scientific research, are to combine modern medical methods and experimental methods and modern pharmacology and medicine efficient methods. After seven years of more than 4000 cancer-bearing animal models, the so-called 200 kinds of commonly used anti-cancer herbs are screened in batches in tumor-bearing animals, then screened out of 48 kinds of anti-cancer effect of good medications.

Then these 48 kinds of natural medication are composed of XZ–C1 ~ 10 number which according to the respiratory, digestive, urinary, gynecological, endocrine system animal models of liver cancer, stomach cancer, colon cancer, breast cancer, Kennedy bladder cancer, lung cancer are built, then tested and selected XZ–C1, XZ–C2, XZ–C3, XZ–C4, XZ–C5, XZ–C6, XZ–C7, XZ–C8, etc. series of immune regulation anti-cancer medication for in vivo efficacy in tumor-bearing animal experiments and toxicological experiment.

The material basis of the traditional recipe playing its unique clinical efficacy is chemical composition. The changes of quality and quantity of the chemical composition directly affect the clinical efficacy of prescriptions. So the research of the changes of quality and volume of chemical composition in medications to find out the main active ingredients and to explore the mysteries of the unique effect on the molecular immunology can make traditional prescription research reach a new level.

The formulation of XZ-C immune regulation medication is Chinese medicine innovation and reform which is not mixed boiling liquid compound, but particles per herb concentrates or powders, which every membrane in every flavor raw pharmaceutical drug retains its original composition, pharmacological effect, molecular weight, constant structure and is made by using modern scientific methods to keep the original flavor of each ingredient and function in order to evaluate the efficacy of affirmative actions.

XZ-C1: Smart Anticancer medication

1. Pharmacodynamics 96%-100% inhibit cancer cell without affecting the normal cells

2. Pharmacology: righting, taking away of harm things, inhibiting cancer cells strongly without affecting the normal cells

3. Toxicology: acute toxicity experimental shows: No obvious side effects, the median lethal dose(LD50) is difficult to make, is pretty safe medication.

XZ-C4 "protect thymus and increase the immune function"

1. Pharmacodynamics on Liver H22 mice the effect of inhibition: XZ-C4 55% on 2 week, 68% on 4 week, 70% on 6 week

2. Pharmacology: promote the lymphocyte conversion, increase the cells immune functions, increase the white cell functions, inhibit the cancer cells, protect the immune organ functions, and protect the thymius without atrophy and increase the immune functions.

3. Toxicology: XZ-C4 may be used for a long period. Acute toxicity experimental shows: No obvious side effects, the median lethal dose(LD50) is difficult to make, is pretty safe medication. Some patients live more than 3-5 years, even more than 8-10 year so that maintain the body immune function and protect the cancer metastasis and recurrence. This medication can be used for a long period and is safe to take by month.

Face the future of medicine, look forward, after 20 years of long and hard work, practice the scientific concept of development, face the frontiers of science, for innovative, forward. To fight against cancer must come from the clinic through experimental study , then go to clinic again in order to solve practical problems of patients; must be realistic with the facts to speak with the data; must be constantly self-transcendence and self-advancement; scientific research should emancipate the mind in bandage and get rid of the traditional old ideas based on independent innovation and original innovation; our decades of research line is to find the problem →research the problem →ask a question→ solve the problems or explain the problem; the road works out step by step with the difficult journey; we hope to walk out a Chinese characteristics way with innovative and anticancer metastasis.

Our medical oncology research model is based on patient-centered to discover questions from clinical work on the basis of in-depth study of animal experiments , then turned to the clinical application of basic research results to improve the overall level of health care and ultimately benefit patients

Our medical oncology research model, based on patient-centered, discovery and questions from clinical work, on the basis of in-depth study of animal experiments, and then turned to the clinical application of basic research results to improve the overall level of health care, and ultimately benefit patients.

Part III XZ-C immune regulation control anticancer medications: Pharmacology

Table of Contents

Preface

Immunomodulatory drug looks promising

No matter how complex the mechanism behind cancer is , immune suppression is a key cancer progression. Removal of immunosuppressive factors and restoration of recognition system cells to cancer cells can effectively resist cancer. More and more evidence shows that by regulating the body's immune system, it is possible to achieve the purpose of controlling cancer. Treating cancer by activating the body's anti-tumor immune system is the field that many researchers are currently excited to. The next major breakthrough in cancer is likely to come from this.

In order to investigate cancer etiology, pathogenesis, pathophysiology, we conducted a series of animal studies. From the analysis of these experimental results, we obtain new discoveries and new revelations: thymus atrophy and immune dysfunction is one of the cause of cancer and pathogenesis, therefore Dr. Xu Ze professor proposed causes of cancer at international conferences, one of the mechanisms that may be thymus atrophy, central immune sensory dysfunction, immune dysfunction, decreased immune surveillance and immune escape ability.

As results of experimental studies we found: progressive thymus atrophy, central immune sensory dysfunction, decreased immune function, decreased immune surveillance in cancer-bearing mice so that its treatment principle must be to prevent atrophy of the thymus, to promote thymic hyperplasia , to protect bone marrow function and to improve immune surveillance. All of these studies provide the theoretical basis and experimental evidence for immune regulation treatment.

Based on the above revelation about cancer etiology, pathogenesis of experimental results, the new concept and new methods of XZ immunomodulatory therapy is put forward to. After 16 years of oncology clinical validation in more than 12,000 cases of advanced cancer patients, it was confirming that the treatment principle of protection of thymus and increasing immune function is reasonable and its efficacy is satisfactory. Application of immune regulation control medications achieved good results and improved the quality of life and prolonged the survival time.

XZ-C(XU ZE-China) immune regulation law is first proposed by Professor Xu Ze in 2006 in his monograph <<new concepts and new methods of treatment of cancer metastasis>>. He believes that under normal circumstances the body's defenses and cancer are in a dynamic equilibrium and the cancer is caused by the dynamic balance disorders. If this unbalance status has adjusted to normal levels, cancer growth can be controlled and it makes cancer subside.

As we all know, the incidence of cancer development and prognosis depends on the comparison of two factors, namely the biological characteristics of cancer cells and the host defense against the body's own cancer cell. If these two are balance, the cancer in controlled; if these are imbalances, the cancer will develop.

Under normal circumstances the host organism itself against cancer cells has a certain capacity constraint, but in cancer these constraints are subject to different levels of defense suppression and damage leading to the loss of the immune surveillance of cancer cells and immune escape occurred so that cancer cells further develop and metastasize.

Basic experimental study investigated the recurrence and metastasis mechanism by more than four years, and after three years from the inherent natural medicine herbal test experiment in vivo anti-tumor cancer-bearing mice, anti-cancer immune regulation medications XZ-C are composed of herbs selected from a group of traditional Chinese medications with better anticancer inhibition rates.

I. Overview

XZ-C immunomodulatory anti-cancer medications from China's traditional herbal medicine are selected 48 kinds of anti-tumor Chinese herbal medication which have better inhibitory rate in cancer-bearing mice experiments, after the composition of the compound, , and then to be verified in mice antitumor experiments which the compound inhibitory rate inhibition rate is much greater than single herbs. $XZ\text{-}C_1$ and $XZ\text{-}C_4$ are composed of God grass, Agrimony, Shu Yang Quan and other 28 Chinese herbal medications, of which $XZ\text{-}C_{1\alpha}$ and $XZ\text{-}C_{1\beta}$ 100% inhibit cancer and 100% don't kill normal cells, with righting and enhancing the body's immune function. From our experiments of XZ-C pharmacodynamic study the results show: XZ-C medication has better inhibition rate on Ehrlich ascites carcinoma(EAC), S180 and hepatocellular carcinoma; there are obvious synergy and attenuation; the experiments also demonstrated that XZ-C Chinese immune regulation medication significantly improve immune function.

After acute toxicity test on mice, no significant side effects; in clinical long-term oral taken a few years (2--6 years) it has no significant side effects. While oral taken XZ-C immune regulation medication during chemotherapy can significantly reduce the toxicity of chemotherapy drugs; intermittent oral taken XZ-C during chemotherapy can recover the number of leukocytes and hemoglobin. In advanced cancer patients there are mostly weakness, fatigue, loss of appetite, after taking XZ-C anticancer immune regulation medication 4-8-12 weeks, the patients' physical strength and sleep are more significantly improved and the pain is relieved and the patients gradually recuperate.

2. We have been carried out experimental studies and clinical validation work

(A) Experimental studies

In our laboratory conducted the following experiment study new cancer screening from traditional Chinese medication and anti-metastatic drug:

1. An in vitro screening test: in vitro cancer cells we observed anti-cancer drugs directly to cancer cells damage. Cultured cancer cells in a test tube were placed raw meal drug products (500ug / mI) to observe whether there is inhibition or not and what the inhibition rate of cancer cells is.

2. Screening test of cancer-inhibition in vivo: cancer-bearing animal model was manufactured for the screening of anti-cancer Chinese herbs. Each batch has 240 mice. They were divided into eight experimental groups, each group has 30. Group 7 was the normal control group, Group 8 with a 5-Fu or CTX was control group. The whole group of mice was inoculated with EAC or S_{180} or H_{22} cancer cells, after 24h of inoculation each rat oral was fed by crude drug powder for long-term screen to observe survival time and the inhibition rate was calculated.

    In this way we conducted experimental study for four consecutive years and each year used more than 1000 tumor-bearing animal models , a total of nearly 6,000 tumor-bearing animal models for four years which pathological autopsy was done to test liver, spleen, sheets, pituitary gland, kidney etc after each mice died and a total of 20,000 times slices was made.

3. Experimental results: In our laboratory animal experiments after screening 200 kinds of Chinese herbal medicine, the screening must know certainly has some, even excellent inhibitory effect on cancer cells, inhibition rate of more than 75-90%. The note by animal experiments screened-out to 152 kinds of no significant anti-cancer effect.

(B) Clinical validation

Based on animal experiments successfully, clinical validation was tested:

1. Methods: oncology clinics and combination anti-cancer, anti-metastasis, relapse research collaboration group, keep medical records, establish and improve the follow-up observation system to observe long-term effects. From experimental study to clinical verification, new problems are found during the clinical application, which need fundamental experimental studies. Afterwards new experimental results are applied to clinical verification. Experiments → clinic → experiments once more → clinic once more, recurrent ascent continuously; through eight-year clinical practical experiences, knowledge also continues to improve. Summation, analysis, reflection and evaluation ascend to theory, putting forward new knowledge, new concept, new thought, new strategy and new therapeutic route and scheme.

Clinical criteria are: good quality of life, longer survival

Results: XZ-C immunomodulatory anticancer medicine was observed in many advanced cancer patients and found that the results was significant.

2. Clinical information

Anti Carcinoma Metastasis and Recurrence Research Office and Shuguang Tumor Specialized Outpatient Department had treated 4, 698 carcinoma patients in Stage III and IV or in metastasis and recurrence with Z-C medicine combined with western medicine among which there were 3, 051 men patients and 1,647 women patients. The youngest one was 11 years old and the oldest one was 86 years old. All groups of the patients were entirely subject to the diagnosis of pathological histology or definitive diagnosis with ultrasonic B, CT and MRI iconography. According to the staging standard of UICC, all the cases were entirely the patients in medium and advanced stage over Stage III. In this group, there were 1,021 hepatic carcinoma patients, among which there were 694 primary lesion hepatic carcinoma patients and 327 metastatic hepatic carcinoma patients; there were 752 patients suffering from carcinoma of lung, among which there were 699 patients suffering from the primary carcinoma of lung and 53 patients suffering from the metastatic carcinoma of lung; there were 668 gastric carcinoma patients, 624 patients suffering from esophagus cardia carcinoma, 328 patients suffering from rectum carcinoma of anal canal, 442 patients suffering from carcinoma of colon, 368 patients suffering from breast carcinoma, 74 patients suffering from adenocarcinoma of pancreas, 30 patients suffering from carcinoma of bile duct, 43 patients suffering from retroperitoneal tumor, 38 patients suffering from oophoroma, 9 patients suffering from cervical carcinoma, 11 patients suffering from cerebroma, 34 patients suffering from thyroid carcinoma, 38 patients suffering from nasopharyngeal carcinoma, 9 patients suffering from melanoma, 27 patients suffering from kidney carcinoma, 48 patients suffering from carcinoma of urinary bladder, 13 patients suffering from leukemia, 47 patients suffering from metastasis of supraclavicular lymph nodes, 35 patients suffering various fleshy tumors and 39 patients suffering from other malignancies.

3. Drugs and administration methods: Treatment rule was to protect thymus and to increase immune function and to protect bone marrow and to recover blood so as to enhance the host's immune surveillance and control cancer escape. From the Chinese medicine the rules are : keep righting and remove bad , soften hard and solution of bump, blood double up and the drugs are XZ-C$_1$, XZ-C$_2$, XZ-C$_3$, XZ-C$_4$, XZ-C$_5$, XZ-C$_6$, XZ-C$_7$, XZ-C$_8$.....XZ-C$_{10}$, depending on different cancers, illness and metastasis condition, according to the disease dialectical to select these drugs. Both oral taken and topical anticancer ointment are applied for metastatic or solid tumor mass; topical analgesic cream is used for cancer pain; jaundice, or ascites is treated with soup of reducing jaundice or eliminating water soup.

4. Treatment Results: Symptom improved, quality of life is improved and survival time prolonged. (Seeing Part I chapter 9)

3. Immune pharmacology of XZ-C immune regulation control medication

Compared with western medication immunity pharmacology, traditional Chinese medication pharmacology has own characteristics and advantages which long-term clinical experience of Chinese medicine has accumulated a large number of prescriptions regulating body's immune function, especially beneficial Chinese medications generally have dynamic regulation of the immune benefits.

Whether single herb medication or prescription will have a variety of active ingredients, and unlike western medication(synthetic drugs) is a matter of a single structure. The roles of Chinese medication are many aspects, in addition to the regulation of immune function, which has a certain role on the whole system function.

The main role of XZ-C immune regulation control medications regulate cell-mediated immune response, including various cytokines or lymphokines. Immune function of XZ-C medication has the major role on stem cells immunity, such as the thymus, gonads and lymphatic systems and T, B cells and various cytokines.

China ancient medicine has the concept of that righteousness isn't false and evil doesn't go into which constitutes an integral part of traditional Chinese medicine theory. Its essence is to maintain the balance of the overall function and to enhance resistance to disease. Its main role is to enhance immune function, in fact, the tonics medication is based on immunity pharmacology. Immunity pharmacology is an emerging interdisciplinary and serves as a bridge contact between pharmacology and immunology. XZ-C immune control regulation medication has obvious immune function, as an effective immune enhancers, this area should be vigorously developed to get a new type of immune accelerator, making them become reliable, efficient and safe drugs. various Chinese herbs in $XZ-C_4$ has substantially immune enhancer effects. In animal experiments $XZ-C_4$ has been proven to significantly promote thymus function. The main role of Chinese medication immunomodulator is to regulate cellular immunity and various cell-mediated immune response, including cytokines or lymphokines.

4. Pharmacological research of immune regulation anticancer Chinese medications

1. To sum anticancer pharmacology and experimental cancer-bearing animal solid tumors in vivo anti-tumor experiments, XZ-C drugs have significant anti-tumor effects. The inhibition rate of antitumor activity $XZ-C_1$ medication was 58% in the first six weeks; the inhibition rate of $XZ-C_4$ was 70% in the first six weeks; the inhibition rate of cyclophosphamide amine (CTX) was 49% in the first 6 weeks in liver cancer H_{22} bearing mice. Life span in $XZ-C_1$ was 9.8% which indicates XZ-C drug has a good anti-cancer effect.

2. XZ-C drug has synergistic effect of attenuated toxicity from chemotherapy drugs, as said anti-cancer pharmacology above, $XZ-C_4$ has been shown to have better function to reduce the toxicity from chemotherapy.

3. XZ-C anti-cancer medication protects immune hematopoietic function. Chemotherapy drugs such as MMC or CTX cause bone marrow hematopoietic system suppression such as WBC↓, PLT↓, and then served $XZ-C_4$ for 4 weeks Hb, WBC, PLT were improved significantly in cancer-bearing mice.

4. XZ-C immunomodulatory anticancer medication has a role in protecting the immune organs and improving human immune function.

CTX caused leukopenia, reduced immune function and kidney damaged on pathologic slices ; after taking $XZ-C_4$, it can significantly improve immune function and can recover white blood cells and red blood cells in H_{22} cancer-bearing mice. There is no thymic atrophy but a little hypertrophy, lymphocytes intensive, increased epithelial reticular cells in XZ-C treatment group.

5. The research on cytokine induction factors of XZ-C anticancer immune regulation and control medication

1. XZ-C$_4$ induces endogenous cytokines

   (1). Through the experiments: XZ-C$_4$ has many immune strengthening functions and has closely relationship to the induced endogenous cytokines

   (2). XZ-C$_4$ can recover the reduction of the white blood cells, granulation cells and platelets.

   (3). XZ-C$_4$ can have the direct function on GM-CSF production from granulation cell (GM) through IL-1β, also increase TNF, IFN etc all of kind of the cell factors, which are possible the indirect function.

   (4). XZ-C$_4$ can increase the Th1 cell factors, which were decrease in the cancer patients. There are the curative effects on the anemia and the white blood cells decrease due to the chemotherapy.

   (5). The experiment analysis showed that XZ-C$_4$ not only protects the bone marrow function, but also has direct function on the tumor cell division.

In brief, XZ-C$_4$ can induce the tumor division and natural death through the autocrine which produce all of kind of factors. The autocrine is the secretory things from the host to affect the host's function. XZ-C$_4$ probably will become the induction therapy to the tumor division in the future.

2. XZ-C$_4$ inhibiting cancer development and metastasis

The malignant development is defined as tumor cells accepting invasion and metastasis characters during the proliferation. Cancer research need to have good repeated animal models. Then the good repeated animal model was made from the mice fibrosis cancernoma QR-32. QR-32 cannot proliferate after inoculation in the skin, and will completely disappear; there were no metastasis lump after injecting into the vein. However, if QR-32 was injected with Gelatin sponge together under the skin in the mice, QR-32 will become the proliferating tumor cells QRSP.

In vitro culturing QRSP and then transfer into another mice, even if there is no foreign thing, the tumors will grow such as the lung metastasis will happen after injection in the vein.

XZ-C$_4$ was used in the animal models to search the effects of the tumor development. To divide this animal models into two steps: the process from QR-32 to QRSP(early progress) and from the QRSP to tumor(later progress). After using XZ-C$_4$, the tumor development will be inhibited in these two models, especially the former will be inhibited significantly. And this has relationship with the dose of the medication.

On the survival experiment the animal models of the inoculation of the QR-32 AND Gelatin sponge died during 65 days, however in XZ-C group the mice survival rate for 150 days was 30%. XZ-C$_4$ can increase the immune effects and reduce the side effects of other anticancer medication.

This research proved that XZ-C$_4$ has inhibition of the cancer progression function and inhibit cancer invasion and metastasis.

6. XZ-C immunomodulatory anticancer medicine toxicology studies

$XZ\text{-}C_1$ can be long-term use. Acute toxicity experiments showed that: 100 times the adult dose to mice fed (10g / kg) were observed at 24, 48, 72, 96 hours in 30 purebred mice without a death. The median lethal dose (LD50) is difficult to make and is a quite secure prescription.

According to WHO "cancer medicine and acute toxin Classification Standard" assessment patients with different measurement, different forms of treatment, changes in the peripheral blood, liver and kidney function in order to understand its toxicity and adverse circumstances, XZ-C medication was oral taken in more than 6000 cases, continuous medication at less 3 months, some for years. The patients have no abnormal phenomenon before and after treatment and blood tests such as WBC, RBC, Hb, PLT are checked and the results are improvement. In order to control cancers the patients with advanced cancer in our specialty clinics took XZ-C for a long-term such as using $XZ\text{-}C_{1\cdot_4}$ 10 or more years and the patient didn't have metastasis and non-proliferation, the disease condition is stable, and lived with cancer. Adhere to long-term medication XZ-C medication can stabilize condition , inhibit cancer proliferation, improve the quality of life and prolong their lives, did not show toxicity, we insist on a longer-term experience serving XZ-C medicine and can help prevent the patients from short and long term recurrence and metastasis after radical surgery.

7. Active ingredient of XZ-C anticancer immune control and regulation medications

$XZ\text{-}C_{1\cdot4}$ is a compound consisting of 28 Chinese herbs. The extraction work of total effective ingredient compound is extremely difficult, the technology is complex and it was exceedingly difficult to extract the active ingredient compound. Active ingredients of a single herb can be extracted. Thus, XZ- C series drugs except $XZ\text{-}C_1$ outside is boiling agent, and the rest are used every herb of fine powder or capsules in order to remain independent of each herb's active ingredients which can play its antitumor effects. The powders are mixed fine powder and the active ingredient can remain independent of each drug; however, after the drug is boiled, the chemical element changes so as to inevitably change the active ingredient of the drug and make it difficult to know the active ingredients after boiling.

But overall the active ingredients of various medications in the prescription are:

1.Alkaloids

2. Glycosides: saponins and glycosides

Each herb in the prescription has anti-tumor active ingredient, for example prescription Ganoderma lucidum, its anti-tumor component A is Ganoderma lucidum polysaccharides, antitumor effect is: with a hypodermic method, graft inoculation 7 days of S_{180} ascites carcinoma on mouse right groin, at a dose 20% mg / kg 10 days the inhibition rate is 95.6-98.5%. The inhibition rate of treatment of leukopenia was 84.6%, the treatment of leukopenia, recent efficiency 84.6% and total WBC increases 1028 / mm^3. Anti-tumor component B is Fumaric acid. Its anti-tumor effect: with Gavage 60mg / kg 10 days in S180 cancer mice , then weighed tumors: the inhibition rate was 37.1% -38.6% and the body weight of mice did not decline.

Another example is the prescription FRUCTUS LIGUSTRI LUCIDI, its anti-tumor components of ursolic acid (Ursolic acid). Its anti-tumor effect on liver cancer cells in vitro with a very significant inhibition rate, can prolong life Ehrlich ascites carcinoma in mice. Pharmacological experiments show its flooding agent capable of inhibiting certain animals transplanted tumor growth. This product contains oleanolic acid with enhancing immune function, recovering peripheral leukocytes, enhancing phagocytes in reticuloendothelial cells, recovers white blood cells of the reduction induced by radiation or chemotherapy , strengthens cardiac functions and diuretic function and protects liver function.

Another example is the prescription of Sophora, its anti-tumor component A: Sophocarpine. Its anti-tumor effect: In vitro experiments showed that Sophocarpine have a direct killing effect on Ehrlich ascites tumor cells: the inhibition rate was 30 to 60% on mice transplanted U_{1_4} or S_{180}. There is clinical application effect. Sophora antitumor component B is Oxymatrine. Its anti-tumor effects: for S_{180} mice there is significant activity, 500ug and 250 ug per day administration, a total of five days, in treatment groups, respectively tumor weight was 26.1% and 57.9%.

3. Another example is the prescription of bamboo ginseng, its anti-tumor component A, as β-Elemene. Its anti-tumor effects: on the EAC, ARS etc two kinds of ascites cancer there is significant anti-graft tumor effect; also it has effect on YAS and S180 ascites. Its anti-tumor components: ginseng total polysaccharides. Its anti-tumor effects of animal experiments show: total ginseng polysaccharides has a stimulating effect on immune function for Ehrlich ascites cancer in mice at 400-800mg / kg with significant cancer inhibition. Ginseng polysaccharide on many tumor cells doesn't have directly killing effect and its anti-tumor effect may be due to the adjustment of the body's immune function so that cancer-bearing host enhanced antitumor capacity. Its anti-tumor component C is Ginsenoside which has inhibition for S180 cancer cells which its tumor weight inhibition rate was 36.4% in 120mg / kg 7d . Ginsenosides may act directly on cancer cells to inhibit cancer cell growth; also available through effects on metabolism and regulation of immunity so that the body's resistance to disease increased and tumor growth was inhibited. Ginseng extract can inhibit Marine tumor, sarcoma S_{180} and lung cancer T_{55}.

8. XZ-C Prescription Principles

XZ-C1,XZ-C$_4$ of XZ-C immunomodulatory anticancer medications are compound as a powder, or capsules, the compound is a mixture rather than multi-flavored powder, so each herb's active ingredients, pharmacological effects are alone Each herb can be individually separated.

XZ-C compound is completely different with traditional Chinese medicine. After A, B, C, D compound are boiled, the component is completely changed, like eating, "pot", the original pharmacological effect of every taste was widowed after boiling together, and the original pharmacological effect of each flavor was lost after boiled, and after cooking it is difficult to know what the pharmacological effects and what the active ingredient is. It is very difficult and very complex technology to extract the active ingredient after boiling the compound. Our XZ-C drugs are completely different, not boiling, every individual taste is grinded into fine level, and then mixed in different amounts (cannot afford a compound effect), the pharmacological effects of each herb and its active ingredient completely do not change while retaining all herbs and pharmacological effects of the active ingredient. This is the reform and innovation for traditional Chinese medicine formulations.

Why use compound rather than single herb? Because the role of power is not enough, more herbs together have stronger effects such as A = a + b + c + d .. then there must be A> a, A> a + b, A> a + b + c, etc., such as the inhibition rate of its single flavor was 20%, another flavor was 30% , and then another 31%, which totally the inhibition rate of this mixed serving may be 20 + 30 + 31 which may reach 81%. To improve the immune system, such as one flavor is 19%, the second flavor is 40%, the third flavor is 24%, then the mixed one together may be 83%. Holding constant every individual taste is the most important; each herb play its independent role in anti-cancer and increasing the role of immunity function.

Furthermore, XZ-C prescription principles also are followed the biological characteristics of cancer and cancer metastasis multi-link, multi-step characteristics so over the years we achieved remarkable results on anti-recurrence and anti-metastasis for the patients with long-term XZ-C immunomodulatory medications. Many patients with advanced cancer are inoperable and also should not have radiation and chemotherapy; however after long-term taking XZ-C immune regulation medication can achieve stable condition, control metastasis, improve quality of life and significantly prolong survival time. Every herb in XZ-C immunomodulatory anticancer medication was selected by two step in solid tumor-bearing mice in vivo anti-tumor screening: the first step is screening a single flavor for the better inhibition rate, and the second step is to select prescription which there are three indicators: 1). it has a good anti-tumor effect; 2).without damage the normal cells of the body 3).increase immune function. If it has a high inhibition rate, but reduced immunity, it will not be chosen. In "new concept and new methods of cancer treatment," recently published a book written specifically for 16 years in our laboratory experiments work in cancer research confirmed cancer development and recurrence, metastasis and host immune organ function and immunity have certainly clear relationship. The medication which protects the immune organs and enhances immunity function are more important than the medication which inhibit or kill cancer drugs. XZ-C anti-tumor immune regulation medicine through experimental research and clinical validation observations show that:

1. There is significant anti-tumor effect, a higher inhibition rate;

2. Better improve the body's immune function, it can be cancer mouse experiments showed incomplete atrophy of the thymus and improve immune function;

3. Protect the hematopoietic system of the role of the chemotherapy drugs inhibit the outer periphery of the bone marrow after the white blood cells, platelets, red blood cells have been significantly improved;

4. Have a good effect for advanced cancer patients. Can significantly change the patient's appetite, sleep, physical and mental state, can significantly improve symptoms, improve quality of life;

5. Have a role in reducing the toxicity in advanced cancer patients with chemotherapy drugs. Its efficacy is superior to the treatment of chemotherapy drugs;

6. In animal experiments there is no toxic side effects. In clinics for 16 years on 16000 patients, especially in many cases of advanced cancer patients the medication were used for a long-term 3--5 years, and some patients even served 8--10 years, it showed no toxic side effects. If the patients have long-term medication adherence, their spirit, appetite, physical strength are good, significantly prolonged survival.

9. Molecular level immune function of XZ-C Immunomodulator anti-cancer medicine

With more and deeper researches on traditional Chinese medication, it has been proved that many kinds of traditional Chinese medications can regulate and control the production and biological activity of cytokine and other immune molecules, which is meaningful to explain the immunological mechanism of XZ-C immunologic regulation and control anti-carcinoma medication from the level of molecule.

I. Protecting Immune Organs and Increasing the Weight of Thymus and Spleen

1. XZ-C-T (EBM): Using its 15g/kg and 30g/kg extracting solution (equivalent to 1g original medicine) along with 12.5mg/kg, 25mg/kg ferulic acid suspension to feed the mice for seven days in a raw can increase the weight of thymus and spleen obviously, especially the effects of the group with high dose are more apparent. Intraperitoneal injection of EBM polysaccharide can also alleviate thymus and spleen atrophy obviously caused by prednisolone.

2. XZ-C-O (PMT): Extract PM-2, feed the mice with 6g/kg PMT decoction for successive seven days which can increase the weight of thymus and celiac lymph nodes and antagonize the reduction in the weight of immune organs caused by prednisolone. Drenching the mouse of 15 months old with 6g/kg decoction (with the concentration of 0.5g/ml) for 14 days can increase the weight and volume of thymus, thicken the cortex and raise cellular density apparently. The combined use of PM and astragalus root can promote non-lymphocyte hyperplasia and benefit the micro environment of thymus.

3. XZ-C-W (SCB): SCB polysaccharide can gain weight of thymus and spleen of a normal mouse. Lavage with it enables cyclophosphane to control the gain in the weight of thymus and spleen.

4. XZ-C-M (LLA): Drench a mouse with LLA decoction for seven days resulting in increasing the weight of thymus and spleen.

5. XZ-C-L: For a 15-month old mouse, its thymus degenerates obviously. Astragalus injectio can enlarge the thymus significantly. The cortex under microscope is thickened and the cellular density increase obviously.

II. Effects on Proliferation, Differentiation and Hematopiesis of Marrow Cells

1. XZ-C-O (PMT): Extract PM-2

2. XZ-C-Q (LBP): (1)Effects on the proliferation of hematopoietic stem cell (CFU-S) of a normal mouse: inject PM-2 with the dose of 500mg/kg ×3d or 10mg/kgx3d LBP into the experimental mice respectively by venoclysis and kill them in the ninth day. It can be found that the number of spleen CFU-S in the group with administration increases obviously. The number of CFU-S in group PM-2 is 21% higher than that of the control group and it is 36% in the group with LBP;(2)Effects on colony forming unit of granulocytes and macrophages (CFU-GM): the experimental results indicate that LBP with the dose of 5~30mg/kg×3d can increase the number of CFU-GM and PM-2 can also strengthen the effect of CFU-GM with the effective dose of 12.5~50mg/kg×3d. In the early stage of cultivation, most CFU-GMs are units of granulocytes and then units of macrophages increase gradually. In the anaphase units of macrophages take over the dominance.

   From the above experiment, it can be found that PM-2 and LBP can promote hematopiesis of normal mice obviously. The experiment proves that during the process of restoring hematopiesis damaged by CTX, PM-2 and LBP stimulate the proliferation of granulocytes at first, and then marrow karyocytes multiply; at last these two promote the restoration of peripheral granulocytes.

3. XZ-C-D (TSPG):Ginsenoside, which is the active principle of ginseng to promote hematopiesis, can bring the recovery of erythrocyte in peripheral blood, haemoglobin and myeloid cell of thighbone in the mice of marrow-inhibited type, increase the index of myeloid cellular division and stimulate the proliferation of myeloid hematopoietic cell in vitro so as to make it into cell cycle with active proliferation (S+G_2/M stage). TSPG can promote the proliferation and differentiation of polyenergetic hematopoietic cells and induce the formation of hemopoietic growth factor (HGF).

4. XZ-C-H (RCL):Steamed Chinese Foxglove can promote the recovery of erythrocyte and haemoglobin for animals with blood deficiency and accelerate the proliferation and differentiation of myeloid hematopoietic cell (CFU-S) with the effect of predominance and hematosis significantly. Peritoneal injection of rehmannia polysaccharides for successive six days can promote the proliferation and differentiation of myeloid hematopoietic cells and progenitor cells as well as increasing the number of leucocytes in peripheral blood.

5. XZ-C-J (ASD):ASD polysaccharide has no effects on erythrocytes and leucocytes of normal mice, but for those damaged by radiation, injection of ASD polysaccharide can influence the proliferation and differentiation of both polyenergetic hematopoietic stem cells (CPU-S) and hemopoietic progenitor cells. But its decoction has no obvious effects.

6. XZ-C-E (PEW):Poria cocos (micromolecule chemical compound extracted from Tuckahoe polysaccharide) is the active principle that can strengthen the production of colony stimulating factor (CSF) and improve the level of leucocytes in peripheral blood inside the mouse's body. It can also prevent the decline in leucocytes caused by cyclophosphamide and accelerate the recovery with the effects better than sodium ferulic which is used to increase leucocytes.

7. XZ-C-Y (PAR): Its polysaccharide can obviously resist the decline in leucocytes caused by cyclophosphamide and increase the number of myeloid cells to promote the proliferation of myeloid induced by CSF as well as the recovery and reconstitution of hematopiesis for the mice irradiated by X ray. It can also increase the number of hematopoietic stem cells and myeloid cells along with leucocytes.

III. Enhancing Immunologic Function of T Cells

The active principles of XZ-C traditional Chinese medicine and their effects are following.

1. XZ-C-L (AMB): It can raise the percentage of lymphocytes in peripheral blood obviously. The LBP in small dose (5~10mg/kg) can cause the proliferation of lymphocytes, indicating that LBP can promote the proliferation of T cells apparently. 50mg/(kg·d)×7d is the best dose in that it will have no effects if lower than the level and it will bring the effects down if higher than the level. Oral administration of LBP can raise the conversion rate of lymphocytes for the sufferers who are weak and with fewer leucocytes.

2. $XZ-C_4$: It can regulate immune system and active T cells of aggregated lymphatic follicles, as well as stimulate the secretion of hemopoietic growth factor in T cells. Among the crude drugs of $XZ-C_4$, the extract from the hot water of atractylodes lancea rhizome can obviously stimulate the cells of aggregated lymphatic follicles, which is regarded as the base of $XZ-C_4$ immunoloregulation.

IV. Activating and Enhancing NK Cell Activity

Natural killer cell, NK cell is another kind of killer cell in lymphocytes for human beings and mice, which needs neither antigenic stimulation, nor the participation of antibodies to kill some cells. It plays an important role in immunity, especially in the function of immune surveillance as NK cell is the first line of defense against tumors and has broad spectrum anti-tumor effects.

NK cell is broad-spectrum and able to kill sygeneous, homogenous and heterogenous tumor cells with special effects on lymjphoma and leucocytes.

NK cell is an important kind of cells for immunoloregulation, which can regulate T cells, B cells and stem cells, etc. It can also regulate immunity by releasing cytokines like IFN-α, IFN-γ, IL-2, TNF, etc.

The active principles in XZ-C traditional Chinese medicine and their effects are following.

1. XZ-C-X (SDS): Divaricate Saposhniovia Root can strengthen the activity of NK cells of experimental mice. When combined with IL-2, it can make the activity of NK cell higher, indicating that its polysaccharide can give a hand to IL-2 to activate NK cells and improve the activity. LBP can strengthen T cell mediated immune reaction and the activity of NK cells for normal mice and those dealt by cyclophosphamide. Peritoneal injection of LBP can improve the proliferation of spleen T lymphocytes and strengthen the lethality of CTL increasing the specific lethal rate from 33% to 67%.

2. XZ-C-G (GUF):Glycyrrhizin can induce the production of IFN in the blood of animals and human beings and strengthen NK cell activity at the same time. Clinical tests made by Abe show that after intravenous injection of 80mg GL, the raise of NK cell activity reaches 75% among 21 sufferers. Peritoneal injection of 0.5mg/kg GL on mice can strengthen the activity of NK cells in liver.

3. XZ-C-L (AMB): Its bath fluid can promote NK cell activity of mice both in vivo and in vitro, and can also induce IFN-γ to deal with effector cells under the certain concentration of 0.1mg/ml. Cordyceps sinensis extract can strengthen NK cells activity of the mouse both in vivo and in vitro. Fluids with the concentrations of 0.5g/kg, 1g/kg and 5g/kg can strengthen NK cell activity of mice.

V. Effects on LAK Cell Activity

Lymphokine activated killer cell, namely LAK cell can be induced by IL-2 cytokine. LAK cells can kill the solid tumors that are both sensitive and insensitive to NK cells with broad anti-tumor effects.

The active principles in XZ-C anti-carcinoma traditional Chinese medicine and their effects are following:

1. XZ-C-L (AMB): Its polysaccharide can strengthen LAK cell activity within a certain range of dose with 0.01mg/ml being the most effective, which is three times better than the damage effects of LAK cells. The concentrations of both higher and lower than this level can not achieve the effects.

2. XZ-C-U (PUF):It can significantly strengthen the spleen LAK cell activity of killing tumor cells and improve the activity of erythrocyte C3b liquid. PUF and IL-2 are synergistic that can be used as regulator for biological reaction in tumor biological therapy based on LAK/Ril-2.

3. XZ-C-V:ABB polysaccharide can also raise LAK cell activity for the mouse and inhibit tumors remarkably. Its anti-tumorous mechanism relates to its strengthening immunity and changing cell membrane features.

VI. Effects on Iterleukin-2 (IL-2)

The active principles in XZ-C anti-carcinoma traditional Chinese medicine and their effects are following:

1. XZ-C-T:EBM polysaccharide can enhance obviously the production of IL-2 for human beings when the concentration is 100ug/ml. At higher concentration (2500ug/ml and 5000ug/ml), it will lead to inhibition. Hypodermic injection of barrenwort polysaccharide for seven days in a row can significantly improve the ability of thymus and spleen of the mouse induced by ConA to produce IL-2.

2. XZ-C-Y:PAR polysaccharide has strong immune activity and is able to promote the production of IL-2. For the mouse bearing S-180 tumor, it can raise the ability of spleen cells to produce IL-2 obviously。

3. XZ-C-D: Ginseng polysaccharide has great promotion on IL-2 induced by peripheral monocytes for both healthy people and sufferers with kidney troubles. The effects are relevant to the dose positively.

VII. Function of Inducing Interferon and Promoting Inducement of Interferon

IFN are broad-spectrum in resisting tumors and can regulate immunity. It can also inhibit the proliferation of tumor cells and activate NK cells and CTL to kill tumor cells. Meanwhile, IFN can cooperate with TNF, IL-1 and IL-2 to enforce anti-tumorous ability.

The active principles in XZ-C anti-carcinoma traditional Chinese medicine and their effects are following:

1. XZ-C-Z: 250mg/kg or 500mg/kg CVQ polysaccharide can improve significantly the level of IFN-γ produced by mouse spleen cells.

2. XZ-C-D: Ginsenoside (GS) and panaxitriol ginsenoside (PTGS) can induce whole blood cells and monocytes of human beings to produce IFN-α and IFN-γ. It can also recover the low level of IFN-γ and IL-2 to the normal. The IFN potency of ASH polysaccharide on S-180 cell line of acute lymphoblastic leukemia and S7811 cell line of acute myelomonocytic leukemia produced after acanthopanax polysaccharide stimulation is 5~10 times more than that of normal control group.

3. XZ-C-E

Hydroxymethyl Poria cocos mushroom polysaccharide has many kinds of physical activity like immunoloregulation, promoting to induce IPN, resisting virus indirectly and alleviating adverse reaction resulting from radiation. Do IFN inducement dynamic experiment on S-180 leukaemia cell line by using 50mg/ml Hydroxymethyl Poria cocos mushroom polysaccharide. The results indicate that its potency to induce interferon at all stages is better than that of normal inducement.

4. XZ-C-G (GL): It can induce IFN activity. Make peritoneal injection of 330mg/kg GL on mice. IFN activity reaches the peak after 20 hours.

VIII. Function of Promoting and Increasing Colony Stimulating Factor

Colony stimulation factor, namely CSF is a kind of glucoprotein with low molecular weight that can stimulate the proliferation and differentiation of marrow hematopoietic stem cells as well as other mature blood cells. Cells that can produce CSF include mononuclear macrophages, T cells, endothelial cells and desmocytes. CSF not only take part in the proliferation and differentiation of hematopoietic stem cells and regulating mature cells, but also play an important role in anti- tumorous immunity of host cells.

The active principles in XZ-C anti-carcinoma traditional Chinese medicine and their effects are following:

1. XZ-C-Q:PAR polysaccharide is able to promote to produce CSF by spleen cells of experimental mice. 100~500ug/ml PAP-II can encourage spleen cells to produce CSF depending on the dose and time with the fittest dose of 100ug/ml and best time of 5d. Moreover, lentinan can also increase the amount of CSF.

2. XZ-C-Q:Injection of LBP can facilitate the secretion of CSF by mouse spleen T cells and improve the activity of CSF in serum.

3. XZ-C-T:EBM icariin can promote the proliferation of mouse spleen lymphocytes induced by ConA and bring CSF activity.

IX. Function of Promoting TNF

Tumor necrosis factor, namely TNF is a kind of cytokine that can kill tumor cells directly. Its main effect is to kill or inhibit tumor cells, which can kill some tumor cells or inhibit the proliferation both in vivo and in vitro.

The active principles in XZ-C anti-carcinoma traditional Chinese medicine and their effects are following:

1. XZ-C-Y (PEP):It can induce the production of TNF, so as PEP-1. Inject 80~160mg/kg PEP-1, once every four days. Collect peritoneal macrophages (PM), add 10ug LPS into culture medium to cultivate PM. Take the supernatant to determine TNF and IL-1. It can be found that PEP-1 can parallelly increase the auxiliary production of TNF and IL-1. The time of TNF inducement reaches the peak on the 8th day after the second intraperitoneal injection. Compared with the known startup potion BCG, the inducement of TNF has no difference.

2. XZ-C-E:Carboxymethyl-pachymaran (CMP) is the principle essential component distilled from traditional Chinese medicine Tuckahoe. It can not only strengthen the ability of mouse spleen to create IL-2 and macrophages and promote the activity of T cells, B cells, NK cells and LAK cells; but also encourage the production of TNF. The experiment proves that CMP is an effective potion to promote and induce cytokines.

3. XZ–C–V:ABB polysaccharide can promote the production of TNF-b in mouse cells induced by ConA. It can also induce the synthesis of peritoneal macrophages and secrete 20ug/ml TNF-αachyranthes bidentata polysaccharides. The time of TNF-α to reach its peak is 2~6 hours after effects. Peritoneal injection of 100mg/kg achyranthes bidentata polysaccharides can accelerate the production of TNF-α, whose intensity of effects is comparable to that of BCG.

X. Effects on Cell Adhesion Molecule

Most adhesion molecules are glycoproteid and are distributed on cellular surface and extracellular matrix. Adhesion molecules take effect in the corresponding form of ligand-acceptor, resulting in the adhesion between cells, or between cell and stroma, or the adhesion of cell-stroma-cell. These molecules take part in a set of physical pathologic processes, like cellular conduction and activation of information, cellular stretch and movement, formation of thrombus as well as tumor metastasis, etc. Intercellular adhesion molecule-1, namely ICAM-1 is one kind of adhesion molecules in the super family of immune globulins.

The effect of corn stigma as an active principle in XZ-C traditional Chinese anti-carcinoma medicine: Hobtemariam has proved that alcohol extract from corn stigma has significant inhibition on the adhesion of endothelial cells to inhibit effectively the expression of ICAM-1 and the adhesive activity with TNF, LPS as agents.

10. XZC immunomodulatory anticancer medications: structural formula; antitumor ingredient; present site; anti-tumor effect

Z-C1 - A ApL
Anti-tumor components: agrimonniin
Effective parts: the whole plant for the plants.

Anti-tumor effect: Okucla other scholars isolated out agrimonniin from ApL grass which has proven to be the main anticancer component. Before and after inoculation of MM2 breast cancer cells, 10mg / kg of this product is given by ip, the results were that all cancer are rejected. No matter how it was given by P.O. or I.P., it can prolong survival time in tumor-bearing animals. Agrimonniin can inhibit MH 134 liver cancer and sarcoma Meth-A cellulose growth. With or without calf serum medium, MM2 breast cancer cells and agrimonniin together for 2h, then for 48h at 37 humidified CO_2 incubator, and found time without calf serum, agrimonnii on MM2 breast cancer cells showed strong cytotoxicity, and its IC50 is 2.66ug / ml, but adding fetal calf serum in the culture medium, then weakened to around 4% of the original, namely an IC50 of 62.5% ug /ml, after intraperitoneal injection of agrimonniin 4d, the absorption of H3-thymine was obviously inhibited on MM2 breast cancer and MH134 hepatoma cells .

These results indicate that agrimonniin is a potent anti-tumor acid and its anti-tumor effect may be due to the drug action on tumor cells and enhance the immune response. ApL grass produces 1: 1, PH6.5 (1g crude drug / ml) solution by water extraction method to inhibit S_{180}, cervix U_{1_4}, brain tumors B_{22}, Ehrlich EAC, melanoma B_{10}, rats W_{256} cancer. The results show that for more than transplanted tumors better inhibition, the inhibition rates were between 36.2 -6.59%, $P<0.05$, there is a significant difference .

ApL grass water extract has a strong inhibitory effect on human JTC-26 cancer cells in vitro and inhibition rate reaches 100% and meanwhile it promotes the normal cell growth 100%. While 30mg / kg ApL grass phenol was injected daily in intraperitoneal cavity, it has a significant therapeutic effect on rat sarcoma S_{37} and cervical cancer U_{1_4}. The inhibition rates on tumor growth were 47.0% and 38.7%, The inhibition rate was 47.4% on sarcoma S180 mice with 0.625g / day and was 52.6% on liver cancer.

Fluid extracted from liver cancer ascites was diluted with sterile physiological water 1-2 $\times 10^7$/ml , then inoculated into mice, each mouse by intraperitoneal injection O.2ml, the next day were randomly divided into treatment group and control group. 30mg / kg ApL grass phenol was injected in intraperitoneal cavity once daily for 7 days, saline was injected in control group, then observed 30 days to calculate life span. Results: the mean survival day was 26.2 disabilities 0.9 in 24 animals treatment group; the average survival was 17.5 + 1.3day in control group. Life span prolonged above 49.6%. ApL grass phenol has significantly prolong life in animal liver cancer ascites carcinoma..

Z-C1 - B SLT
Anti-tumor components: β-SoIamarine
Effective parts: the SLT whole plant.

Anti-tumor effect: the whole plant has anti-tumor effect, in many countries for a long time as a folk medicine to cure cancer, β-Solamarine its active ingredient, at 30mg / kg on S_{180} mice the tumor weight from control group 1285 mg reduced to 274mg, the inhibition rate was 78.6%.

The whole plant has anti-cancer effects on human lung cancer.

Studies have reported recently, extracted from the SLT anti-tumor active ingredient into health foods, it has given anti-tumor effect and almost no toxicity. SLT also contain solanine Australia which has inhibitory activity on S_{180} mice.

Recently it has been reported: an effective anti-tumor ingredient was extracted from SLT through water or an organic solvent or a mixture of water capacitive solvent, then can be made into oral or parenteral medication: the oral dose serving as 1g /d; the parenteral drug as 60mg / d. The drug can inhibit a variety of tumors, such as S180 and neck cancer with its low toxicity. Murakami Kotaro etc isolated two different body sugar from SLT, each with some anti-tumor effect.

SLT can inhibit S_{180}, cervical cancer U_{14} and Ehrlich ascites carcinoma. In vitro the product of hot water extract can has inhibition rate 100% on human cervical cancer JTC-26 system. And there was no effect on normal cells; in vivo experiments on mice S180 inhibition rate was 14.57%. This product contains an effective anti-cancer ingredient β-bitter solanine which significantly inhibited mice S180 and W256 mouse cancer.

Z-C1-C SNL

Antitumor A: Vitamin A Vitamin A

Existing parts: the whole plant for an amount of 9666 IU%.

Anti-tumor effects: Va has anti-tumor activity. Wald had conducted a survey in 1975-1979 , indicating Va having anti-tumor effect in vivo; Bontwell found that Va can stop cell membrane mucopolysaccharides aggregate effect induced by tumor promoters and block the receptor which bindstumor promoters. A new method for cancer treatment: normal sugar plus LETS (large cells are transferred outside sensitive protein from), two of which are affected Va material synthesis, which shows Va is important in cancer treatment. Meanwhile, Va and their derivatives can reverse cancerous cells inducedy by chemical carcinogens, viruses, and ionizing radiation.

Antitumor Component B: Vitamin C. Vitamin C

Existing parts: the whole plant for the plant, its content is 20mg%

Anti-tumor effects: Vc is antioxidants in anti-tumor effects in blocking nitrite and primary amine to synthesize carcinogenicity compounds in vivo. Cameron will use 10g / day Vc to hundred cancer patients from long-term, 42 times of higher efficacy than control group and has better effect in gastrointestinal cancer. Murata use Vc high-dose to treat cervical cancer and its effect is 5.7 times higher than the effect of small doses. Malistratos induced sarcoma growth with benzo, then treat them with lots of Vc. Vc inhibited sarcoma growth and occurrence. For bladder cancer and skin cancer, it has the preventive effect. In epidemiology cancer occurrence is also related with the intake of Vc.

Vc with various anticancer drugs in combination can increase the efficacy of the drug. As with Vincristine (VCR) it has a synergistic effect and V + CCNu have higher treatment efficacy than single CCNu in leukemia . The survival time extended twice, but also alleviate the condition of patients with advanced cancer. Cisplatin anticancer drugs, because of its toxicity and the larger application subject to certain restrictions, if Vc their combination, can reduce toxicity. New Jersey now Englehard company Hollis developed a cisplatin and Vc mixture composition which has better efficacy.

The whole plant contains Solasonine and solanine which also have activity against S180 sarcoma. Nigrum extract of dried green fruit of total alkali Solanum nigrum can inhibit animals transplanted tumor system by 40- 50%. In tissue culture 50-500mcg/ml 24h total alkali Solanum nigrum inhibit meningioma cells growth. Alkali component isolated from total alkali Solanum nigrum has the strongest antitumor activity and there are significant cytotoxicity. 10mcg / ml 15h concentration causes HeLa cells to collapse. A total extract also has inhibition effect on mice ascites sarcoma 180. Solamine also be used as hematopoietic system stimulant, increasing leukocyte. With barbata and comfrey it was used to treat malignant mole and the result is good. With surgery, chemotherapy, radiation it was used to treat uterine choriocarcinoma, ovarian cancer, liver cancer and had effectiveness.

This product can inhibit cervical cancer, U_{14}, S_{180}, Ehrlich ascites carcinoma and lymphosarcoma, Ehrlich ascites carcinoma, L_{615} lymphatic leukemia, S_{180} , gastric cancer cells and leukemia in mice, etc

SNL has anti-cancer effect on nuclear division. Extract of SNL has inhibition rate of 40% -5O% on animal transplanted tumor. In tissue culture 50-500ug/ ml 24 hr total alkali SNL can inhibit brain tumor cell growth.

Z-C-D PGS
Anti-tumor components A: β-Elemene
Existing parts: the root of the volatile oil and flowers of about 10%.

Antitumor effects: The product has significant anti-tumor effect on ECA and ARS etc two transplanted animal ascites and S180 ascites.

Anti-tumor component B: PGS total polysaccharides:

Antitumor effects: animal experiments show: PGS total polysaccharides have a stimulating effect on immune function. It inhibit mice transplanted tumor S180 to a certain extent and significantly inhibited Ehrlich ascites tumor cells in mice at 400-800mg / kg. PGS polysaccharide doesn't directly kill many tumor cells; its anti-tumor effect may be due to the adjustment of the body's immune function so that tumor-bearing hosts enhance antitumor capacity. There are also reports: PGS total polysaccharide is administered at 460.620mg / kg / d in S180 abdomen the inhibition rate of tumor weight was76.81% (P <0 001.).

Another report, PGS total polysaccharides have some anti-tumor activity, its system may be induced tumor necrosis factor: PGS total polysaccharides on normal mice and tumor-bearing mice can enhance immune function and activation, PGS total polysaccharides also inhibit cancer cell growth.

Anti-tumor components C: PGS saponin Ginsenoside
Formula formula :
Anti-tumor effects:

On mouse sarcoma S180 it had significant inhibition at 120mg / kg/d x7 and the inhibition rate of its tumor weight was 60.48%; on Ehrlich ascites carcinoma (ECS) at a dose of I00mg / kg / d x70, its inhibition rate was 36.40%; on S180 at a dose of 100 mg / kg / dx10 its inhibition rate was 41-61% (P <0.05); large doses on U14 also have some anti-tumor effect.

With chemotherapy drugs CXT used in conjunction, it can enhance the anti-tumor effects of chemotherapy drugs.

Its anti-tumor effect is more complex; one, it can act directly with the cancer cells so that the cancer cell growth was inhibited or be reversal. Second, it can also regulate the body metabolism and the immune function to resist diseases so that the tumor growth was inhibited. National and international clinical trials have proved: it has a therapeutic effect on gastric cancer, not only reduces tumor; but also increases appetite, improves immunity and prolongs patients' survival time.

PGS soap component as a human anti-tumor agents, adapt to a wide range, almost no side effects. The application ranges: gastric cancer, colorectal cancer, breast cancer, uterine cancer, mouth, esophagus, gallbladder cancer, kidney cancer, lung cancer, brain cancer, liver cancer, skin cancer, etc., are valid for almost all tumors. The mode of administration: it can be taken orally at 100-300mg/day x2-3 doses. It can also be used 1-I0% of hydrophilic or hydrophobic ointment topically.

Korea Atomic Energy Research Institute Nguyen and other reports: Application of carcinogens in laboratory animals treated, serving long red ginseng can reduce the incidence of cancer and inhibit tumor growth. Small Tajima and other reports: on cultured hepatoma cell PGS soap can change the cancer cell structures indicating PGS can induce cancer cells to be reversed. Hiroko Abe and other reports: PGS saponin induced reversal to hepatic cancer cells. Li xianggao believes: PGS soap can inhibit 3-O- methyl glucose through the cell membrane and overflow on liver cancer cells so presumably the inhibition of membrane transporters of PGS saponin may be non-specific.

In addition to the relevant ginseng root soap antitumor activity studies, ginseng soap flower total inhibition has also been reported: Yuyongli and other scholars studied the effect of a total ginseng flower soap on NKC-IFN-IL-2 regulatory network and inhibition of tumor Effect. The results showed that: PGS total promote natural killer (NKC) activity in vitro mouse spleen, and in the presence of Con-A induces the production of Y-IFN and IL-2 , indicating the total soap flower PGS has regulation on NKC-IFN-IL-2 network to regulate the immune function by this adjustment extensive network.

Liang Zhongpei etc applied PGS to study how dimethyl buttery yellow sugar induced rat liver cancer. The results showed that: PGS can increase the percentage of ANAE positive lymphocyte cells, reduce the incidence of liver cancer, the tumor is smaller, a higher degree of differentiation of cancer cells, the longitudinal fibers hyperplasia and lymphocyte infiltration around tumor tissue, indicating that PGS should be able to promote immune function so that it has prevention or control action to the chemical carcinogen-induced liver cancer.

Ginseng inhibits variety of experimental animals. Ginseng had reduced tumor incidence and tumor growth inhibition after rats and mice were fed with ginseng long-term for aflatoxin-induced rat lung adenomas, urethane-induced lung cancer in mice. Its main active anti-tumor ingredient is Ginseng saponin of which ginseng saponin Rg3 can strongly inhibit tumor formation of new organs, inhibit tumor recurrence, proliferation and metastasis in mouse melanoma and S180 tumor. The inhibition rate was 60% and on a variety of animal and human tumor lung metastasis, liver metastasis the inhibition rate reached 60% -70%. Ginseng saponin Rg3 is promising as anti-metastatic drugs.

Z-C-E PCW
Antitumor points A, Adenine
The presence of areas: plant sclerotia.

Anti-tumor effect: for the prevention and treatment of various leukopenia, particularly caused by chemotherapy, radiotherapy and benzene poisoning. Its phosphate stimulates white blood cell hyperplasia. It was found that Leukocyte recovered about 2-4 weeks after administration. It can extend the time of chemotherapy and prevent the occurrence of leukopenia if used before chemotherapy or simultaneously.

Antitumor B: Pachyman
Structural formula; [13-D-Glcp- (1.-3) a 13-D.-Glcp- (1 - 3)] n

Antitumor effects: Studies have shown that: new Pachymaran: in 1970 Chihara etc slightly transform pachyman structure into pachymaran of removing the side chain β (1--6) with significant anti-tumor activity, but the poor water-soluble activity.

Carboxymethyl Pachymaran was synthesized by Hamuro etc. in 1971 with pachymaran carboxymethylation which has significant anti-tumor activity in animal experiments.

Hamuro, J and other experiments proved: new biological Pachymaran of pachyman such as CM-pachymaran and HM-pachyman 2-4, have significant anti-tumor activity. Anti-tumor activity of its agents and routes of administration have a great relationship and the appropriate route of administration of the optimal dose must be selected.

About pachyman antitumor mechanism of action and its derivatives, it has also been reported: think no direct cytotoxicity; however through the host's intermediary it played anti-tumor roles which enhance the body's immune system.

Chaoqiaoli etc. observed inhibition of carboxymethyl Pachymaran mouse lung metastasis of inbred uterine cancer U615. The results show that the non-transfer of 64% tumor control group were 94%; metastasis inhibition rate of 75.68%, significantly higher than the control group, the experimental group tumor weight, inhibition rate was 23.58%, the above results suggest that: indeed carboxymethyl Pachymaran has some anticancer activity.

Data reported also: carboxymethyl tuckahoe polysaccharide is a good immune enhancer and apply the treatment of various tumors.

Patent No. 4339435 reports: A Poria sclerotium obtained cultured mycelium, then the mycelium of the water or that the water-soluble organic solvent such as ethanol extraction, to obtain an anti-cancer medicament "A-1", it is not only very good anti-cancer activity and no toxicity, 92% inhibition of the S180, this anti-cancer substance accounted for 24.2% cultured mycelia. Xu Jin et al reported that a group of fat-soluble organic tetracyclic three, collectively known as Poria factors was isolated from Pachyman and significantly inhibited Ehrlich ascites carcinoma, S180 metastasis of Lewis lung carcinoma in mice. When administered with Cyclic amines and phosphorus, there is a certain synergy and it proved Poria increases immune function.

In 1986 Japanese scholars Jinshan isolated a water-soluble anti-tumor polysaccharide, called Pachymaran H_{11} from cultured mycelia of Poria, accounting for about 0.6% of dry mycelium. With 4mg / kg injection JCR / TCL mice subcutaneously x10 days on S180 the inhibition rate was 94%, this report shows that there have been polysaccharide which has anti-cancer activity with no structural transformation in Poria.

There are also reports, after Poria cocos contained β- polyester (β-pachyman) was treat and approached to obtain Poria cocos glycan complex (abbreviated UP), it had a significant anti-tumor effect and the inhibition rate was 57%. It can extend Tumor-bearing mice survival time, improve the spleen index, and it has a direct effect on cancer cells.

Wu Bo and other scholars also conducted experiments to observe PPS's anti-tumor effect and mechanism on mouse S180 cells and human leukemia cells K5G2. It was found that PPS has a strong suppression effect and discusses its anti-tumor mechanism of S180 cell membrane composition. The results showed that after PPS contacts with the cells 24h, the membrane phospholipid content decreased and cell membrane sialic acid content increased, but the membrane cholesterol content, membrane fluidity and membrane fatty acid composition is not affected. When PPS membrane put together with S180 under appropriate conditions, it was found that PPS interference of membrane of inositol phospholipid metabolism is critical step. Changes related to PPs antitumor mechanism and biochemical characteristics also have some reports. PPS significantly inhibited DNA synthesis in mouse L_{1210} cells with irreversible inhibition and increased with the dose.

Poria has anticancer drug synergistic effect : on mitomycin and using inhibitory (mouse sarcoma S180) was 38.9% (5-Fu alone 38.6%) ; in mouse leukemia L1210 cyclophosphamide alone amines life extension of 70%, combined with phosphorus Thalidomide was 168.1%.

PPS and thymus-related anti-tumor effect. Polysaccharides can nonspecifically stimulate the reticuloendothelial system function and enhance the host of cancer-specific antigen immunity to resist the effects of cancer.

Pachymaran with Poria known significant anti-tumor effect, can inhibit the growth of solid tumors , extend survival time in mice S180 and Ehrlich ascites carcinoma. Pachymaran has distinct anticancer roles on cultured mouse sarcoma S180 cells and human chronic myelogenous leukemia K562 cell. Antitumor mechanism includes two aspects of increased immune system and direct cytokine roles. Antitumor mechanism may be suppressed by inhibiting tumor cell nuclear DNA synthesis and enhance production of tumor necrosis factor (TNF) from macrophage and the ability to enhance tumor cell killing effect.

Intraperitoneal injection of polysaccharides (PPS) 5-200mg / kg continuous 100, above 10mg , it inhibited S180 significantly. On S180 sarcoma in mice and Ehrlich ascites carcinoma (EAC) orally taken 8d, it can enhance tumor necrosis factor (TNF) levels and significantly increased natural killer (NK) cell activity.

It significantly inhibited lung metastasis from U_{1_4} after mice were fed carboxymethyl tuckahoe polysaccharide (250mg / kg/d) 25d. The mouse sarcoma S180 cells were seeded in ICR / JCL mice subcutaneously, 24 hours later 5mg / kg polysaccharides once daily once 10 days injected intraperitoneally. The results showed that inhibition rate was 95%.

Carboxymethyl Pachymaran strongly inhibited U_{1_4} in mice. Using 500mg / kg, 100 mg / kg, 50mg / kg, the result of inhibition rate was 75.5%. 92.7% 78.7%, respectively, of which 100 mg / kg dose was the best. Intraperitoneal injection carboxymethyl tuckahoe polysaccharide 100mg / kg/ d 10d extended lifetime was 23.49% compared with the control in Ehrlich ascites carcinoma. It reduced the amount of ascites 7%, reduced total number of cancer cells 139.20%. PPS can inhibit DNA synthesis in Ehrlich ascites tumor cells. The inhibition role of PPS is related to the dose which using 100 / kg., 50mg / kg, 5mg / kg 3 the results of tumor inhibition rates were 92.3%, 96.1%, 53.4%.

Z-C1-G GuF
Anti-tumor components A: Glycyrrhiza acid
Existing parts: wooden grass roots, rhizomes.

Antitumor effects: The product can produce morphological changes on rat hepatoma and Ehrlich ascites carcinoma (EAC) cells and inhibit subcutaneous Yoshida sarcoma. Licorice as raw material soluble Monoaniniornum glycyrrhetate, namely licorice acid amine, can inhibit Ehrlich ascites carcinoma and muscle tumor. Meanwhile, licorice acid amine has some detoxification for certain toxic of anti-cancer drugs. Natural products, such as having a certain anti-tumor effect: Caniptotliecine causes toxic reactions and limits the use of drugs, but a licorice acid amine can lower camptothecin toxicity by not reducing its efficacy and having a certain synergy. On animal experiments: the number of white blood cells caused by camptothecin, Glycyrrhizinate amine has a protective effect.

This product is hot-water extract on human cervical cancer cells JTC-26 and the inhibition rate is 70%- 90%.

Anti-tumor component B: Gycyrrhetinic aicd

Existing parts: the herbal roots, rhizomes.

Antitumor effects: glycyrrhetinic acid inhibited transplanted Oberling-Guerin myeloma on rat. Its sodium salt has been inhibition on the growth of mouse Ehrlich ascites carcinoma and sarcoma -45 , even orally.

Anti-tumor components: Liguirtin

Structure:

Existing parts: the root herbal.

Antitumor effects: The product can inhibit morphological changes and also have anti-tumor effect on rat hepatoma and Ehrlich ascites carcinoma cells and rat mammary tumor. It has the preventive effect on rat stomach cancer, can reduce the incidence of gastric cancer. In addition, grass sweetener has inhibited aflatoxin B1-induced hepatic precancerous lesion.

Z-C-K LwF
Antitumor points: (Tetrainethylpyrazine, TTMP)

Anti-tumor effects: TTMP can inhibit TXA2 synthetase activity. Li Xue Tang et al reported: TTMP administered once has a certain anti-metastatic effect on hepatoma cell metastasis. Jin Rong and other reports: TTMP anti-tumor effect and its mechanism, the experimental results show that: TTMP at 20mg/d x 18d could significantly inhibit the artificial lung metastasis in B16-F10 melanoma and TTMP can enhance normal and tumor-bearing spleen NK cell activity in isotope incorporation assay in mice and antagonized cyclophosphamide inhibition of NK cell activity. TTMP anti-metastatic effect may be related to reduce plasma TXB content and to enhance NK cell activity.

Some academics have also been reported: isolated from this plant gland (Adenine), its pharmacological activity has been confirmed that stimulate white blood cell proliferation, prevent fine thrombocytopenia, particularly for leukopenia caused by radiotherapy or chemotherapy. TTMP has a certain anti-metastatic effect on liver cancer cells.

Z-C-L AMB
Anti-tumor component B: β-Sitosterol
Existing parts: The root of the plant.

Anti-tumor effects: β-Sitosterol has an edge activity for lymphocytic leukemia P134; has effect on mouse adenocarcinoma 715, which inhibition rate of tumor weight (TWI) was> 58%; it has effects on Lewis lung carcinoma ,its TWI was > 58%; for the rat carcinoma Wacker cancer 256 its TWI was > 58%.

Reports: AMB roots have in a certain amount of polysaccharide; AMB polysaccharide contains 1.34-2.04% and there are several polysaccharides. It has broad biological activity and has anti-tumor effect in vivo, but does not directly kill cancer cell in vitro which means that AMB polysaccharide works by enhancing immune function.

AMB can improve human and mouse plasma cAMP levels, can inhibit tumor growth, and make tumor cells even reversed; can promote animal leukocytosis; can recover leukopenia induced by chemotherapy or radiotherapy; can promote immune function and inhibit tumor cell killing effect. The inhibition rate of its water extract was 41.7% in vivo experiments on mice sarcoma -180. The alcohol extract AMB is currently used clinically as an anticancer drug righting.

ZhouShuYin reported: the results of AMB polysaccharide show in vivo experiments: APS 2.5mg/kg, 5mg/kg, 10mg/kg, 20mg/kg significantly inhibited on transplanted tumor S180 liver cancer; in vitro results showed that: APS and interleukin-2 can significantly improve the compatibility of applied rate LAK cell killing target cells P851 and Yae cells. Its anti-tumor mechanism is related to increasing immune function.

In vivo the inhibition rate of AMB hot extract was 41.7% on mice sarcoma S180; was 12.25% on human lung adenocarcinoma SPC-A- 1. The inhibition index Iodized oil was induced with MCA human-mouse lung which the injection group with MCA was 16.28%, the control group was 51.52% cancer, the difference is very significant. MCA can inhibit DNA synthesis in human ovarian cancer cells. When the drug concentration increases, the inhibition will strengthen and the duration of action of the drug will prolong and inhibition of DNA synthesis of cancer cells also will be enhanced. MCA polysaccharides have synergies on T lymphocyte activation of malignant ascites.

Z-C-M LIA
Fight tumor components: Ursolic acid
Exist parts: the leaves of the plant.

Anti-tumor effect: it has a very significant inhibition rate on cancer cells in vitro culture and can prolong the life on Hershey ascites carcinoma mice.

Pharmacological experiments show that: the goods flooding agent can inhibit certain animals transplanted tumor growth; it can increase immune function; it can recover leukopenia induced by chemotherapy and radiotherapy. There are also reported that the active ingredient in this product is Oleanic acid.

Z-C-N CzR

Anti-tumor component A: Turmeric alcohol Curcumol

Structure:

Exist parts: roots for the plants.

Anti-tumor effects: Curcumol has anti-tumor effect. At 75mg/kg the inhibition rate was 53.47-61 .96% on mice sarcoma S37; at 75ug/kg the inhibition rate was 45.1-77.13% on mice cervical cancer U14; the inhibition rate was 65.8- 78.9% at the same doses on EAC. There is better effect on treating cervical cancer.

Antitumor Component B: Turmeric dione /Curdione

Structure:

Exist parts: roots for the plants.

Antitumor effects: turmeric significantly inhibited mouse sarcoma 37, U_{1_4} and neck cancer and mouse Ehrlich ascites carcinoma and can make cancer cells degeneration and necrosis. This product is processed in Ehrlich ascites carcinoma can be successfully immunized mice to obtain initiative. The clinical results indicate that cervical cancer has a good effect.

There are also reports: In its same plant Curcuma wenyujin Y.H. Chen etc isolated β-elemene which has anti-cancer activity. The research proved that β-elemene could significantly prolong the survival time on Ehrlich ascites carcinoma and ascites reticulocyte cell sarcoma in mice and has strong killing effect on liver cancer cells in vitro. It also reduced nucleic acid content on EAC , especially in RNA content decreased more significantly. On leukocyte and bone marrow nucleated cells and Immune test: β-elemene has relatively small toxicity.

100% 0.3-0.5ml of Curdione has a good effect and the inhibition rate reached over 50% when it was injected to mice abdominal in S180.

Z-C-Q LBP

Antitumor components:. Lycium burbarum Polysaccharides LBP

Structure: The main components are arabinose, glucose, galactose, mannose, xylose, rhamnose and other components.

Exist parts: to have come from the fruit.

Anti-tumor effect: Wangbekung etc proved: LBP enhanced immune function on normal mouse cells. At 10mg / kg it can improve the immune function and have inhibitory effect on S18O tumor-bearing mice, and synergistic anti-tumor effect with chemotherapy cyclophosphamide. There are also reports: LBP has a certain influence on the immune function. Lu Changxing and other reports: LBP showed significant radiosensitization with radiotherapy.

In addition, its roots and skins have Betaine, which also have anti-cancer function: with D-isoascorbic together it can inhibit mitosis in vitro on sarcoma 37, Ehrlich cancer and lymphoid leukemia L1210 which is stronger than alone medication. LB P contained β- sitosterol, ascorbic acid, etc. which has anti-tumor effect.

There are also reports: LBP and interleukin-2 have the regulation effect on two anti-tumor LAK activity.

Z-C-R
Panax pseudo-Wall, var.notoginseng Hooet Tseng
Anti-tumor components: Notoginsenoside R1
Effective parts: that the roots of plants.

Antitumor effects: 180 µg/ml 5 days Panax saponin R can induce 68% HL-60 cell differentiation which proved Panax saponin R1 is a strong inducer of HL-6 0 cell lines and can induce HL-60 neutrophil cell differentiation. H-TdR incorporation assay results show: notoginsenoside R1 can induce differentiation of HL-60 cells while it affects DNA and RNA synthesis. There are also reports: during Cr release assay with soap studied Panax test it induced mouse spleen activity against tumor; have a strong anti-tumor effect with ConA / PHA together. Further experiments showed that soap Panax has no stimulation on proliferation of splenocytes, but changes the level of intracellular CAMP in spleen cells.

Z-C-Z1
Corioius versicolor Quel.
Anti-tumor components: Polysocohaitibe-piptide

Structure: α, β (1-4) dextran as main chain of Polysaccharide with 15% protein and 18 kinds of amino acids

The presence of site: mycelium body

Antitumor effects: target cells: human gastric cancer cell lines (SGC79O1); human lung adenocarcinoma fine lines (SPC); human monocytic leukemia cell line (SLY); human skin cell lymphoma cell lines (MEI)

In vitro inhibitory test of PSK Application the results showed that: PSK has moderate inhibition of proliferation at a concentration dose 1000ug / ml on human lung adenocarcinoma cell line (SPC) . The Japanese scholars shared PSK (Kiestin) has effects on sarcoma 180, liver AH-13, AH-7974, AH-66F, leukemia P388 in vivo by intravenous, intraperitoneal, subcutaneous, or oral administration and has almost no toxicity. Its mechanism is to improve the immune function through "host agency" role.

Li Jian and other scholars in the report: versicolor extract has no inhibition on ascites hepatoma on subcutaneously transplanted mouse while it has significant effects on the subcutaneous mouse ascites sarcoma S180.

In clinical the extracellular polysaccharide PSK is used on primary liver cancer and alone can improve the clinical symptoms and prolong life, anticancer drugs; in combination with antitumor drugs it also reduces the toxic side effects of antitumor drugs. Japanese wood has developed into proteoglycan "PSK" anti-cancer drugs.

Lentinus edodes Sing
Anti-component A: Lentinan

Structure: The structure of β-D- (1 3) glucan backbone, C-6 has two fulcrum of every five D- glucosyl, connecting β-D- (1 6) and β-D- (13) glucose branched-chain, also containing small amounts β-D- (16) branches.

Existing parts: its fruiting bodies.

Anti-tumor effects: Lentinan has some anti-tumor effect and improve the body's immune function. At a dose of 0.2, 1, 5, 25mg /kg, the daily cavity injection for consecutive 10 days, the inhibition rates were 78, 95.1, 97.5 and 73% on S180. It can increase their compatibility anti-tumor effect with chemotherapy drugs .

Lentinan can induce DNA synthesis and immune globulin and interferon-inducible, and non-specific cell-mediated cytotoxic effect in human peripheral mononuclear cells (PMNC, mainly lymphocytes); can enhance the cytotoxic response of NK cells of. NK cell activity is very low and even absent in Leukemia patients; the general immune enhancer treatment increases the risk of cancer of the white blood cells. Lentinan can increase the activity of NK cells. It induced r-IFN which has stronger anti-cancer effect than α and β -IFN, can enhance the phagocytic activity of white blood cells in patients with hormone production. At the same time, it can prevent patients with cancer from bacteria and viruses infection.

Shiio T et al reported: LNT and chemotherapeutic agents together can inhibit tumor metastasis in mice which the effect is the best when it is administrated after the surgery. Fachet T et al found Lentinan and their preparations A/ph(A/ph B10) F1 hybrid mice A/ph, MC, S1 fibrosarcoma have significant anti-tumor alivity; however, Lentinan does not directly affect tumor growth in vitro. Shiio T et al also studied the inhibitory effect of Lentinan on cancer lung metastasis; intravenous Lentinan can inhibit Lewis system cancer (3LL), melanoma (B6) and fiber sarcoma (ML-CS-1) transfer.

11. Survey of Study on XZ-C Medicine for Immunologic Regulation and Control

In 1985, the writer made system follow-up statistics to more than 3,000 patients who had accepted cancer operations of chest and abdomen performed by the writer himself. The results show that 2~3 years after the operation, most patients suffer from relapses or metastases. To reduce the relapse rate and increase the curative rate, the clinical fundamental research is a must. If there is no breakthrough of fundamental research, the clinical effect is hard to improve.

Current anti-cancer drugs are cell toxicants that kill both cancer cells and normal cells. The untoward reaction is intense. Now a kind of anti-cancer drug is extracted from traditional Chinese medicine, such as vinblastine, which is extracted from vinca rosea as alkaloid, has been used as anti-cancer drugs for clinical practice. But it will also kill normal cells. So the untoward reaction is intense too. While we hope that anti-cancer drugs have fewer untoward reactions, may be taken by mouth and can build up patient's strength and resistance. Then scientific research is being designed. The plan is to adopt animal experiments of tumor-inhibition in tumor-bearing mice, and from natural drugs to find new anti-cancer drugs, anti-metastasis and anti-relapse drugs, traditional Chinese medicine that only inhibit cancer cells but not normal cells, and new drugs that can adjust the regulation and control relation between host and tumor.

According to cell proliferation cycle theory, anti-cancer drugs must maintain long-term application and make cancer nidi chronically and continuously immerse in drugs. Only in this way can the cell division be inhibited and relapse and metastasis be prevented. Drugs have to be used for a long term, which is the only way to control existing cancer nidi and prevent the

formation of nascent cancer cells. But current used anti-cancer drugs induce intense untoward reaction, and therefore they cannot be used chronically and continuously but only be applied as per the treatment course for a minor cycle. All the current anti-cancer drugs have a series of untoward reactions, such as suppressions of immunologic function, bone marrow hematopoietic function and thymus gland, etc. the formation and development of cancer is due to the loss of immune monitoring caused by the reduction of patient's immunity. Therefore, all the anti-cancer drugs must improve immunity and protect immune organs, but should not suppress immunity.

To this end, our laboratory has carried on the following experimental studies for screening of new anti-cancer and anti-metastasis drugs from traditional Chinese medicine.

1. Adopt the method of cancer cells cultured in vitro to carry on the screening experimental study of tumor inhibition rate of traditional Chinese medicine

Screening test in vitro: adopt the method of tumor cells cultured in vitro; observe drugs' direct damage to tumor cells.

1. Method

(1) Preparation of crude drugs' agentia: dry crude drugs; add sixty times of water; heat and extract filtering liquid; decompress filtering liquid; distill it to dryness; form coarse dust; then it can be applied.

(2) Screening test in culture dish: 1×10^5/ml cells of Ehrlich ascites tumor (FAC), or fleshy tumor 180 (S-180), or ascites liver cancer (H_{22}), or carcinoma of uterine cervix, fetal calf serum 10%, coarse crude drugs 500μg/ml, based on the above proportion to inject 20ml solution in culture dish of 10cm×15cm. Place it at 37 centi- degree for a given time. Then compare the quantity of surviving cells with those of control group. Measure suppression ratio of cell proliferation caused by cytotoxicity.

(3) Drug screening: put crude drugs respectively into test tubes that used for culturing human cancer cells. Observe them whether crude drugs have inhibiting action on cancer cells. For 200 kinds of anti-cancer traditional Chinese medicines identified by traditional Chinese doctors, the writer carries on the in vitro screening test in sequence. Also under the same condition, use those medicines to carry on fibrocytes culture of normal person. Measure this medicine's cytotoxicity to fibrocytes, and then compare it with that of control group.

2. Experimental Result after animal screening tests by the writer in laboratory, 48 kinds of crude drugs (totally 200) certainly have and even hold sovereign inhibiting action on cancer cells proliferation. Tumor inhibition rate is above 90%. But some

commonly used traditional Chinese medicines, which are generally considered to have anti-cancer effects, are verified by experiments to have no or little anti-cancer effects. The suppression ratio of another 50 kinds of traditional Chinese medicines is below 30%, such as Chinese clematis, selfheal, earth worm, akebia stem, cortex lycii, rosa multiflora and so on.

2. Make animal model, carry on the experimental study of tumor inhibition rate of traditional Chinese medicine in cancer-bearing animals

1. Screening test of tumor-inhibition in vivo tumor-bearing animal model: each batch of experiment needs 240 Kunming mice, divided into 8 groups. Each group has 30 mice. For the first, second, third, fourth, fifth and sixth experimental group, each group chooses one kind of traditional Chinese medicine. The seventh group is set as the blank control group. The eighth group selects fluorouracil or cyclophosphamide as control group. All the mice are inoculated with 1×10^7/ml EAC or S-180 or H_{22} cancer cells through right front axillary subcutaneous injection. After three days, green gram-sized subcutaneous tumor nidi grow. 24 hours after inoculation, each mouse is fed orally with coarse dust of crude drugs, as per the weight 1000mg/kg. The feeding time is once a day for eight weeks. Mice's weights and sizes of tumor nidi need to be measured daily. After eight weeks, 20 mice of each group are executed. Measure their weights of body, tumor, liver, spleen, lung, thymus gland and other organs. Make pathological section to observe tissue condition and know metastatic condition. Another 10 tumor-bearing experimental mice are chronically fed with the screening traditional Chinese medicine. Observe the surviving time and untoward reaction. Calculate prolonged survival rate and tumor inhibition rate. Each batch (i.e. screen each kinds of traditional Chinese medicine) of experimental cycle is three months. Each batch of experiments can simultaneously screen and study six kinds of traditional Chinese medicines or prescriptions. One group of experiments can simultaneously get screening results of six kinds of traditional Chinese medicines.

This research institute can test three experimental groups over the corresponding period. Three master or doctor postgraduates manage one experimental group. In this way can tumor inhibition experiments with eighteen single traditional Chinese medicines or prescriptions be simultaneously studied. In this year, 72 kinds of single traditional Chinese medicines screening experiments which are used for in vivo tumor-inhibition of tumor-bearing mice can be carried on and completed. Thus the writer has continuously carried on four-year experimental studies and another three-year study on pathogenesis and metastatic compound mechanism of tumor-bearing mice and exploration of reasons that why cancerous protuberance can cause the death of host. 1000 tumor-bearing animal models are used every year. A total of about 6,000 tumor-bearing animal models have been done during four years. Each experimental mouse is performed with pathological anatomy on liver, spleen, lung, thymus gland and kidney after death. More than twenty thousand pathological sections have been accomplished to explore and seek cancerogenic micro-pathogens. Use microscopes to observe tumor micrangium establishing and microcirculation condition of 100 tumor-bearing mice. Through experimental studies, the writer firstly finds in China that traditional Chinese medicine TG has obvious effects on suppressing the formation of tumor micrangium. Now this medicine has been used for clinical anti-metastasis treatments on over 200 patients. Curative effects are being observed.

2. Discussion

(1) Through experimental studies, put forward new thought, new knowledge, new concept and new strategy for resisting against cancer: over a period of seven years; over 6,000 tumor-bearing animal models; in vivo tumor-inhibition experiments for anti-cancer, anti-metastasis and anti-relapse in sequence with 200 kinds of natural traditional Chinese medicines; have cognizance of train of thought, knowledge and experience to renew concept, thought, traditional principle and method for traditional anti-cancer work.

Use tumor-bearing animal models to carry on scientific, objective and strict experimental screening, analysis and evaluation on 200 kinds of traditional Chinese medicines in sequence with so called anti-cancer curative effects by Chinese Medicine Literature. Results show that only 48 kinds of medicines have better anti-cancer effects. Although another 152 kinds of medicines are the commonly used anti-cancer medicines by veteran practioner of TCM, they have been verified by this group of experimental screenings to have no anti-cancer effects or little tumor inhibition rate. These 200 kinds of traditional Chinese medicines used for experimental screening are chosen from over ten books with TCM anti-cancer famous prescriptions. They are also common medicines with anti-cancer effects described in Journal of Traditional Chinese Medicine and literature reports. While the experimental study results prove that 152 kinds of medicines have no tumor inhibition rate or low anti-cancer effects. The reason might be that Chinese Medicine Literature has no distinction between lump, abdominal mass of Chinese medicine and cancer of modern medicine. 48 kinds of medicines in this group, which are screened through animal experiments, really have better tumor inhibition rate. Through optimization grouping and repeated trials, different medicines are composed to XZ-C$_{1\sim10}$ immunoregulation anti-cancer Chinese materia medica preparation. It has been verified clinically for sixteen years. Over 12,000 cancer patients have used this preparation and obtained better curative effects.

Through experimental screening study results of this group, we have realized that TCM prescriptions are gained from prolonged experience. The prescription matches symptoms of disease and is the synthesis composed with various kinds of crude drugs. As seen from Chinese Medicine Literature, symptoms of abdominal mass and accumulation seem similar to those of cancer. Traditional Chinese medicines are used to treat abdominal mass. Sometimes symptoms can be improved, but not all abdominal mass are cancers. In general, TCM has no effect on cancer. So we should adopt modern scientific methods to verify, observe and reevaluate cancer resistance and carcinogenicity of various crude drugs in prescriptions of traditional Chinese medicine, and avoid unscientific parts of traditional Chinese medicine and pharmacology.

In medicine screening experiments, it's found that single crude drugs have worse tumor-inhibition effects than optimization grouping compound of many kinds of crude drugs. The reason may be that single crude drugs can only suppress tumor proliferation. While optimization grouping compound of many kinds of crude drugs not only can suppress tumor proliferation of tumor-bearing mice, but also can build up strength, improve immunity, promote to produce cancer-inhibition cytokines and protect normal cells.

Since 1992, over seven-year scientific experiments, different medicines are screened and composed to XZ-C$_{1\sim10}$ immunoregulation anti-cancer Chinese materia medica preparation. This medicine owns curative effects on anti-cancer, supporting healthy energy to eliminate evils, clearing away heat and toxic materials and activating blood circulation to dissipate blood stasis.

From experimental study to clinical verification, and then from clinic to experiment again, the writer has organized to set up the joint breakthrough research coordination group for cancer prevention and resistance. This coordination group has experimental study base and verification base of clinical application. The former is in medical college and medical university laboratory; the latter is in clinical medical department of nationwide coordination group for cancer prevention and resistance studies combined with traditional Chinese and western medicine. From experimental study to clinical verification means the clinical application on the basis of successful experimental study. Then new problems are found during the clinical application, which need fundamental experimental studies. Afterwards new experimental results are applied to clinical verification. Experiments → clinic → experiments once more → clinic once more, recurrent ascent continuously; through eight-year clinical practical experiences, knowledge also continues to improve. Summation, analysis, reflection and evaluation ascend to theory, putting forward new knowledge, new concept, new thought, new strategy and new therapeutic route and scheme.

Breakthrough research experience of coordination group includes: ① Choose the way that professors, experts and postgraduates of universities and colleges coordinate to carry on scientific researches and joint breakthrough; advocate large-scale coordination of scientific researches; give prominence to concentrate scientific research and technology strength of all parties; enrich anti-cancer strength. ② Cancer prevention and resistance should make use of nation-wide advantages; give full play to the advantage of traditional Chinese medicine; conform to actual conditions in China. ③ Fundamental studies are important, but application and development research are more important. It should be observed that fundamental research → applied research →development research. Emphases are application and curative effects. Focus on increasing life quality of cancer patients, improving symptoms and prolonging survival time. ④ Restore the conservation of outpatient records (since 1976, Hubei province cancels conservation system of outpatient records and sends them to patients.); fill in full and detailed outpatient records. Therefore, full information of clinical verification is obtained to be convenient for analysis, statistics and follow-up survey (Generally, 80%~90% patients accept outpatient service, 10%~20% patients receive hospital treatment. At present hospital records are reserved to analyze and study clinical data. That 80%~90% patients accept outpatient service leads to the inexistence of outpatient records. Analysis, statistics and follow-up survey of patients' curative effects in out-patient department, and follow-up statistics of scientific researches may become impossible. Hospital records can only observe short-term curative effects; while the conservation of outpatient records can observe long-term curative effects.) Restoring and reserving outpatient records data is favorable toward outpatient clinical research to improve medical quality.

(2) Experimental work of finding new anti-cancer drugs, anti-metastasis and anti-relapse drugs from natural drugs: it's aimed at screening new anti-cancer drugs with non-tolerance, no untoward effect and high selectivity that can chronically be taken by mouth. As known to all, although current anti-cancer drugs can suppress cancer cells proliferation, due to their severe untoward effect, while using many patients have to stop administration. Afterwards cancer cells proliferate again and begin to have drug tolerance. Such as the famous anti-cancer drug formyli sarcolysine quinine, as seen from ongoing cancer cells tissue cultures, drug tolerance is up to 20,000 times. Before the appearance of drug tolerance, the dosage is usually only several milligrams.

While when drug tolerance is produced, such dosage cannot meet the demand. Then it is necessary to increase the dosage. But when its dosage increases to ten times, it will cause the death of patient. Therefore, drug tolerance of cancer cells on anti-cancer drug and untoward effect of anti-cancer drug on host are long-standing problems that puzzle tumor treatment researchers. Our purpose of finding new drugs is to avoid those disadvantages and screen anti-cancer drugs with non-tolerance, no untoward effect and high selectivity that best can chronically be taken by mouth. Western anti-cancer drugs have single ingredient. Micro dosage is effective, but it will suppress normal cells. Its toxic reaction is quite strong. Some current anti-cancer drugs are extracted from traditional Chinese medicine, such as vincristine, camptothecin and colchicine; these alkaloids are similar to traditional anti-cancer drugs, i.e. micro drug is effective, but toxicity is very high.

The question is whether anti-cancer traditional Chinese medicine, which can suppress the growth of cancer cells but not kill normal cells, can be extracted from TCM. Through several years' experimental screening, the writer finally finds such kind of TCM with rather ideal anti-cancer effects. Usually when the dosage reaches $500\mu g$/ml, it has inhibiting action on cancer cells. The writer also finds $XZ-C_1$ and$XZ-C_4$ drugs that can 100% suppress cancer cells and never kill normal cells. $XZ-C_1, XZ-C_4$ and $XZ-C_8$ also can improve the immunologic function of host, which is a superior feature of anti-cancer TCM.

As seen XZ-C series of TCM, its anti-cancer effect changes as the change of dosage. When the dosage is $250\mu g/ml$, it can only suppress 60% cancer cells; when the dosage is $125\mu g/ml$, suppression ratio is zero. Micro A-type drugs will be effective, such as vinblastine, berberine in Chinese goldthread, and myrobalan fruit in alkaloid, etc. But they can also suppress normal cell proliferation, which is same to traditional anti-cancer drugs. B-type drugs are other anti-cancer TCM. Only high concentration is effective. That is, micro dosage has no inhibiting action on cancer cells. Effect is directly proportional to dosage. If the dosage is larger, curative effects will be better, such as $XZ-C_{1A}$ and $XZ-C_{1B}$.

3. Verification of clinical effects

Over the past ten years, the writer has applied experimental crude drugs to clinical medicine. XZ-C series drugs have distinctive clinical effects. That is, a certain period after the administration of B-type drugs, cancer cells neither proliferate nor shrink, while the patient begins to restore vigorous energy. Several months later, the physical strength recovers gradually. The tumor starts to shrink slowly. That is probably not toxic effect on cancer cells, but the result of creating a circumstance that is adverse to cancer cells proliferation in organisms. The long-term administration has no toxic cumulative effect on normal cells. Many patients have taken XZ-C$_1$ and XZ-C$_4$ drugs for 3~5 years, there is still no relapse, metastasis and untoward effect. The long-term plentiful administration can obtain unexpected good results.

Different types of XZ-C preparation match with various kinds of cancers, such as cancer of alimentary canal, lung cancer and cancer of uterus, etc. Compound prescriptions must be made from symptoms. Only in this way can good results be obtained.

Different from traditional medicinal broth, what the writer chooses is the mixture with every kind of single crude drug through 100 mesh screening. These crude drugs are composed as compound prescription, which is not the decoction of combined preparation, but is the mixed preparation. This kind of mixture can preserve pharmacological characteristics of each crude drug. Prolonged use of this drug will not produce the untoward effect. Probing into the application way of crude drugs is quite significant.

In actual clinical medicine, will the prolonged use cause any problems? Patients can be divided into two kinds of cases: one type of patients take considerable amount of drugs with no abnormalities. The curative effects appear slowly. Many patients have taken XZ-C$_4$ drugs for 3~5 years. They have high spirits and good appetites. Physical strength recovers better; body condition strengthens; state of an illness is stable; patient's condition is good. The daily clinical dosage is about 20g of coarse drugs, in which the basic remedy is anti-cancer drugs, accounting for about 10% (equal to 40g crude drugs). It is considerably different from the dosage of traditional Chinese medicine.

When will curative effects present after taking medicine? Usually 1~3 months reach peak. Therefore if patients can survive for more than six months, then about 90% patients' symptoms can be improved remarkably; 50% patients' cancer proliferation will stop; about 80% patients' survival time is lengthened.

The completely significant thing is that XZ-C$_{1~4}$ crude drugs preparations have favorable abirritation. Medium and advanced stages of liver cancer and cancer of pancreas both produce severe pain. Patients who have used this kind of crude drugs preparation for over one month hardly feel any pain. They even don't have to be injected with analgesic drugs. This is extremely amazing.

Extracts of single crude drugs and compounded crude drugs almost produce the same curative effect. But when decocted with traditional compound prescription, extracts of single crude drugs are less effective. Presumably this is caused by the existence of interaction among drugs. In terms of cancer treatment, the better choice is compounded medicinal preparations.

Please note that some crude drugs can also promote the reproduction of cancer cells but suppress normal cells' growth, especially mineral drugs and animal drugs. Such as pallas pit viper, hairy antler and others, even the microdosis can promote above reactions. The centipede can damage renal tubules.

Akihiko Sato says that cancer resistance of natural drugs can be divided into three categories. The first category is that ingredients of natural drugs have the effect on killing cancer cells, such as vinblastine. The second one is that polysaccharides of some drugs (e.g. purple ganoderma lucidum and evodia rutaecarpa), due to the action on enhancing immunologic function, is very popular as immunotherapy. While there is a limit that polysaccharides almost have no effect on progressive stage and advanced stage of cancer. But because of fewer untoward effects, they can be used as favorable adjuvanticity drugs. The third one is B-type anti-cancer drugs, whose active mechanism is not yet clear. When B-type drug is in high concentration, it can suppress the proliferation of cancer cells but not normal cells. Also it has fewer untoward effects and can be taken for a lone time. But it can neither kill cancer cells nor promote immunologic function. The B-type anti-cancer drug is considered as a kind of new drug.

In nearly a decade, with the intensive study, the writer has contacted with a large number of patients monthly, and collected much information that is not recorded in books and literature. And the writer has an intimate knowledge of many patients' epidemiology, clinical symptom, evolution of physical sign and analysis, evaluation and reflection on progress. Therefore the writer can carry out the following theoretic discussions.

II. Theoretic Discussion

1. Research on anti-cancer netustasis of traditional Chinese medicine from the level of modern molecular biology

In recent years, on the level of molecular immune pharmacology, domestic scholars have been carrying out a great deal of research on looking for traditional Chinese medicine and new drugs for anti-cancer, anti-metastasis and anti-relapse.

1. From the perspective of increasing immunologic function to study traditional Chinese medicine with anti-metastasis Tumor metastasis is a complex process, which is affected by many factors, such as wet ability and adhesiveness of cancer cells, hypercoagulable state of blood and low immunologic function, etc. Hypercoagulable state of blood plasma and low immunologic function play the major role in carcinomatous metastasis. While in microcirculatory system, detention of cancer cells is the key link in the formation of metastasis. Therefore, research is a must to exploit the traditional Chinese medicine, which can improve hypercoagulable state, low immunity and microcirculatory disturbance on the molecular level. While XZ-C anti-cancer mixture can obviously suppress experimental lung metastasis in mice with Lewis lung cancer. The mechanism may be to enhance organism immunity, improve microcirculation and adjust immunologic function. Blood-activating and stasis-dissolving drugs, such as Elemene and others, can enhance immunologic function, reduce blood viscosity, eliminate microcirculatory disturbance and then decrease the formation and metastasis of cancer embolus.

2. From the perspective of resisting platelet aggregation to study traditional Chinese medicine with anti-metastasis Studies in recent years show that tumor metastasis is closely related to blood platelet. That cancer cells in blood circulation causing platelet aggregation of host is a critical step in the formation of metastasis. After cancer cells into blood circulation, they will activate platelet to produce cancer embolus. Some blood-activating and stasis-dissolving drugs have effects on resisting platelet aggregation, suppressing cancer cells and withstanding metastasis. Chen Jianmin has observed 440 cancer patients, in which 82.7% patients have high viscosity states in various degrees and are treated with stasis-dissolving prescription-xiong long decoction. Its curative effect is better. The effective rate is 65.2%. Some scholars combine red peony root and red sage root with small dose of chemotherapeutic drugs to obviously decrease metastases of cancer cells to lung. Cui Wei and other scholars use experimental studies to prove that leatherleaf milletia can obviously suppress platelet aggregation. Depolymerization rate is high. Observation under electron microscope shows that leatherleaf milletia can promote the increase of dispersive platelets. Clinically leatherleaf milletia is used to resist hematogenous metastasis of cancer embolus.

3. From the perspective of anti-adhesion therapy to study traditional Chinese medicine with anti-metastasis During the process of carcinomatous metastasis, cancer cells will adhere to various cells of host (e.g. endothelial cell, platelet and lymphocyte, etc.) and (or) extracellular matrix and basement membrane components. The above is also one of key factors for the occurrence of metastasis. Therefore, anti-adhesion therapy may be a new target for anti-metastasis. In recent years, studies discover that red sage root can suppress the adhesion of red blood cells in vitro with endothelial cells and platelet aggregation. It can also change tumor cell membrane to affect the affinity between tumor cells and host tissues. It has damaging effect on cancer cells. Results of animal experiments show that red sage root can decrease cancer cells into circulatory system, lessen the adhesion of cancer cells and vascular endothelial cells, reduce the capability of forming cancer embolus and lower the chance for cancer cells escaping from circulatory system.

Pilose asiabell root and large headed atractylodes can obviously suppress metastases of cancer cells in tumor-bearing mice. Qiu Jiaxin and other scholars discover that large headed atractylodes can suppress Lweis tumor metastases to lung. This writer adopts BALB/C nude mice as models. 30d after inoculating with SGC-7901 human gastric cancer cells beneath the splenic envelope, nude mice are executed. Metastatic rate of control group is 83.33%. That of traditional Chinese medicine group is 16.67%. In clinical trials, the writer randomly classifies patients who have accepted radical operation for gastric carcinoma into two groups, involving group of taking traditional Chinese medicine that mainly invigorats the spleen and regulats the flow of qi and chemotherapy group. After one year, 35.87% patients of control group (chemotherapy) suffer from metastases of cancer cells. While metastatic rate of traditional Chinese medicine group is only 3.33%. Two years later, metastatic rate of traditional Chinese medicine group rises to 4.76% while metastatic rate of control group rises to 36.84%.

4. From the angle of regulating signalling pathway of cancer cells to study traditional Chinese medicine with anti-cancer and anti-metastasis Since 1980s, the study of signal system has always been the leading edge of cell biology. That is, various drug molecules in organism cannot directly enter into cells to take effect. They must combine with correlative receptors of cells. Then through signal transference, the correlative second signal system generates in cells. Finally information is transmitted to target location to take effect. In recent years, that through regulating and controlling cellular signal system to design and develop new anti-cancer and anti-metastasis drugs has caught redoubled attention from scientists.

Cuttlebones (white dragon tablets) have obvious effects on gastric cancer, lung cancer and bladder cancer, and also can obviously suppress the growth of animal solid tumor (liver cancer, lung cancer and cervical cancer). When cuttlebones are used in combination with chemotherapies, they also have effects on synergic action, toxin reduction and increase of immunologic function, etc. Liu Jun and other scholars have observed cuttlebones' regulating and controlling function to two sets of signal systems CAMP-PKA and DAG-PKC in human gastric cancer cells MGC80-3, cuttlebones' effect on suppressor gene of gastric cancer cells BGC80-3 in G_1 phase and their correlation with PKA signalling pathway. Scholars have found that cuttlebones have obvious inhibiting actions on proliferation of human gastric cancer cells. As seen from the signal system, 3h after cuttlebones' acting on MGC80-3 cells, they can increase cAMP level and PKA activity in cells, while decrease DAG content and PKC activity in cells. This indicates that cuttlebones' effects on MGC80-3 cells are realized by antagonistic regulation of two sets of signal systems.

2. Discussion on mechanism of action that effective elements of traditional Chinese medicine inhibit and kill cancer cells

1. Traditional Chinese medicine that can inhibit and (or) kill cancer cells Experimental studies prove that effective elements of some traditional Chinese medicines can inhibit or kill cancer cells. Such as curcumin has the cytotoxicity with concentration dependent to human gastric adenocarcinoma cells SGC-7901. It can obviously suppress the proliferation of SGC-7901 cells, and also have certain damaging effect. The electron microscope observation shows dissolution and necroses of cells.

There are effective elements of other traditional Chinese medicines that can also suppress cancer cells, such as trichosanthin, elemene, glycyrrhizin, β-carotene and general ginsenoside, etc.

Alcohol extractable matters of vietnamese sophora root have inhibiting effects on the proliferation of human liver cancer cells SMMC-7721 and mitochondrial metabolism.

Elemene can obviously suppress the growth of leucemia HL-60 and K562 cells, prevent cancer cells to grow from S phase to G2/M phase and finally induce apoptosis.

2. Traditional Chinese medicine that can affect cells in proliferative stage of cell cycle Most anti-cancer traditional Chinese medicines are cell cycle specific drugs, which mainly kill cells in the proliferative stage. Especially cells in S and M phases are most sensitive to traditional Chinese medicines. Tanshinone experiments in vitro show that it has obvious inhibiting effect on DNA syntheses of cancer cells. Tanshinone acts on S phase of cell division cycle, suppresses DNA syntheses and has cytotoxic effect. Another example is American ginseng polysaccharides. They can effectively block DNA syntheses of cancer cells in S phase. Laiyang ginseng and fiveleaf gynostemma herb mainly act on G2/M phase of SPC-A-1 cells and block cancer cells to proceed with mitoses. It can clearly be seen that those drugs affect proliferation and differentiation of cancer cells by changing cancer cell DNA and protein metabolism.

3. Traditional Chinese medicine that can induce apoptosis of cancer cells Along with the development of gene studies, it has been proved that the rapid growth, diffusion and metastasis of cancer cells are caused by too few dead cells and excessive cell proliferations. Disorder at this rate is due to the decline or loss of apoptosis ability. It is fully necessary to strengthen the research on apoptosis of cancer cells induced by drugs. Effective elements of some traditional Chinese medicines can induce apoptosis of cancer cells, such as trichosanthin has obvious inhibiting effect on melanoma cells of mice. It can cause the increase of tumor cells in G0/G1 phase and the decrease of cells in S phase, which show the obvious Blocking phenomenon for G0/G1 phase. That is, trichosanthin prevents the proliferation of cancer cells and induces apoptosis of cancer cells. Another example is the taxol. It is a kind of anti-cancer drug that is abstracted from the bark of natural drug—yew. Its cytotoxicity on cancer cells is relevant to its induction of apoptosis. Pharmacody and clinical experiments of elemene prove that it has exact curative effect on cancer. The flow cytometry proves that elemene can prevent cancer cells to grow from S phase to G2/M phase and finally induce apoptosis.

4. Traditional Chinese medicine that can affect genes of cancer cells and inhibit cancer gene expression p53 gene is the cancer suppressor gene and can inhibit cell proliferation. Wei Xiaolong and other scholars have studied the effect of rehmannia root polysaccharide (LRPS) with low molecular weight on p53 gene expression. They have found that when optimal anti-cancer doses of LRPS are 20mg/kg and 40mg/kg, expression levels of p53 gene in Lewis lung cancer cells are respectively 1.52 and 1.48. While that of control group is 0.46, which explains that LRP can promote the obvious increase of p53 gene expressions in Lewis lung cancer cells. The conclusion is that the effect of LRPS on p53 anti-cancer gene expressions belongs to one of its anti-cancer mechanisms. Also icariin can decrease expression levels of bcl-2 and c-myc genes. Arsenic oxide in arsenic trioxide and arsenic disulfide can obviously lower bcl-2 gene and lead to the reduction of bcl-2/bax ratio.

5. Traditional Chinese medicine that can induce the differentiation of cancer cells Inducing differentiation therapy of tumor cells is a tumor research hotspot in the world. Its feature is not to kill tumor cells but induce cancer cells to differentiate into normal cells or cells that are similar to normal cells. In the past decade and more, domestic scholars have started the research on the differentiation of tumor cells induced by traditional Chinese medicine. Until now, they have found dozens of traditional Chinese medicine extracts show the effect on inducing the differentiation of tumor cells in experiments. Yi Yonglin and other scholars adopt general ginsenoside (GSL) to act on 58 cases of acute non-lymphocytic leukemia. The result shows that GSL has inducing differentiation effects with different degrees on various cells of this disease.

Another example is notoginseng saponin R1. It has the strong induction to make HL-60 cells (human promyelocytic leukemia cell strain) differentiate toward granulocyte series. The effective element—poriatin (F101) extracted from poria cocos has effects on inhibiting the proliferation of tumor cells and activating macrophage in mouse' abdominal cavity. Many experiments have found that there is a certain link between effective induction of leukemia cell differentiation and proliferation inhibition. Han Rui and other scholars have found that traditional Chinese medicines belonged to the sort of cassia have cassic acid and ramification. Cells of cloning high-metastasis giant cell carcinoma of lung (PGCL3) are treated with cassic acid. Experimental results show that the form, proliferation rate, divisional index, agglomeration reaction and others of tumor cells totally convert to normal cells. At the same time, invasion and metastasis abilities of tumor cells are obviously weakened. Xu Jianguo and other scholars have found that water extracts of 22 kinds of traditional Chinese medicines have inducing differentiation effects with different degrees on HL-60 cells. For the emulsifying agent of effective elements of β-elemenum emulsion radix curcumae, Qian Jun and other scholars inject 30μg/ml emulsifying agent into human lung cancer cells in vitro culture. Then they discover that the growth of lung cancer cells is inhibited. The flow cytometry analysis shows that 72h after injection, the proportion of lung cancer cells in G0/G1 phase increases. While proportion of lung cancer cells in S phase decreases. Observations under light microscope and electron microscope show that after the injection, the proliferation of cancer cells slows down, cells shrink and turn around, the number of microvilli decreases, nucleo-cytoplasmic ratio reduces and the number of heterochromatin increases. The above prompts that this medicine can reverse into lung cancer cell phenotype on the level of cytobiology and morphology. And finally these cells are induced to tend to differentiation.

Traditional Chinese medicines and their effective elements discovered in the above studies provide instructive train of thoughts and references for searching and preparing tumor differentiation inducer and studying the differentiation inducing mechanism in the future. And they also provide new idea, method and therapeutic evaluation standard for cancer treatment with traditional Chinese medicines. In the past, regulating dysfunction of organism with traditional Chinese medicines only means to regulate dysfunction of viscera. While inducing differentiation therapy with traditional Chinese medicines is on levels of cell, molecular organism and gene to regulate dysfunction of proliferation and apoptosis and dysfunction of proliferation and differentiation control. Cancer cell is the immature cell with incomplete differentiation. Differentiation inducer of traditional Chinese medicines promotes its further complete differentiation. Cancer cells grow to mature cells and lose malignant features. As seen from the level of cells, it can be called a kind of "strengthening vital qi" therapy. The therapeutic standards are the appearance of differentiation index, disappearance of tumor malignant features and survival time prolongation of tumor-bearing organism. The standard is not only the change of lump size. The appearance of differentiation index and prolongation of survival time are the most vital factors.

Tumor inducing differentiation therapy is the continuing discovery that develops the differentiation inducer with higher effective and lower toxic features. In this respect, traditional Chinese medicines have a big advantage. That is because that traditional Chinese medicines are rich in natural resources, traditional Chinese medicine and pharmacology have a long history. In several thousand years, abundant invaluable experience has been accumulated to provide extremely favorable conditions for developing and preparing Chinese materia medica preparation with higher effective and lower toxic features.

In studies, besides referring the above chemical structure of traditional Chinese medicine, effective elements and other factors, there are some other ideas for consideration, such as interferon (IFN). Especially IFN-γ can induce the differentiation of cancer cells. While many traditional Chinese medicines can induce IFN-γ in vivo. In conclusion, tumor inducing differentiation therapy is receiving more and more attention from foreign and domestic scholars. The research and application of traditional Chinese medicines in this field have an extensive future.

12. Observation of Experimental and Clinic Curative Effect on Z-C Medicine Treating Malignancy

In order to look for the traditional herb medicine with actually curative effect and without toxication and adverse reaction, this surgical tumor research institute has screened 200 kinds of Chinese herbal medicines with so-called anticancer reaction recorded on Chinese herbal medicine books for tumor-inhibition reaction on the solid carcinoma in the tumor-bearing animal models one by one in the past 4 years. Through long-term in-vivo tumor-inhibiting animal experiments, we have screened 48 kinds of Chinese herbal medicines with relatively good tumor-inhibition rate that can prolong the survival time, protect the immune organ and obviously improve the immunologic function. According to the clinical conditions, the anticancer medicines screened are combined into 2 compounds including $Z-C_1$ and $Z-C_4$ with better anti-cancer reaction than each single medicine. In the original screening, we carried out the tumor-inhibiting animal experiment for each single medicine and now we further carry out the experimental study on these two groups of compounds for the tumor-inhibiting reaction in the solid tumor of the tumor-bearing rats.

1) Experimental Study on Animal

1. Materials and Method

   (1) Experimental animal: 260 Kunming clon white rats, half of male and female respectively, weight:21 ± 2g, 8~10 weeks.

   (2) Cell strains and inoculation: hepatic carcinoma H_{22} cell strains, the fresh tumor bodies from the rats with tumor were prepared into the single cell suspended liquid, after dyeing and counting of the cancer cells (1×10^6/ml), 0.2ml normal saline of cancer cell was subject to subcutaneous vaccination at the front axilla at the right side of each rat.

   (3) Drugs and experimental group: the traditional herb medicines $Z-C_1$ and $Z-C_4$ were entirely developed and prepared by Hubei Branch of China Anti-cancer Research Cooperation of Chinese Traditional Medicine and Western Medicine, the former was a compound and the latter was a medicinal powder.

The chemotherapy control medicine used by the chemotherapy group was cyclophosphane (CTX).

Experimental group: the animals with H_{22} cancer cell transplanted were divided into four groups randomly: ① traditional herb medicine $Z-C_1$ group (90 rats). The rats were subject to gastriclavage once every day after 24h of transplantation of cancer cells, 0.8ml per rat every time, equivalent to 1.4mg of the dried medicinal herbs. ②Traditional herb medicine $Z-C_4$ group (90 rats), as to the dose and gastriclavage method, ditto. ③Chemotherapy group (50 rats), from the next day after transplantation of cancer cells, they were subject to gastriclavage with CTX50mg/kg weight every other day. ④Control group (30 rats), they were subject to gastriclavage with normal saline every day from the next day after transplantation of the cancer cells, 0.8ml/rat.

(4) Observation of indexes: measure the weight of the rats every 3d, measure the diameter of the tumor with vernier caliper, measure the immunologic function and blood picture. Half of each group as Group A, subject to tumor-bearing experiment, regular killing of the rats in batches, separation of tumor and weighing of the tumor and then calculation of tumor-inhabiting rate. The tumor was subject to the pathological section and a few of the specimens were subject to the observation of ultra-structural organization. The rest half of each group as Group B. The tumor-bearing experimental rats were drenched for a long time until they met with natural death. Then the tumor was separated and weighed, the long-term inhibition rate and life elongation rate of the tumor was calculated.

2. Experimental result

(1) The tumor-inhibition effect of Z-C Medicine on Rats bearing hepatic carcinoma H_{22}: in the second week after administration of $Z-C_1$, the tumor-inhibition rate was 40% and the one in the fourth week was 45% and 58% in the sixth week. The tumor-inhibition rate after administration of $Z-C_4$ was 55%, 68% in the fourth week and 70% in the sixth week. ($P<0.01$) the tumor-inhibiting rate after administration of CTX was 45% in the second week, 45% in the fourth week and 49% in the sixth week.

(2) The effect of Z-C medicine on the survival time of the rats bearing hepatic carcinoma H_{22}: the average survival time of $Z-C_1$, $Z-C_4$ and CTX was longer than the one of the normal saline control group ($P<0.01$); Z-C medicine played a role in obviously prolonging the survival time. Through comparison with the control group, the life

elongation rate of Z-C_1 group was 85%, the one of Z-C_4 group was 200% and the one of CTX group was 9.8%. The rats in Z-C_1 and CTX in Group B met with death in 75d. 6 rats bearing carcinoma in Z-C_4 survived after seven months.

(3) Both Z-C_1 and Z-C_4 medicine improved the immunologic function and Z-C4 obviously improved the immunologic function, increased the white blood cells and red blood cells, without any effect on the hepatic function and kidney function and without damage to the hepatic and kidney section. CTX decreased the white blood cells and reduced the immunologic function with the renal damage to the kidney section. The thymus in the control group was obviously atrophic while the one of Z-C_1 and Z-C_2 therapy group was not atrophic but a little hypertrophic.

Pathological section of thymus in the control group: the cortex of the thymus was atrophic, the cells were discrete and the blood vessel met with sludge. The pathological section of the thymus in Z-C_4 therapy group displayed that the cortical area of the thymus built up, the lymphocyte was dense, the epithelium reticulocyte increased and the thymus corpuscles increased.

II. Observation on Clinic Application

1. Clinical information

(1) Hubei Branch of China Anti-cancer Research Cooperation of Chinese Traditional Medicine and Western Medicine, Anti Carcinoma Metastasis and Recurrence Research Office and Shuguang Tumor Specialized Outpatient Department had treated 4, 698 carcinoma patients in Stage III and IV or in metastasis and recurrence with Z-C medicine combined with western medicine from 1994 to Nov. 2002, among which there were 3, 051 men patients and 1,647 women patients. The youngest one was 11 years old and the oldest one was 86 years old, the high invasion age was 40~69 years. All groups of the patients were entirely subject to the diagnosis of pathological histology or definitive diagnosis with ultrasonic B, CT and MRI iconography. According to the staging standard of UICC, all the cases were entirely the patients in medium and advanced stage over Stage III. In this group, there were 1,021 hepatic carcinoma patients, among which there were 694 primary lesion hepatic carcinoma patients and 327 metastatic hepatic carcinoma patients; there were 752 patients suffering from carcinoma of lung, among which there were 699 patients suffering from the primary carcinoma of lung and 53 patients suffering from the metastatic carcinoma of lung; there were 668 gastric carcinoma patients, 624 patients suffering from esophagus cardia carcinoma, 328 patients suffering from rectum carcinoma of anal canal, 442 patients

suffering from carcinoma of colon, 368 patients suffering from breast carcinoma, 74 patients suffering from adenocarcinoma of pancreas, 30 patients suffering from carcinoma of bile duct, 43 patients suffering from retroperitoneal tumor, 38 patients suffering from oophoroma, 9 patients suffering from cervical carcinoma, 11 patients suffering from cerebroma, 34 patients suffering from thyroid carcinoma, 38 patients suffering from nasopharyngeal carcinoma, 9 patients suffering from melanoma, 27 patients suffering from kidney carcinoma, 48 patients suffering from carcinoma of urinary bladder, 13 patients suffering from leukemia, 47 patients suffering from metastasis of supraclavicular lymph nodes, 35 patients suffering various fleshy tumors and 39 patients suffering from other malignancies.

(2) Medicine and medication: the treatment aims to support healthy energy to eliminate evils, soften and resolve the hard mass and supplement qi and blood. $Z-C_1$ is the compound, 150ml to be taken on the daily basis, $Z-C_4$ is powder, 10g to be taken on the daily basis. According to the analysis and differentiation of the diseases, anti-cancer powder shall be taken orally and the anti-cancer apocatastasis paste shall be applied externally for the solid tumor or the metastatic tumor. In case of being in pain, anti-cancer aponic paste shall be applied externally. Icterus removal soup or dropsy removal soup shall be taken orally for the patients suffering from icterrus and the ascites.

(3) Therapeutic evaluation: it pays attention to the short-term curative effect and iconography indexes as well as the survival time of long-term curative effect, quality of life and immunologic indexes. Attention shall be paid to the changes in subjective signs in administration of drugs. It will be effective when the subjective signs are improved and last over one month; otherwise, it will be ineffective. As to the quality of life (Karnofsky Performance Status), it will be effective when it is improved and lasts over one month, otherwise, it will be ineffective. As to the evaluation standard of the curative effect of solid tumor, it can be divided into four levels according to the changes in size of tumor: Level I: disappearance of tumor; Level II: tumor reduces 1/2; Level III: softening of tumor; Level IV: no change or enlargement of level tumor.

2. Curative results

(1) The symptom was improved, the quality of life was improved, the survival time was prolonged: among the 4,277 carcinoma patients in medium and advanced stage who took Z-C medicine with the return visit over 3 months, the case history had the specific observation record of the curative effect. It improved the quality of life of the patients in an all-round way. (See Part I chapter)

III. Discuss about Z-C Medicine Experiment and Clinic Curative Effect

1. Tumor-inhibition effect of Z-C$_{1\sim4}$ Medicine on hepatic carcinoma H$_{22}$ rats bearing tumor

It was found that after the medicine was taken to H$_{22}$ tumor-bearing rats for two weeks, four weeks and six weeks, the tumor inhibition rate increased with the prolongation of the administration time, the tumor inhibition rate of Z-C$_4$ in the 6th week reached up to 70%. Through two repeated experiments in succession, the results were stable, which indicated that the tumor-inhibition effect of Chinese herb medicine was slow and it would increase gradually, that is to say, the tumor-inhibition effect was of positive correlation to the accumulated dosage of Chinese herb medicine.

The effect on the survival time of hepatic carcinoma H$_{22}$ tumor-bearing rats from Z-C$_1$ and Z-C$_4$ medicine: it was proven by the experimental results that Z-C$_1$ and Z-C$_4$ medicine could obviously prolong the survival time of the tumor-bearing rats, especially Z-C$_4$, it could prolong the survival time as long as 200%, more than that, Z-C$_4$ could remarkably improve the immunologic function of the organism, protect the immune organ and the bone marrow, alleviate the toxic action and side effect of the radiotherapy and chemotherapy medicines. Furthermore, no toxic action or side effect had been found in the past 12 months after the rats took the medicine. The above-mentioned experimental study offered the beneficial basis to the clinical application.

2. Clinical curative effect

Based on the experimental study, it had been applied to various clinical carcinomas, most of the patients were the ones over Stage III and IV, namely: the ones suffering from the cancer of late stage that could not be removed with exploratory operation; the ones with the exploratory operation without operation indication; the ones meeting with metastasis or reoccurrence in short term or long term after operation of the carcinoma; the ones suffering from hepatic metastasis, lung metastasis or brain metastasis in late stage or the ones accompanied with carcinoma hydrops and hydrops abdominis; the ones suffering from various carcinomas conservative removal operation with the exploratory operation only for the anastomosis of intestines and stomach or colostomy but not for removal and the ones not suitable for the operation, chemotherapy and radiotherapy and so on. Through over 10 years' clinical application and systematic observation, Z-C$_1$ and Z-C$_4$ medicine had obtained remarkable curative effect and no toxic action and side effect had been found after long-term administration. It had been proven by the clinical observation that Z-C$_1$ and Z-C$_4$ medicine could improve the survival quality of the carcinoma patients in medium and late stage in an all-round way, improve the whole immunity, control the hyperplasia of the cancer cells, consolidate and enhance the long-term curative effect. The oral-taken and external-applied Z-C medicine had good curative effect in softening and shrinking body surface metastatic tumor. With the assistance of intervention or treatment with cannula spray pump for medicine, it could protect liver, kidney and bone marrow hemopoietic system and the immune organ and improve the immunity.

3. Good pain alleviation effect of Z-C anti-cancer pain alleviation paste

Pain is the relatively remarkable and painful symptom of the carcinoma patients in late stage, the common pain reliever had no remarkable effect on carcinoma pain, the stupefacient pain reliever had the addiction and dependence, Z-C anti-cancer pain alleviation paste had strong pain alleviation effect with a long maintenance time. It was proven through 298 cases of clinical verification that the effective rate was 78.0%, the total effective rate was 95.3%, after repeated application, there were no toxic action or side effect, without addiction. The paid alleviation effect was stable and it was an effective therapeutic method for the carcinoma patients to get rid of the pain and improve the quality of life.

IV. Z-C Medicine is a Modern Production of Traditional Herb Medicine

Z-C medicine was neither the experiential prescription nor the prescription made by the famous doctor of traditional Chinese medicine, but 48 kinds of traditional herb medicines screened from 200 kinds of common Chinese herbal medicines with so-called anticancer reaction after the animal screening test in batches and vitro screening and screening of tumor-inhibition rate in the tumor-bearing animal body one by one through over 4000 tumor-bearing animal models in the past 7 years with the modern medical method, experimental tumor study method and modern pharmacody and drug effect study method.

The substantial foundation of the traditional prescriptions that bring its unique curative effect into play in clinic was its chemical compositions. The changes in quality and quantity of the chemical compositions would directly affect the curative effect of the prescription in clinic. Therefore, it is necessary to study the changes in quality and quantity of the chemical compositions in the prescription and find out the main effective compositions in the prescription. Z-C medicine basically finds out its effect of medicine, action, molecular weight and constitutional formula and makes the study on the traditional prescription on a new step.

The prescription of Z-C medicine is the innovation and reform of the traditional herbal prescriptions, it is not the bonded solutions through mixing and boiling, but the granular concentration or powder of the medical compounds. The dried medicinal herbs in the medical compound still remain its original compositions without any change in pharmacological action, molecular weight and constitutional formula. It is made with modern scientific method but not through chemical combination, in this way, the original compositions and functions are remained for assessing and affirming the action and curative effect of the medical compounds.

13. The role and efficacy which are similar to BRM in XZ-C anticancer immune medications

Biological response modifier (BRM) explores the new field of the tumor biological therapy. Currently BRM as the fourth methods of the tumor treatment gets widely attention in the world.

1. BRM theory

Oldham in 1982 built BRM theory. In 1984 based on this he advanced the fourth modality of cancer treatment-----biological therapy again. According to this, in the normal condition, there is the dynamic equilibrium between the tumor and the body. The development of the tumors, and even invasion and metastasis, completely is caused by the loss of this equilibrium. If this imbalance situation is adjusted to the normal level, the tumor growth can be controlled and will disappear. The anticancer mechanism of BRM in detail as the following: 1.) Improve the host defense abilities or decrease the immune inhabitation of the tumors to the host to reach the immune response to the tumors 2.) Look for the biological active things in natural or gene combination to enhance the host defense abilities 3.)Reduce the host response induced by the tumor cells. 4).Promote the tumors to division and mature to become the normal cells 5).Reduce the side effects of the chemotherapy and radiation therapy and enhance

The biological therapy is to adjust inherent BRM through from the outside of the body to add, induct or activate the cell toxic biological active factor inside the cell. The biological therapy is different from the previous three therapy models such as surgery, radioactive and chemotherapy, to directly attack the target of the tumors.the biological reaction systems inside the host bodys. The therapy ranges of BRM is beyond the traditional immune therapy concepts, which the equilium between the body and the tumors is not limit to the immune reaction, but involved in all kinds of the regulation genes and cell factors related to the tumor proliferations.

The tumor biological therapy mainly includes: 1). The injection of the immune active cells 2).The production /application of the cytokines and cell factors. 3).Specific autoimmune including the application of Monoclonal Antibody, Vaccine, and its crossing-things.

The cytokines and liquid factors in the host immune system is in subtle control . If the balance of them was lost, the body response or the answer abilities will be affected significantly so that BRM can recover this unbalance condtion to the normal equilianume to reach the goal of treating the tumors.

BRM is a group of medicine which can adjust the host body immune function, recovering the immune function from the inhibition conditions, the function mechanism of which are active the immune function systems. Which are mainly from the microbiology agents and the plants, the former is the drugs as the immune strengthener and immune active agents and immune regulator, now the new name is the BRM.

Recurrently there are some BRM-similar medicine from the traditional Chinese medicine, which have excellent results.

2. The classifications of BMR

1). Cytokines: is the production from the immune effective cells and related cells, which are the cell-mediated proteins with the important biological activities. The types of their biological activities as the following: a. Interleukin 2(IL-2) is the molecules between the immune cells and active the killer cells such as T cells, B cells proliferation, and active the NK cells etc. b). IFN has three types of IFN-α,β,ϒ which are groups of glycoproteins. c). CSF is the factor which stimulated the blood stem cells growth an division into GM-CSF, M-CSF and G-CSF.d). TNF.

2).The immune active cells: so far there are four immune cells which are used to the tumor therapy:

  a. LAK

  b. TIL

  c. PWH-LAK and OKT3-LAK: The PBL or TIL from pwh, okt can stimulated LAK proliferation activity.

  d. CD8 CTL which can recognized the MHCI tumor groups has the strong activities which killed the tumor cells.

3).The vaccines of the tumor molecules: currently the main research on the tumor vaccination is the unique vaccine of antitumor monoantibodys, which can produce the anticancer response after imitating the antigen stimulation.

4). The natural medicine with BRM function: XZ-C have BRM function.

3. The function mechanism of BRM

BRM has the effects on the regulation of the host immmun response to the timor and killing the tumors. The mechanism are the following five aspects:1).Directly regulating the growth and division of the tumors 2).Increasing the sensitivies of the tumors to the anticancer mechnisum in the body to benefit of killing the tumor cells. 3).Acting on the tumor vessels and affects the tumor's nutrition, blood supply so as to lead the death of the tumors and not damage the normal tissues. 4).Stimulating the immune response to host antitumors. 5).Stimulating the production of the blood to improve the inhibited bone marrow function to increase the tolerance of the damage from the tumor therapy.

BRM can improve the body immune response and can strengthen the body immune surveillance to the tumors. The patients with the smallest size have good response to the BRM. BRM have very good effects on the early patients or the remaining tumor after surgery, or the tiny tumors.

BRM is one of the combination therapy methods to treat the malignant tumors, which some scientists said that immune therapy just treat the 10^5 tumor cells such if the tumor cells formed clearly, the RRM functions will be limit the tumors to growth.

Even if the immune therapy have great development and attacted the whole world attentions, the mature degree of the tumor immune therapy is still in controevent., Currntly this is a worth research and there are some questions as the following:

1). It is difficult to have effects to the big tumors, only as the supply therapy to the therapy of the operation, chem. And radiation

2).Because the tumor antigen is specific, it is very difficult to produce the specific antibody.

Some researchers showed that the antitumor therapy doesn't need absolute specificity, therefore , even if the tumors don't have the specific antigen, the immune therapy of the tumors is still acceptable. The concentration of the tumor relative antigens in the malignant tumor cells is higher than the normal cells, which this difference can make it possible for these antigens to become the effective attacked target. In addition, because the patients with cancer almost have the decreases of the immune function, and the increase of the immune inhibition factors, and the decrease of IL-2, TNF, and IFN etc , therefore, it is necessary to increase the immune function.

Because of the immune function decrease in the tumor patients, during the therapy it should try to improve the immune function in the patients with the tumors. Because of the increaser of the immune inhibiting factors in the tumor patients, it should be treated to black ; because of the decrease of the IL-2, TNF and IFN etc, it should try to stimulate the production of these factors.

In order to improve the effects of the immune therapy, it is necessary to investigate how to get the best combination forms of these therapies with the current therapy.

4. The research survey on the XZ-C anticancer medication of immune regulation control similar to BRM

XZ-C immune regulation anticancer medicine have the functions and curative effects similar to BRM after four years experimental research and 16 years clinical research which are the drugs similar to BRM selected from traditional Chinese medicine.

XZ-C is the drugs that XU ZE in China professor selected from two hundreds of the anticancer herbs after the experiments. At first the culturing tumor were done. The in vitro was done One by one to select and observe the direct damage to tumor cells in the culture setting and the control groups of the rate of the anticancer are the chemotherapy CTX and the normal culture tube cells. The results are to select the a series of the medicine of the anti-cancer proliferation, then made the animal modes which 200 drugs were used on one by one . These experiments of the analysis and evaluation are steps by steps, scientific, practical and strict, etc. The results proved that48 of them have the excellent tumor inhibition effects, however the rest 152 of the tumors anticancer medicine are all common old anticancer medicine which proved no anticancer or less inhibition of the tumors in the animal models during these medicine selection experiments.

In the process of the experiments, the main work were conducted on the tumor animal models: one medicine was experienced on one group to observe them about three months and then selected 48 of the effective anticancer medicine, then combination of two or three medicine to do experiment on these animal models so that the single medicine has less effects than the multiple compound effects , which seems that the single medicine has the inhibition only on the tumor cell proliferation, however the multiple combination not inhibition to the tumor proliferation, but have the immune regulation control function of the body regulation, strengthen the energy, improvement of the immune system, promoting the production of the inhibiting cell factors, protecting the normal cells and promoting the anticancer factors etc.

Based on the author's experiments during four years of the single traditional medicine selection in the animal models, then the combination of the experiment, then set up again XZ-C $_{1-10}$ recipes of anticancer, anti-metastasis and anti-recurrence and last conducted the clinical verification. From 1992 the wide clinical tests were set up. After 16 years of the tumor specialty in outpatient centers there were 12000 cases of the tumor patients who were tested and showed the excellent effects which their medical condition are stable; their symptoms are improved , their life quality are improved and the survival time prolongs. The medical condition in many metastasis patients was stable and didn't further spread. Some of the patients with leukopenia couldn't have chemotherapy and radiation therapy; however after taking these medication, there were no further metastasis and have excellent effects.

5. The function and curative effect of the XZ-C traditional Chinese anticancer medicine for the immune regulation control similar to BRM

In 1982 BRM was first described by Oldham, which the reaction or response ability to foreign attack is through the BRM.

The cell-mediated and antibody mediated immune response is in subtle control situation. In the imbalance situation the host response or the response ability will be significantly affected. The application of the BRM regulator can recover the normal equilitiun from the loss of the equilitium to reach the goal of the disease prevention .

BRM explored the new field of the tumor biology therapy, which currently was used as the fourth model which got great attentions from all over the world.

BRM regulates the body's immune function, recovers the immune function which was inhibited. These classes of medication function mechanism are multiple, however no matter what mechanism theirs, they are function through the activating the body immune systems.

BRM , mainly from the microorganism and plants, is called as immune strengthener, immune stimulator, immune exciting factors or immune regulation in the past, now called as BRM.

Authors selected the excellent anticancer XZ-C medication through animal experiments in his lab. XZ-C can improve immune function, protect the central immune organs such as thymus , improve the cell-mediated immune functions, protect thymus function and bone morrow function, recover the red blood cells and white blood cells number, activate the immune factors, improve the immune surveillance in the blood etc. The main pharmacology function of XZ-C anticancer medication is anticancer and increase of the immune function. After four years of the animal experiments of the selection of the medication, 48 medications were selected as the single medication for the high anticancer medication, then after the immune and cell factors level tests, 26 medications of them separately have phargocyte functions; increase immune cells function; increase the antibody- humoral immune functio; increase the thymus weight; promote bone marrow proliferation; improve T cells function; increase the activities of the LAK cell function, increase IFN activities levels and TNS activity level; strengthen CSF factors; inhibit the platelet anticoagulation to inhibiting the cancer thromobosis; inhibit metastasis, or clean free radicals etc.

XZ-C has the following function as :

1). activating the host immune system to promote the host immune function to reach the immune respond to the tumors.

2). Activating the host immune factors of the anticancer systems to strengthen the host immune function and improve the immune surveillance of the host immune systems.

3). protecting the thymus and bone marrow, improving the immune function, and stimulating bone marrow function to reduce the inhibition of the bone marrow and recovering the white blood cell and red blood cells etc.

4). Reduction of the side effects of chemotherapy and radioactive therapy to increase the tolerance of the hosts.

5). Cancer development is imbalance between the biological characteristic of the tumor cells and the inhibition of the host to tumor. XZ-C improve immune system function and recover the balance of both them.

6). Directly regulating the tumor cell growth and division to have the regulation function of the growth and division.

7). Increasing thymus weight and stop the shrink of thymus because when the tumor develop thymus goes on shrink.

8). Stimulating the host immune response to the tumors and strengthening the host anticancer abilities and strengthening the sensitivities of the host anticancer mechanism so as to benefits of killing the tumor cells on the ways of the metastasis.

XZ-C can make the body to produce the strong immune reaction to the tumor cells so that it can treat the tumors, which can produce the following immune response: 1). Strengthen the regulation or recover the host immune response to the tumors;2). stimulate the host immune system to active the host immune defense system;3)recover the immune functions.

As the above statement, the basic mechanism of XZ-C is similar to BRM and the clinical application is similar to those of the BRM.

6. The clinical application principle and the application range of the XZ-C anticancer immune regulation traditional medicine

1).The clinical application of XZ-C: BRM and XZ-C similar to BRM can increase the immune response and strengthen the host immune surveillance function. When the cells started the mutation or the tumors are small, the effects are good. After the surgery or radioactive therapy, the medicine therapy make the tumor shrink to the smallest size which therapy effects are the best.

For the patients who cannot have the operation and are weak and cannot have the chemotherapy and radioactive therapy, the immune therapy has some effects and reduce the symptom and prolong the survival time.

After the removal of the tumor in order to reduce the mestastas and reccurency , the XZ-C can be used . After the operation removed the big tumors XZ-C can be use to get rid of the remaining tumr cells and the tumor which already spred further away.

IF the tumor is not removed, the chemotherapy or the radicaotive therapy can be used first, which kill the most of the tumor cells to reduce the number of the tumor cells , then XZ-C can be used to supply.

2).The clinical observation and application ranges of XZ-C

1). Antimestastasis after the operation: recover and improve the immune response after the surgery to improve the life quality and kill the remaining tumor cells after the operation to prevent the metastasis and inhibit the cell proliferation to prevent the recurrence and strengthen the long term curative effects.

The ranges of the application: a.)all kind of the middle, and advanced tumor after the surgery. b.)All kind of the tumor after the surgery c.) the advanced tumor which cannot be removed after the operation investigation d.) only can have the intestine recombination or the opening of the colon during the operation. e.) cannot removal the advanced tumors and lost the indication for the surgery. f.)the removed tumors plus the intubation drug pump surgery.

2). Improving the life quality , prolonging the survival rate, inhibiting the division of the tumors, control the tumor cell proliferation, improve the body immune response , mainly anti metastasis

Application ranges: a). all kinds of the tumors including the new, further metastasis after the operation; b). all of the cancer with the later metastasis such as the liver, lung, brain, chest cavity, abdominal cavity.

3). Reducing the tumor pain: XZ-C can treat all kind of the pain from the advanced tumors and soft and reduce the tumor size.

4). Supply with the chemotherapy or the tube pump therapy to protect the liver, kidney and bone marrow and thymus etc immune organs to improve the immune response and change the whole body immune condition, to support and strengthen and increase the period and long time curative effects to prevent the metastasis and spreed and recovery and to improve life quality, prolong the life time after the liver cancer patient had the tubes and chemotherapy etc.

5). Combination with the chemotherapy and radiation therapy, can reduce the side effects and increase the curative effects to protect the liver, kidney and bone marrow and other immune organs function to increase the white cell numbers.

6). the combination of the application of XZ-C and the traditional Decoction: such as the using with soap of liver elimination of water for the liver cancer and ascite or the metastasis of the abdominal cavity ascite; used the soap of reducing jaundice for the treatment of liver cancer and jaundice; used with JiangMei negative Soup for the liver tumor with high transaminase and HbsAg positive. Used with soup of increasing blood to treat Leukopenia caused by the chemotherapy.

3. The application time of XZ-C:

The tumor patients mostly have the immune function decreases after the diagnosed, the treatment should be done soon, however the three therapy of the operation, chemotherapy and radiation therapy all can cause the immune function decrease and lead to decrease tolerance of the patients to the surgery or chemotherapy, or radiation therapy and decrease the immune surveillance in the host immune system. Therefore, it is necessary to start the immune therapy during the operation or radiation therapy and chemotherapy. XZ-C can take by oral as long as the patient can eat and this is can be taken by oral. After the 1-2 week of the operation, the patient can start to take them. Before chemotheray and radiation therapy, or during the rest peroids between radiation therapy and chemotherapy, after radiation therapy or chemotherapy the patient can take XZ-C so that decrease or control the cancer recurrence and metastasis. Therefore, XZ-C decrease the side effect of the radiotherapy and chemotherapy; prevent the immune system from decrease induced by chemotherapy and increase immune function; promote the bone marrow function; protect bone marrow functions; activate immune system and immune cytokines function to improve the immune surveillance and prevent the recurrence and metastasis.

14. Immune function in patients with advanced cancer in Chinese herbal medication

1. The medication which should be used and can improve immune function in advanced cancer

  a. The discovery from the tumor experimental research Advanced cancer are immunocompromised mice and thymus atrophy.

(1) In 1986 in our laboratory to manufacture tumor-bearing animal models removal of the thymus (THC) can be produced tumor-bearing animal models and injection of immunosuppressive agents can also contribute to the establishment of tumor-bearing animal models. Results of the study show that the incidence and development of cancer and immune function of the host and immune function of organs and tissues is certainly a significant relationship. No removal of the thymus is difficult to manufacture cancer animal models. Repeating several experiments, results were confirmed.

(2) Whether the prior immunocompromised then easy to get cancer, or cancer happens then lead immune function to decrease. The results of our experiments are: first, unocompromised and then tend to have a carcinoma; in the absence of immune function decline, the inoculation of cancer is not successful. The results of this study tips: to improve and maintain good immune function and to protect the immune organs Thymus (TH) can prevent cancer.

(3) The animal model of liver metastasis were divided into A, B groups, A with immunosuppressive agents, group B without our laboratory studies of cancer metastasis and immune relationship. Results: A group was significantly more than the number of liver metastases group B. The results suggest that: the transfer of immunization-related immune dysfunction or immunosuppressive agents, may promote tumor metastasis.

(4) In our laboratory of tumor impacting on the immune organs it was found that with the progress of cancer, TH namely cell proliferation was progressively blocked, volume was significantly reduced. These results suggest that: the tumor can inhibit TH, resulting in atrophy of immune organs.

The above experimental results prove: cancer occurrence, development, metastasis and host immune function decline have significantly affirmative relationship, mice with advanced cancer are immunocompromised and Thymus atrophy. Thus, in advanced cancer treatment should be used Increasing immune function drugs, but cannot be used to reduce or suppress the immune immune drugs.

2. Natural herbal medications: from experimental study to find elevated tumor immune suppression drugs

Our results demonstrate that, with the progress of the tumor, the host has thymus atrophy so that we can use some ways to prevent a host Thymus atrophy.

In order to stop atrophy of immune organs when tumor is progressing , we investigated the ways of making recovery of TH function and the immune reconstruction method and searched to look for anti-cancer drugs increased immune from natural herbal medications. Our laboratory over a long period, a batch of 200 kinds of traditional considered to be "anti-cancer medicine," the herbal flavor carried by tumor-bearing animals in vivo anti-tumor screening experiments. It was found that 152 kinds of invalid, only 48 kinds do have some even better inhibit the proliferation of cancer cells, while increasing the role of immunity, including 26 kinds of Chinese herbal medicine (HM) with enhanced macrophage function or stimulate the animals thymus weight increase, or elevated white blood cell; or promote spleen lymphocyte proliferation, enhance lymphocyte transformation rate of T cell immune function enhancement of NK cell activity enhancement of the role of interferon induced pro , the optimal combination, and then liver cancer, stomach cancer, S180. And other tumor-bearing animal models in vivo anti-tumor experiments, further screening, out of no stabilizing effect of further screening and formed a c z suppressor immune regulation medicine, may protect the chest rise Free, nursing marrow and blood, improve immune function. In animal experiments, based on the success of screening, clinical practice, clinically proven in 10 years a large number of cases, zc immune regulation medicine, can improve the quality of life in advanced cancer patients, increased immunity, enhance physical fitness, improve appetite, prolong survival period, more significant effect.

2. Experimental research of the medication inhibitory on S180 mice and enhancing the immune effects righting training

1. Objective:

40 years of Integrative cancer prevention research and practice, found that many traditional Chinese medicine for the treatment of cancer does have a certain effect; in particular, studies of the efficacy of traditional Chinese medicine righting training for the treatment of malignant tumors showed righting The multi-class medicine can enhance health and improve immune function, improve quality of life and prolong survival. But Chinese medicine treatment of tumors were observed in clinical experience, without experimental research. In order to explore Chinese medicine righting training the spleen, and kidney medicine whether BNI can inhibit tumor growth, and therefore, the following experiment.

2. Method

(1) Experimental animal: Kunming mice 160, 5-6 weeks old, weighing 27 persons 2. 0g, male and female.

(2) Tumor-bearing animal models: S180 ascites tumor lines, press 1X1O7X0.2ml tumor cells were seeded in each of the mice was the right forelimb armpit skin.

(3) Experimental groups. The experimental animals were randomly divided into, A Group: Yiqi treatment group ((n = 20); Group B: blood double up treatment group ((n = 20); Group C: nourishing yin treatment group ((n = 20); D Group: Warming kidney treatment group ((n = 20); E Group: ATCA mixture treatment group ((n = 20); F Group: Xiaochaihutang treatment group ((n = 20); Group G: Compound Capsule treatment group ((n = 20); H Group: tumor-bearing control group ((n = 20) of each group in the first two days after inoculation, respectively, herbal oral 0. 4ml / (only · d),. tumor-bearing control group with normal saline control treatment.

(4) Preparation of the groups of traditional Chinese medicine: the original party in terms of modern dose decoction made from concentrate, crude drug concentration of 200%. And oral doses of the drug concentration above the normal human dose based on dose into mice come. In this study, the righting training the deficiency of qi and blood make up, nourishing yin, warming yang, supplementation and attack ATCA agent, Xiaochaihutang and compound capsules and other medicine to treat mice bearing S180.

(5) Observation: systematic observation of the mice in each group had time to tumor, tumor survival time measured their serum protein content, the weight of peripheral blood T lymphocyte counts and immune organs.

3. Results righting training and to righting training is a major component of ATCA agent can significantly delay tumor inoculation mice appeared time, inhibition of tumor growth (A, B, C, D, E group inhibition rate was 40 percent, respectively, 45 %, 44.5%, 31% and 36%), to extend the survival time of tumor-bearing mice, (A, B, extend the lifetime of the CDE groups were 27.6%, 45% .38 5%, 25% and 26.5%). Quxie based Xiaochaihutang, compound capsules not significantly inhibited tumor growth and prolonged survival (compared to E group, P> 0. 05) increase 0 A, serum protein B, C, D, E group content , A / G ratio increase, peripheral T lymphocyte counts increased (and G group P <0. 05, B, C groups P <0. 01), thymic atrophy was significantly inhibited.

4. Conclusion This study shows that the righting training or righting training based medicine treatment can inhibit tumor and enhance immunity, can improve varying degrees of peripheral blood T lymphocytes, are more effective treatment than with Quxie.

5. Discussion

(1) The traditional Chinese medicine righting training inhibitory and prolong survival role. Many cancer patients clinically shown "imaginary" symptoms, such as qi deficiency, blood deficiency, yin deficiency, yang deficiency and the like. Righting training should be adopted on the treatment of traditional Chinese medicine. This study investigated the inhibitory effect of all phenomena and righting training supplementation and attack, and the results showed that: deficiency of qi and blood make up, nourishing yin yang, etc. Warming righting training in Chinese medicine and traditional Chinese medicine righting training ATCA-based agent can significantly delay the appearance of tumors in mice inoculated with time, inhibition of tumor growth and prolong survival time of tumor-bearing mice. From each group inhibition rate analysis: blood double up in the experimental group, the inhibition rate was 45 percent; in nourishing yin experimental group, the inhibition rate of 44.5%, followed by deficiency of the inhibition action is also up 40 percent, the effect is also good: Once again, ATCA agent inhibitory rate of 36%: but poor Warming kidney treatment group, the inhibition rate of 31%; opinion should be adopted in terms of inhibition of tumor blood double complement and treatment of nourishing yin. From a prolonged survival rate analysis: supplement qi and blood group of 45%, in order to extend the lifetime of the longest group; followed by nourishing yin group, up 38.5 percent, the effect is also good, as deficiency of warming yang and supplementation and attack the ATCA mixture treatment group, but also to prolong survival, but less nourishing yin qi and blood complement and treatment groups. Quxie based Xiaochaihutang, compound capsule treatment group, shown in

this set of experiments not significantly inhibit tumor, we can not prolong survival of tumor-bearing mice, the effect of the worst. Therefore, from the extension of terms of survival to double up and nourishing yin blood treatment is preferred, followed by the deficiency of warming yang and supplementation and attack. From both inhibition of tumor and prolong survival analysis of both qi and blood complement the optimal places, followed by nourishing yin, then followed Buzhongyiqi and ATCA mixture, Warming kidney treatment ineffective. As for Quxie of Xiaochaihutang and compound capsules, from the present experimental results, no significant effect.

In short, each righting training and righting training to varying degrees based treatment inhibited tumor growth and prolong survival role, and to Quxie based treatment had no significant anti-tumor and prolong survival role.

This experiment showed that: righting training to righting training medicine or medicine-based treatment of smaller tumors very significant inhibitory effect, and can significantly prolong survival and improve quality of life, so much as a clinical and postoperative radiotherapy One of adjuvant therapy of chemotherapy. Many reported in the literature using the clinical treatment of malignant tumors righting training have achieved good results, the present results further confirmed that supplement qi and blood, nourishing yin, deficiency of other treatment can suppress tumors and prolong survival, as in Integrative clinical treatment of malignant tumors provide an experimental basis.

(2) Chinese medicine righting training to enhance the immune effect. This experiment showed that the righting training in Chinese medicine and Chinese medicine righting training based treatment could improve in varying degrees of peripheral blood T lymphocytes, such as when the first four weeks, T lymphocyte levels were as follows: 41.5% Buzhong group , blood group, double up 44.8 percent, 38.6 percent nourishing yin group, warming yang group 37. 5%, ATCA mixture group 35.6%; suppression thymus atrophy, as the first two weeks, the deficiency of blood double up, nourishing yin, yang Warming and AT-CA mixture treated thymus index were significant differences with the tumor-bearing control group. Tip righting training anti-tumor effect may enhance immune function. Some people think that a lot of plant polysaccharides have immunomodulatory agents (immunenoclulator) performance, called anti-tumor polysaccharides, these polysaccharides can not directly kill cancer cells, but it can activate the immune system to release cytokines have anti-tumor effects or enhanced LAK cells killing effect on cancer cells. Righting training this drug is rich in plant polysaccharides, such as Zhao Kesheng reported: Huang contempt polysaccharide extract, wherein the molecular weight was found 20 000ˑ -2500. The components of normal and cancer patients peripheral blood mononuclear cells (PBMC) in vitro

secretion of tumor necrosis factor (TNF) has significant role in promoting. Chen Kai reported: traditional Chinese medicine Fuzheng anti-tumor was transplanted tumor S18. Natural killer cell activity in mice and interleukin-2 (IL-2) activity can promote, and promote T lymphocyte activation, and promote peritoneal macrophage phagocytosis, increased spleen and thymus weight. In short, the role of righting training the human immune system is very complex, pending further observation and research.

(3) Chinese medicine righting training can enhance the body resistance to disease, improve blood cells and build up their strength. This experiment showed that: righting training this drug can increase serum protein in tumor-bearing mice, raising clearing / globulin ratio. Our clinical observations cancer specialist clinics showed that: applications of righting training based XZ-C$_4$ immune regulation medications in liver cancer, esophageal cancer, stomach cancer, colorectal cancer tumor can suppress cancer and increase immune function. Red blood cells, hemoglobin were higher, leukopenia was also suppressed. Description righting instinct enhance blood cells and proteins, increase strength, improve resistance to disease.

One rule is righting training as a combination therapy of tumors has been widely used clinically. The results showed that: righting training drug treatment can delay the vaccinated mice tumor occurrence time, inhibit tumor growth, prolong survival time of tumor-bearing, enhance immune function and disease resistance, improve quality of life. It can provide experimental evidence for clinical anti-cancer medicine.

3. The immune function of Chinese herbal medicine for advanced cancer patients

Patients with advanced cancer is mostly deficiency, a common immune dysfunction. Tonic righting medicine can enhance immune function, prevention and treatment of the patient's tumor immune dysfunction has important significance.

1. Enhance non-specific immune function

(1) Can stimulate animal immune organs thymus, spleen to gain weight: Ginseng can increased thymus weight 2.2-fold as the control group of young mice.

(2) Enhance macrophage phagocytosis: such as ginseng, Codonopsis, Astragalus, angelica, medlar (Wolfberry), etc. can promote macrophage phagocytosis, especially the role of qi drug is obvious.

(3) Increased peripheral leukocytes count: for example, ginseng, astragalus , Codonopsis, Rehmannia and Millettia etc can significantly increase white blood cell count.

2. Enhancing immune function

(1) to promote lymphocyte proliferation: such as ginseng, can increase the number of lymphocytes, yams, mistletoe, etc. can increase the proportion of peripheral blood T cells.

(2) increasing the lymphocyte transformation rate: such as ginseng, astragalus, Angelica, white fungus and other tonics, lymphocyte transformation rate were increased role.

(3) to enhance red blood cell immune function: such as astragalus, medlar (Wolfberry) can significantly increase the red blood cell C36 mice receptor (RBC-C36) a rosette rate and RBC immune complexes (RBC-IC) rosette formation rate.

3. Enhanced humoral immunity

(1) the promotion of antibody production: such as ginseng, Huang Jing, Cynomorium, Curculigo, cinnamon, Dodder, Cistanche deserticola, which are to promote the role of antibody production, to varying degrees, increased serum IgG, IgA, IgM and other antibody levels.

(2) increasing the number of antibody-forming cells in the spleen: Longspur bud polysaccharide injection can mouse spleen cell culture antibody production increased more than 1, yam polysaccharides can significantly increase mouse spleen, hemolytic plaque forming cells. However, some tonic medicine immune enhancement and inhibition of double-acting.

4. Enhance the role of Chinese herbal medicine on immune function in tumor-bearing

In medicine, tumor formation and development are inadequate due to the machine off the upright, and that positive qi deficiency associated with tumor occurrence, development, treatment and prognosis of the whole process. Righting training is a basic rule in the prevention and treatment of cancer medicine, and the most prominent is the body's immune function, particularly in the regulation of cellular immune function.

Modern studies have shown that pain occurrence, development and prognosis of tumor-bearing machine off cellular immune status is closely related to cancer patient's immune function is suppressed, the body in immunosuppression. This immune suppression in, terminally ill patients or long after chemotherapy or radiotherapy is particularly evident. Surgery, radiotherapy, chemotherapy or disorders can cause a decline in immune function. By Chinese medicine righting training to enhance immune function, thereby enhancing the body cancer-fighting ability, improve the effectiveness of surgery, radiotherapy, chemotherapy, improve patient quality of life and prolong survival of patients.

1. Chinese herbal medicines immune protection organs of immune organs, increasing the weight of immune organs was found:

(1) Daily respectively fed mice with 15g / kg, 30g / kg extract Angelica and and with 12.5mg / kg, 25mg / kg ferulic suspension for continuous 7d which could significantly increase mouse spleen and thymus weight.

(2) Gavage mice with Polygonum 6g (kg • d) decoction, continuous 7d can significantly increase thymus weight and also antagonize prednisolone-induced immune organ weight decreases.

(3] littoralis polysaccharide 32mg / (kg • d), continuous 7 days can significantly increase thymus weight in mice by intraperitoneal injection.

(4) Cistanche deserticola decoction can significantly increase the weight of spleen and thymus with fed mice.

It must be noted that some herbs can reduce weight of immune organs and prompt immune organ atrophy, such as Hook, cicada, Puhuang, Sarcandrae, rhubarb, etc. Thymus atrophy, thymus cortical thinning, decreased cells and spleen weight was significantly reduced, splenic artery sheath surrounding the central lymphocytes (mostly T lymphocytes) decrease after fed 0.5g / d rhubarb decoction continuous 8d in normal mice . There is no significant effect on mice immune organs after perfusion medication 10mg / kg per day continuous 10d. Generally small dose had no effect, while large doses decreased.

2. Chinese herbal medicine on mononuclear phagocyte system function enhancement

Medicine polysaccharide, ridge type and a variety of other ingredients to enhance the mononuclear phagocyte system, particularly macrophage activity, enhance its function Free recover from illness. Anti-tumor effect of macrophages are activated by tumor antigen-specific T cells release macrophages, activation of macrophages specifically kill tumor cells: macrophages by cytotoxicity mediated cell killing of tumor cells, such as by activating the macrophages secrete tumor necrosis factor (TNF), a proteolytic drunk, interferon (IFN) and other direct killing or inhibiting the growth of tumor cells.

(1) Medlar (Wolfberry) polysaccharides (LBP): Wang Ling etc. summarizes the research of immunomodulatory LBP effects in the second phase of "Shanghai Journal of Immunology"(1995): LBP with 0.125g / (kg • d) mice intragastric 5d can enhance macrophage phagocytosis that LBP has a certain immune function. Zhang yongxiang and other like researched LBP effects on mouse peritoneal macrophages in tumor cell proliferation inhibition activity.

(2) Velvet polysaccharide (PAPS): 0.01ug / ml concentration PAPS can significantly improve macrophage function in immunocompromised mice induced hydrocortisone, namely that is promoted, and a clear dose-effect relationship. PAPS with 0.01ug / ml concentration has the strongest effect.

(3) Gypenosides: Gypenosides with 300mg / (kg • d) once daily for continuous 7d can significantly enhance the ability of peritoneal macrophage cells in normal mice. Shou Zhi Juan reported that anti-alveolar macrophages volume increases and phagocytic digestion increases under the abdominal loose connective tissue when mice were fed by Gypenosides with 50mg (containing 1.21% total glycosides) once daily for a month later in the "Wenzhou Medical College,"(1990) Volume 20(1).

(4) ABPS: can induce the synthesis of IL-1 and tumor necrosis factor(TNF-α) in macrophages. ABPS 25mg / kg or 50mg / kg can improve the LPS-induced IL-1 production by intraperitoneal injection. ABPS with 100mg / kg can promote the formation of TNF-α by intraperitoneal injection and it has the same strength role as BCG .

(5) Psoralen: with carcinogens Urethane cause lung cancer in mice, then intraperitoneally injection of psoralen 1mg / 20g weight, continuous 10d can significantly enhance lung cancer mouse peritoneal macrophage phagocytosis.

3. Chinese medication enhancing the role of T cells immune function

T cells are very important in body's immune cells, not only will lead to specific cellular immunity, and is involved in immune regulation, and other functions. Tumor cells are often accompanied by changes in cell surface antigens. Because of immune surveillance of T cells, tumor antigen sensitized T cells directly or indirectly kill tumor cells by directly or indirectly cytotoxicity and released cytokines.

(1) Epimedium polysaccharide (EPS): EPS with 100mg / Kg/ d for continuous 5d significantly increased peripheral WBC and T lymph cells by subcutaneous injection .

(2) Alfalfa Polysaccharides (MPS): in vitro can enhance lymphocyte proliferation induced by PHA, CONA, LPS and pokeweed (PWM). MPS 125mg / (kg · d) and 250 mg / (kg · d) significantly increased spleen lymphocyte index and the number of lymphocytes by intraperitoneal injection. MPS also partially antagonized lymphocytes decrease induced by cyclophosphamide in intraperitoneal injection.

(3) Medlar polysaccharide (Wolfberry) (LBP): can significantly increase the percentage of peripheral external T lymphocytes in mouse. LBP 5mg / (kg, d) increases peripheral blood lymphocyte count by abdominal injection for continuous 7d. The control group was 65.4%, 81.6% for the treatment group, but increasing the dose does not continue to improve this effect. In T lymphocyte mitogen CONA inducing conditions, a small dose of LBP (5-10mg / kg) can also cause lymphocyte proliferation which means LBP can significantly promote T cell proliferation.

(4) Moutan: 12. 5 / kg and 25g / kg doses orally can significantly improve the mice's T lymph cell transformation. Radix paeonail rubra(TPG): 25g / kg dose orally can significantly improve mice IL-2 activity. Wulingzhi: dose 12.5g / kg and 25 g / kg not only can significantly improve the T lymphocyte function in mice, but also 25g / kg dose also significantly increased IL-2 activity in mice by Gavage.

It must be noted, herbs also have to inhibit T cell immune function, such as Sophora, turmeric, Hook, Millettia, rhubarb, etc. which reduction of T cell immune function must be caution.

4. The role of traditional Chinese medicine on LAK cells

(1) Wind polysaccharide in a certain concentration range can be significantly increased IL-2-induced LAK cell killing activity.

(2) The sea buckthorn increases blood circulation. In tumor-bearing mice sea buckthorn juice (3g / kg) can significantly improve their spleen NK cells and LAK activity by injected intraperitoneally.

(3) Cao wenguang etc. found that three kinds of traditional Chinese medications such as APS, PAS and LBP could significantly promote the proliferation of mouse spleen cells with 5- 30mg / kg intraperitoneal injection in C57BL / 6 mice and. The spleen cells were 2×10^5 / ml with 125-1 000U / ml of rlL-2 induced 4d, APS group found that injections of spleen cells LAK activity of the group increased by 70%) - 120% compared with normal saline; injection PAS group increased by 20 % -90%; injection LBP group by 26% -80%.

(4) Cao wenguang etc treated 79 cases of advanced cancer patients which didn't have good response to radiotherapy and chemotherapy with traditional Chinese medicine LBP combined with LAK, IL-2 from February 1992 to November 1993. LBP with oral dose 1. 7mg / kg, LAK total doses 1. 2-32X 10^{10}, IL-2 with 3. 4- 4. 8X10^7U / person, specific programs in the conventional therapy is stopped after a month, give LBP 3 weeks after injection riL-2, giving LBP 4 week After a large number of patients with autologous PBL isolated LAK cells in vitro, reinfusion after various inspection, and then continue to give LBP and work L-2, 1 weeks. Results : 75 cases of evaluable patients, LAK / IL-2 combined with the efficacy of LBP group (36.36%) than single with LAK / IL-2 effect group (18%), the former combined LBP group before and after treatment and NK activity of PBL 500U / ml IL-2 induced the LAK activity increased level significantly higher than the latter alone LAK / IL-2 group. Show LBP could significantly promote NK and LAK cells antitumor activity.

Strength Spleen, warm yang, supporting kidney,YiQi,Yangyin etc increase LAK activity in vivo.

5. Immune function regulation of traditional Chinese medication on RBC

In 1981 American scholar Siegel and others put forward to the concept of "red cell immunity", illustrates not only the respiratory function of red blood cells, and is involved in a variety of immune and immune regulate the body's: such as the removal of circulating immune complexes, and promote phagocytosis, immune regulation of lymphocyte by red blood cells can recover from illness kill attached phenomena and red blood cell surface type I complement variant (CR1) according with immune complexes (IC) combining facts presented RBC involved in IFN-7, IL2 antibodies and natural killer cells (NK cells), lymphokine-activated killer cells (LAK cells) and phagocytic immune cells regulation and so on.

(1) It was found that Astragalus (Astragalus polysaccharide , APS) enables cancer patients in vitro activity of erythrocyte C3bR attached to the tumor cells

and enables immune function in cancer patients. APS enhances erythrocyte immune function in cancer patients.

(2) In the group of Trichosanthes root(TCS) treatment and of untreated group in Ehrlich ascites carcinoma in mice it was found that in the untreated group RBD-C3 bR rosette rate was significantly lower than the normal group, the treatment group RBC-C3bR rosette rate significantly higher than the untreated group and slightly higher than the normal group, which means mice RBC-C3bR activity was significantly decreased in the cancer mice and Trichobitacin can increase RBC-C3bR activity significantly.

TCS influence on mice erythrocyte SOD activity: After the mice inoculated with cancer cells to 11d, the treatment group erythrocyte SOD activity was significantly higher than the untreated group and the normal group. Late tumor-bearing mice decreased erythrocyte SOD, this experiment shows Chinese medication TCS can restore and enhance the activity of SOD.

TCS influence on red cell immune cat attached the ability of tumor cells: with Ehrlich ascites tumor cells as target cells, to determine the TCS effect on mice red blood cell immunity breast tumor cell attachment capability, found after tumor cell inoculation 11d, treatment mice tumor erythrocyte rosette rate (11.90 Soil 5.00)%, significantly lower than the normal mice (22.13 Soil 6.28)%; while tumors treated mice erythrocyte rosette rate (26. 54 persons 7.27)%, slightly higher than the normal group was significantly higher than the untreated group.

TCS's effect on erythrocyte immune to cancer patients: its cancer patients hemadsorption ability of tumor cells is also a significant enhancement. Tests found that cancer patients directly enhance rosette rate of RBC-C3bR effect, there is a significant difference with normal saline (NS) group, and promote the role and dose-dependent manner.

5. Types of biological medicine and its component response regulator (BRMS) action

Chinese medicine has a very important characteristic which has the role of two-way adjustment for biological therapy which can restore the body immune function to the normal direction.

In 1983 Jingjianping found that Astragalus can significantly increase IL-2 in "spleen false" mice model, but have no effect on normal mice.

In 1991 Xungxiaolin etc studied the effects of Millettia, FruitofPurpleflowerHolly, Psoralen Chinese medication on IL-2 production in mouse spleen cells and found that these drugs in three groups such as immunocompromised, hyperthyroidism, normal showed increased, inhibition, no influence which reflect double-acting medicine. Besides traditional Chinese medicine on the body due to the impact of anti-tumor substance and the amount thereof are closely related. Medlar at low concentrations can promote IL 3-secretion, but high concentrations inhibit IL-3 levels. When total glucosides of peony increase IL-2 production in the low concentrations by a dose-dependent. After the concentration exceeds 12. 5mg, it will inhibit IL 2-secretion.

Chinese medication has been used in our country for thousands of years and many Chinese medications can have the roles of BRMS which the research of anti-cancer immune agents will have a bright future. Chinese medication by oral has mild adverse reactions. Compared with genetic engineering BRMS and exogenous IL-2, IFN TNF, the advantages of traditional Chinese medication similar to BRMS has the whole body anticancer role in the body immune system and can be repeatedly administered with non-toxic side effects, and is available for tumor, chemotherapy, radiotherapy-induced immune dysfunction, boost the immune cell activation so that endogenous cytokines can be released and cause inhibition of tumor growth.

In modern cancer treatment, Chinese medication can at least play a role in three areas: ① enhance the role of inherent anti-cancer member effect in the body, enhance the body's anti-cancer cell system (NK cells, TK cells, LAK cell factor); ② Some traditional Chinese medicine has a direct anti-cancer effect; ③ some medicine ingredients can reduce side effects of radiation therapy, chemotherapy, and reduce the inhabition to the white cells and help to recover , even increase radiotherapy and chemotherapy anti-cancer effect.

15. Anticancer cell-mediated immunity

As we all know, the occurrence and prognosis of cancer development and treatment are decided by two contrast factors: the biological characteristics of cancer cells and the host restrictive ability to cancer cells. If these two are balance, the cancer is controlled; if they are imbalance, cancer will develop.

What are the biological characteristics and the biological behavior of the cancer cells? The previous chapters in this book have been outlined respectively. Under normal circumstances, the host itself against cancer cells have certain constraints defense capability, but in cancer the defense capabilities of these constraints are suppressed and damaged in different degrees so as to lead the loss of the immune surveillance of cancer cells and cancer occurs immune escape, making cancer metastasis.

1. The human body anticancer mechanism and its influencing factors

The human body has a complete anti-cancer immune system: the anti-cancer immune cells series; anticancer cytokine family; humoral immunity series; series of anti-cancer gene.

Anti-tumor immunological mechanism of the body can be divided, ①Cell-mediated immunity

: including T lymphocytes; NK natural killer cells; K cells; LAK cells; monocyte-macrophages. ②Humoral immunity: contains B cells; anti-tumor antibodies. ③ cytokines: interleukin-cell lines have; IFN; TNF; CSF and the like.

These human inherent anti-cancer system and immune substances are their own material in vivo. How biological response modifiers mobilize, activate and enhance the anti-tumor effect occupies an extremely important role in the anti-cancer and anti-metastatic therapy and will have vast work prospects.

Therefore, we have to study which are anti-cancer cells, which are anti-cancer cytokines, which humoral immunity can be activated to enhance the anti-cancer metastasis in the human body.

Here, we first look at the history of the 20th century in the treatment of cancer and several biological therapy have impressive results.

In the 1930s, Willam Coley and their successors Coley nauts treat those with advanced cancer with "Coley toxins". More than 200 cases of various types of cancer patients can be analyzed, which more than 30 cases were cured, and life more than 30 years. In the early 1980s Guesada and others treated hairy cell leukemia with IFN-a, actually treatment effective (CR + PR) are over 90%.

In the mid-1980s Rosenberg and others treat patients with advanced metastatic cancer who cannot be treated with other methods with LAK / IL-2. Some patients can be partial remission (42/228 patients) and complete remission (9 / 228 cases).

"Biological Therapy" (biotherapy) is also known as "biological regulation therapy" (bioregulator therapy). " anti-cancer system" is quite complex. From a structural and functional point it is a fairly large network system and under this system a number of members constitutes a "network learning system."

Because of the rapid development of molecular biology, molecular immunology, molecular immunology pharmacology, genetic engineering, basic and clinical research at the molecular level, "cancer establishment" continues to expand and depth, its anti-cancer metastasis is very lure people.

Currently, the research on anti-cancer immunotherapy molecular biology, are mainly in the "four sub-systems," :"anti-cancer cell therapy," "anti-cancer cytokine therapy", "anti-cancer gene therapy" and "anti-cancer antibody therapy."

The basic characteristics of these molecular biology, molecular immunotherapy are: molecular biology immunotherapy formulations used in vivo are discharged theirselves. The fundamental difference is that chemotherapy: its normal body tissue cells, especially and function of cells of the hematopoietic system and the structure and function of the immune system, not only did not carry out the role of the damage, but mainly there is a regulation and enhance the role of the immune response; we all know, radiotherapy and chemotherapy are completely different. Chemotherapy is a kind of non-selective "treatment injury", both kill cancer cells also kill normal cells, which damage the body's normal tissue cells, bone marrow and immune system structure and function suffered serious damage and lead to serious consequences.

Biological therapy is through the regulation of biological response mechanism to make life stable and balance . American scholar Oldam (1984) proposed biological regulation (BRM) theory, which later on this basis, proposed the concept of biological therapy of cancer.

Immune regulation mechanism of life is very important. Immune structure and function are extremely complex and its essence is to identify themselves by intolerance leaving the body to maintain a stable internal environment. Immune defense, immune surveillance and immune homeostasis are that bodies identify themselves, intolerance of three basic types of functions. From the basic point of biological function, immune regulation is one of the basic biological therapies.

On development of cancer there has always been two different views: one view, the tumor occurrence and development is a basic defense mechanism against any restriction body "independent process" in the treatment for the tumor itself emphatically, Few pay attention to the regulation of the immune system; another view is that the tumor occurrence and development of a variety of factors in vivo, particularly in the regulation of immune factors "involuntary procedure" or "controlled process", is subject to immune surveillance The cancer cells escape the immune surveillance so that cancer was able to develop. Based on these two different views there are two completely different proposition. The former believe that cancer is a largely unaffected by the body's defense mechanism for any restriction "independent process", which targets the treatment with simply killing cancer cells (regardless of the immune status) which the methods of treatment are radiation therapy and chemotherapy.

Caoguang Wen and Du ping presented an important concept which it is about as cancer biotherapy core foundation - the concept of "cancer establishment". And in vivo "cancer establishment" is a fairly large network system, the current basic and clinical research on the anti-cancer organization is expanding and depth, in anti-cancer treatment shift work has an extremely important role and broad prospects.

Network functionality issues concerning anti-cancer mechanism, the current study is more cytokine network structure and function, the other side also studied less, which this is called as "cytokine network". Simply, various cytokines in structure and function have certain correlation.

2. Anti-tumor effect of various immune functions

The cause of the tumor is very complicated, there are environmental factors, but also the organism internal factors, particularly with the gene mutation, oncogene expression and the decreased immune function. Modern immunology immune system proposed three major functions: the immune defense, immune stable immune surveillance i know, there is great significance in the anti-tumor. Immune defenses can resist bacteria, viruses, parasites and other pathogens infection. Immune surveillance function can eliminate mutant cells, prevent tumor occurrence, if the immune dysfunction or loss of immune surveillance monitor, can lead to cancer. After the body's normal cells, cancerous cells on the membrane surface expression of tumor weir, a host of fish-free system recognizes such antigens and immune response; and the exclusion of attack tumor cells. Anti-tumor immune response are many ways, both acquired immune response, but also the natural immune response; both a cellular immune response, humoral immune response there; both participate in immune cells, and other immune molecules have to participate.

(A) anti-tumor effect of cell-mediated immunity

What anticancer human immune cells may be activated, enhanced the anti-cancer cell metastasis to do? Participation in vivo anticancer effects of immune cells:

1. Anti-cancer effect of cytotoxic lymphocytes

Cytotoxic lymphocytes(CTL) play a major role in the anti-tumor immunity and have specific cytotoxicity to the same kind of autologous tumor cells and is one kind of anti-tumor lymphocytes subject to MHCI class and (or) class II antigen restrictions. Human CTL cells are CD3 and CD8. CTL cells in peripheral blood and spleen have high amounts;thoracic duct, thymus, bone marrow contains a certain amount. The ability of proliferation and accumulation in tumors localized is stronger and the body is more sensitive to radiation and chemotherapy drugs such as cyclophosphamide. CTL is an important effector cells in situ treatment of cancer.

Under certain conditions CTL can produce IL-2, IL-4, IFN, etc., to activate other immune cells, such as anti-cancer killer macrophages, NK cells and anti-B-cell joint anti-tumor effect. Such CTL has a potentially important role in anti-cancer, anti-metastasis.

2. Anti-tumor effect of natural killer cells(NK cells)

NK cells are a group of broad-spectrum anti-NK cell tumor cells, killing activity does not require prior sensitization antigen , do not rely on antibodies, does not depend on the thymus, but also no MHC restricted. The main role is to monitor and to remove cancerous cells. Clinical observations: if NK cell activity is deficient , the incidence of malignant tumors is significantly increased. NK cells are important parts of early anti-cancer immune surveillance.

NK cells bind with tumor cells through tumor cell surface receptor to release perforin protein (Perform, PF) or cytolysin piercing on the tumor cell membrane so that cancer cells die within a fluid outflow. NK cells can release natural killer cell factor (natural killer cell factor, NKCF), this factor can lyse tumor cells. NK cells have a small number, only about 3% of lymphocytes so that it have smaller force for later and larger tumors.

In addition, NK cells produce IL-2, TFN-y and TNF-a, enhance the anti-tumor effects of other cellular and humoral factors.

Distribution of NK cells in organs and tissues is the highest concentrations in peripheral blood and spleen, followed by lymph nodes and peritoneal cells. NK cells is also in the lamina propria alveoli, sinusoidal, intestinal epithelium, skin and bronchial wall, interstitial, esophagus, reproductive tract lymphoid tissue. Low NK cell activity is in bone marrow, thymus undetectable NK activity. NK cells accounted for 5% to 7% of the total number of peripheral blood lymphocytes. NK activity among individual patients is quite different and the level of NK activity in vitro and in vivo is often associated with anti-cancer effect. Therefore, NK activity is often used as a strength and prognosis of cancer immunology indicators and assessment body's anti-cancer therapy response. NK activity was reduced or deficiency often occurs in cancer metastasis. NK activity is often associated with improvement or deterioration of the condition in parallel.

Given the important role of NK cells in anti-tumor immunity, so look for a strong enhancement of biological therapy anti-tumor activity of NK preparation is important. Some micro-organisms or their products, such as BCG (BCG), Corynebacterium parvum (Corynebacteri-urn Parvwm, CP) and certain cytokines such as IL-2, IFN, immune adjuvant interferon inducer can significantly enhance NK activity. IL-2 and IFN-y combination of NK cell activity enhancement are stronger than a single factor activation. Multiple cytokines enhance the role of NK activity and eliminate residual cancer cells, reducing metastasis and relapse rates. In addition, we developed medicine XZ-C immune regulation agents which can activate NK, IFN-Y.

3. K cells

K cells are in human peripheral blood, spleen and peritoneal cavity, but not much in the thoracic duct and lymph nodes. Advanced cancer patient's serum contains large amounts of free tumor antigen which antigen binds tumor antibody so that K cells can not bind to the tumor cells, and therefore can not play a role in killing tumor. Remove the free tumor antigen, the addition of anti-tumor antibody, or with a non-specific immune stimulants, can enhance K cell activity.

Anti-tumor effect K cells without prior sensitization, do not need to complement participation, but requires the presence of anti-tumor antibodies, so K cells is one of the main anti-tumor antibody effector cells biological therapies.

4. LAK cells LAK cell is the most important modern biotechnology anti-cancer cell. In 1980 Rosenberg and his colleagues found T cell growth factor (TCGF) can short-term induce mouse spleen cells which can give a strong anti-tumor activity. Human peripheral mononuclear cells (PBMNC) can significantly kill a variety of human tumor cell under IL-2 induced. In 1982 Grimn called this kind of IL-2-activated cells which can kill tumor cells that NK cell cannot kill as Lyrnphokine-activa-ted Killer(LAK) cells . LAK cell is a group mainly consisting of mixed lymphocyte with LGL body which is activated by IL-2 cytokines into anticancer cell ; it not only kills the same kind of passaged tumor cells, more importantly, can kill itself.

LAK cells can kill broader spectrum of tumor than NK cells, which LAK cells can kill tumor cells that NK cells cannot kill.

In fact LAK cells are IL-2-activated NK cells and T cells which have similar activity to IL-2-activated NK cells.

 From a clinical and practical points all of cells , which are activated into anti-tumor cells by IL-2 cytokines , can be called LAK cells.

5. Macrophages Macrophage plays an important role in tumor immunity. It itself is a kind of effector cells capable of dissolving the tumor cells. If there is significant macrophage infiltration around tumors, the tumor spreads in the lower metastasis rate, the prognosis is better. Conversely, when macrophage infiltration around tumors is small, the rate of tumor metastasis will be highter. Prostaglandin E can inhibit the secretion of TNF gene transcription from macrophages, which antagonist was indomethacin and may counteract this effect.

6. Anti-tumor effect of monocyte-macrophage Its anti-tumor immunity, unless involved in recognizing an antigen and presented the antigen information to T cells and B cells, as well as participatory role in killing tumor cells antigen. Pathological biopsy tip: there are a lot of tumor monocyte-macrophage infiltration around the tissues, especially in primary and metastatic tumors. If the incidence of patients with a high degree of infiltration, tumor spread and metastasis is low, the prognosis is good; on the contrary, if there is no obvious monocyte-macrophage infiltration surrounding tumor tissue, metastasis rate of tumor spread is high, prognosis is poor.

Monocyte-macrophage tumor cell killing pathways are nonspecific:

(1) An activated macrophage can contact with the tumor cell directly and play a direct killing effect.

(2) The release of TNF and IL-i and other cytokines.

(3) The generation of reactive oxygen species, such as H_2O_2.

(4) The release of lysosomal enzymes and proteolytic enzymes play killing effect.

(5) The release of arginase. L-arginine is an amino acid essential growth of tumor cells. Mononuclear cells stimulates macrophages to release massive arginase and to decompose arginine so as to inhibit tumor growth.

7. Anti-tumor effect of neutrophils

Massive neutrophil can be observed as aggregation and infiltration around the tumor tissue. After activation neutrophil releases: ① reactive oxygen species; ② fat derivatives; ③ cytokines such as IFN, TNF and IL-i, these substances have tumoricidal activity.

Anti-cancer effects of neutrophils: one inhibiting tumor growth, the second is to play a role in killing. Killing time is several hours similar to macrophages, but longer than the time required lymphocytes and NK cells. Although neutrophils life is short, but are huge amounts so that anti-tumor effect must be paid attention. Neutrophils are non-specific anti-tumor effectors and have effects on a variety of tumors.

(B) Anti-tumor effect of humoral immunity

In cancer patients serum, anti-tumor antibody can be found , but cannot be detected in all cancer patients. Serum antibody is negative in the majority of progressive or metastasis patients; after surgery or radiation therapy, some patients may turn negative into positive.

Anti-tumor antibodies are divided into protective and closed two: the former is beneficial; the latter is harmful.

1. Protective antibodies

The existing of protective anti-tumor antibodies is closely related to tumor growth and decline. A month or one week before metastasis, serum anti-tumor antibody titer tends to fall, or from positive to negative. There are three kinds of protective antibodies: cytotoxic antibodies, lymphocyte-dependent antibody and cytophilic antibody.

(1) Cytotoxic antibodies: These antibodies need complement participation to kill tumor cells, they are mostly IgM or IgG class.

(2) Lymphocyte-dependent antibody (LDA): such antibodies are mostly IgG, after binding to tumor antigens, which Fc fragment binds lymphocyte surface Fc receptor, the lymphocytes and tumor target cells attach to play a killer role. Such lymphocytes are antibody-dependent killer cells, i.e., K cells.

(3) Cytophilic antibody: It is IgG class antibodies and is macrophages specifically kill tumor way. Unlike activated monocyte-macrophage non-specific cytotoxicity, when addicted to cell antibodies present in body fluids, monocyte-macrophage cells surround the tumor to form a large rosette.

2. Closed factor

Animals and cancer patients have serum blocking factors, it may be proved by experiments. Closed factor is closely related to the presence of tumor ; after tumor is resected, closed factor disappears. If the tumor is blocking factor, the tumor appears relapse. Closed factor has specificity and blocks the same type of autologous or allogeneicfor tumor tissues, however, doesn't block different classes of tumor tissue.

3. The unblocking factor

After tumor resection, not only blocking factor disappears from the serum, and the serum also appeared closed factor antagonist, called deblocking factor (unbiocking factor), deblocking factors also have tumor specificity.

(C) Anti-tumor effect of human cytokine

 Which anti-cancer cytokines can be activated, enhanced with anti-metastatic cancer cells in vivo? Cytokines against viruses, parasites, bacteria and cancer immune response in cells plays an important role in the body. It is in clinical trials for cancer treatment and other aspects of bone marrow regeneration. Therefore, cytokine research has a significant increase and there are lots of papers related to the structure and function of cytokine published in the last 10 years. Here is a brief elaboration for interleukins, colony stimulating factor, tumor necrosis factor, interferon and cytokine growth factor 5 categories.

1. Interferon (IFN)

In the 1930s it was discovered that virus-infected cells can protect surrounding cells from virus infection. In 1957 Isaacs and Lindenmann discovered a protein produced by the cells while the body cells are damaged by a virus or stimulation is an interferon. A few years later people realized that the interferon can resist cell differentiation and have immune regulation. Interferon belongs to the cytokine with a variety of biological functions, now known interferon which is divided into three categories: α, β and γ. IFN-α mainly from leukocytes; IFN-β mainly from fibroblasts; IFN-Υ mainly from T lymphocytes.

IFN has anti-proliferative effect on some tumor cells. Its anti-cancer effects may be related to immunoregulatory activity. It increases the activity of NK cells and macrophages.

The main formulations of interferon are: ① a drug name Interferon-alfa-2a, trade names Roferon R -A; ② drug name Interferon-alfa-2b, trade names Intron R -A

Clinical application of interferon: IFN-a is mainly used for ① blood system tumors and lymphomas: for hairy cell leukemia (HCL), chronic myelogenous leukemia, essential thrombocythemia, multiple myeloma, non-Hodgkin's lymphoma. ② solid tumors: Kaposi's sarcoma , renal cell carcinoma, metastatic melanoma. IFN for hematologic malignancies and solid tumors have the effect of slowing its progress; however only part of the role and transient effects.

2. Interleukin (IL)

Interleukin is human immune system natural ingredients, which are a class of cellular kinase, a chemical ingredient is protein, and is a group of molecule family. It mainly works on signal transduction of the immune system and the main function is immune regulation and immune modification. The originally definition of Interleukin is immune system signal transduction between cells. IL is secreted by white blood cells. When they bind to the receptor on the cell membrane, the target cells are activated.

Complex balance between cell activity and immune regulation is kept by the coordination of secretion of IL and immune system cells.

To date, only IL-2 and IL-11 for clinics, their therapeutic effects of cancer treatment and stimulation of hematopoietic cells are under clinical observation.

(1) Interleukin-2 (IL-2):

This lymphocyte line first is described in 1976. It is a T cell growth factor, mainly is produced by activated T helper cells and has a strong regulation immune function.

Biological activity of IL-2: IL-2 is an important material in the body to produce an immune response, which promotes proliferation of all T cel subsets, increases the activity of the cytotoxic T cell lymphocyte, NK cell and monocyte. Lymphocyte in the blood after activated is called LAK.IL-2 can help B cell growth, also promote the release of IFN-a, GM- CSF, TNF.

From 1984 it started to try recombinant IL-2 to treat various malignancies. There are multiple cases reports that IL-2 alone or combined with LAK cells were used to treat renal cell carcinoma and malignant melanoma. In May 1992 FDA approved that IL-2 is used to treat adults with metastatic renal cell carcinoma.

Recombinant IL-2 has been used as a single agent, or in combination with LAK cells, TIL cells, other biological regulatory factors, and other combined chemotherapy for cancer therapy.

(2) IL-4 : IL-4 is produced mainly by activated T cells. ① The effect on B cells: it can stimulate the growth and differentiation of resting B cells, stimulate B cells to replicate DNA, become a B cell growth factor. ②The effect on T cells: it can stimulate T cell growth, increase the production of IL-2 , promote the proliferation of cytotoxic T cells and activate LAK cells. IL-4 promote Til growth, increase the cytotoxic effect on melanoma cells.

The clinical application of IL-4: IL-4 clinical trial has entered Phase II renal cell carcinoma, mainly, melanoma and chronic lymphocytic leukemia, Hodgkin's disease and the like.

(3)Interleukin -12 (IL-12): IL-12 has immunomodulatory and anti-tumor effect. Monocytes is mainly source for IL- 12. Its main role is to: stimulate the activity of T cells and NK cell proliferation; to induce T lymphocytes and NK cells to release IFN-y.

 The clinical application of IL-12: the stage I, II clinical trials have been finished on the treatment of metastatic renal cell carcinoma and melanoma.

3. Tumor necrosis factor (TNF)

In 1975 Old etc isolated a material produced by activated phagocyte cell, monocytes and lymphocytes in the contact to toxin, called tumor necrosis factor (TNF). In 1984 TNF gene was cloned so that people can get a lot of recombinant TNF.

The biological effects of TNF: In vitro tests showed that TNF effect on cells is cytotoxicity, and can affect tumor microvasculature, resulting in the center of the tumor necrosis. In particular, TNF can induce the expression of tissue factor vascular endothelial cells and promote the formation of fibrin deposition and thrombosis.

In the anti-tumor effect of TNF, T lymphocytes play important role. Many observers prove that TNF and IFN-Y have a synergistic anti-tumor effect.

TNF has been tested in the treatment of melanoma, colon cancer, non-small cell lung cancer, ovarian cancer, but unfortunately none of them showed a clear reduction or therapeutic effect .

TNF and IFN-y work together, IFN-Y can increase the expression of cell surface TNF receptors, thus increasing the effect of TNF on cells. TNF and IL-2 together can treat all types of cancers, its strategy is IL-2 can stimulate cytotoxic lymphocyte activity and TNF can expand the effectiveness of anti-tumor. The side effects of the two drugs have emerged and only one case of breast cancer and one case of renal cell cancer in combination therapy have improved after exacerbations.

4. Hematopoietic growth factors (HGF)

HGF is also known as colony stimulating factor in the past because in vitro it can induce specific cell clones formation.

HGF effects on normal hematopoiesis: blood cells are made from pluripotent stem cell (PPSC). PPSC has small number within the bone marrow and can differentiate into any blood cell. In the bone marrow, each one PPSC split into two sub-cells, one will go to differentiation pathway; another return to the cell bank to maintain a static state. PPSC grow and develop in the sinus-like gap around stroma in the bone marrow.

(1) Neutrophils: a granule cells, total white blood cell count of 50% -70%, its maturation process has six steps, namely bone marrow blasts, before bone marrow cells, bone marrow cells, these three steps need 4-5d, then no mitosis, but continued to mature about 6d, and then released into the peripheral blood. Half of cells are free circulation; half of cells attached to the vessel wall. Cells circulating in the blood will remove into the tissue after 6- 8h, where it can survive 2-3d. Generally the number of circulating cells is three times of the number of cells in the bone marrow so there is always reservation of neutrophils in vivo. Once serious injury, a lifetime of neutrophils is reduced to a few hours.

(2) Platelets: its ancestor cells are megakaryocyte colony forming units. In the bone marrow it is the megakaryocytic mother cell, and then differentiates into megakaryocytes which can release platelets. Platelets can form clots in injured blood vessel walls, while activation of the clotting factor. Platelets in the blood can survive 7-8d.

(3) Lymphocytes: lymphoid stem cells differentiate into pre-T or B lymphocytes. Pre- T lymphocytes mature in the thymus before becoming thymocytes, lymphoblastoid cells and T lymphocytes. They can mediate cellular immunity. They can freely circulate in the blood and peripheral tissues. When it is stimulated by antigen, T cell produces a variety of cytokines, which control specific immune response.

Pre-B lymphocytes mature after moving to the spleen and lymph nodes. When the antigen-antibody appear its response on the cell membrane, B lymphocytes has become mature, and eventually become plasma cells. Plasma cells secrete specific immunoglobulins, namely antibodies, responsible for humoral immunity. B lymphocytes accounted for 20%- 25% of total lymphocytes.

Blood cell growth factors control blood cell development by stimulating cell differentiation and maturation.

Particles colony stimulating factor (G-CSF) have been made to pre-clinical animal studies, such as G-CSF was administrated to accelerate neutrophil recovery during the use of 5-FU and after total body radiation. Further research with monkeys show: intravenous injection of GM-CSF (granulosa cells of macrophage colony stimulating factor increased white blood cells after 24-72h.

In 1986 to begin clinical trials, FDA approved the use of G-CSF which can reduce the risk of incidence of infection in bone marrow cancer in patients receiving myelosuppressive chemotherapy in 1991.

16. Sources background and experience of research projects

(A). The source background of the subject and the journal of the completion(Zigzag through)

In fact my three monographs are that I assumed 85 period key scientific and technological project - Project Title: "to further explore the anti-cancer herbs for liver cancer, stomach cancer and precancerous lesions of the Western anti-metastatic combining prevention Experimental and clinical studies". The topic title of 85 period national research programs thematic: "Clinical and Experimental Research of treatment of gastric cancer and precancerous lesions with Chinese and Western medicine," directed by National Science and Technology Commission.

In April 1991 the author made an application to the State Science and Technology Commission, "85" key scientific and technological project, the project name is " The experiment and clinical research to further explore the anti-cancer herbs for stomach cancer, liver cancer and precancerous lesions of gastric cancer prevention". In June Hubei Province Science and Technology Organization Director Tian consisted of 3 project Leaders who applied for State Science and Technology research projects (who I Tongji Medical College, Hubei Medical College, one person, one person in Hubei Medical College) to come to Beijing and to report to the Ministry of Health in Beijing Traditional Chinese Medicine Administration. Two months later provincial Science and Technology Field Director with three people went to Beijing to report further design tasks to the Health Ministry issues and to accept the task. Two months later the project tasks were assigned and "85 national research programs thematic contract" was signed. At that time Professor Xu Ze suddenly had acute myocardial infarction, the front wall and high lateral myocardial infarction. After treatment and hospitalization for six months, he was discharged and rested for another six months, then gradually improved. State Science and Technology research project was suspended.

1993 Professor Xu Ze's physical health gradually recovered, and wanted to continue to carry out the program study because I had follow up a large quantities of cancer patients and found that cancer recurrence and metastasis is the key factors to influent long-term efficacy of the cancer cure and must carry out the research of clinical basis to find an effective way to prevent the recurrence and metastasis and determined to do whatever research work should be done in this area, but only have ideas but they do not research funding so that we began to find ways to set up self-research funding. In 1993 my wife was retired and opened her Clinic office, then she used her meager office income to support Professor Xu Ze animal research funding. We purchased Kunming mice, animal cages, related equipment and instruments to start animal experiments from Animal Medical Center. All of the meager income from the clinics was used to support Professor Xu Ze animal research and budget savings applications. The six rooms on the second floor were used for animal experiments. In 1996 Professor Xu Ze had been 63 years old and also applied for retirement. Since then this modest income support a series of experimental studies and clinical validation. After 16 years of hard work, summer and winter, and finally basically completed the research topics of the State Science Commission. The experimental and clinical research data and data collection summary had been published into three monographs: ① "new understanding and new model of cancer treatment." Author Professor Xu Ze with Hubei Science and Technology Publishing House in January 2001, the Xinhua Bookstore; ② "new concepts and new methods of treatment of metastasis," Author Professor Xu Ze , People's Medical Publishing House, in January 2006, the national Xinhua Bookstore issued. People's Republic of China in April 2007 and Publication Administration issued the "three hundred" original books certificate. ③ "new concept and new methods of cancer treatment," Author Professor Xu Ze, Xu Jie forward, in October 2011 Beijing People's Medical Publishing House. Followed by Dr. Bin Wu etc. in America into English. The English version was published on March 26, 2013 in Authorhouse publication, international distribution.

(B) Experiences

In the past I conducted research work in medical university and there are supervisors and colleagues to help and to guide me: excellent laboratory conditions and taken care of the research projects from National Natural Science Foundation of China, the State Science and Technology Commission issues, topics provincial Science and Technology Commission of which had made two scientific researches, a items for the domestic advanced level, one for the international advanced level, won the Hubei Provincial Science and Technology Achievement Award twice, Hubei Province Health Science and Technology Achievement Award once.

But things are different now, in this particular case, in a clinic or outpatient department, starting with an unconditional, nor equipment condition. How was this national research task carried out and completed? I have a few superficial experience or less:

1. Self-reliance, self-financing. Outpatient services for patients, outpatient revenue as research funding.

2. Retaining patient medical records and fully following-up.

3. Establishing research collaboration topics according to collaborative research projects and cooperation.

4. Establishment of detailed medical information (including epidemiological data of patients), in-depth analysis of the disease particularity of each patient treatment through the successful and failures experience.

5. Sharing the use of common instruments, equipment sharing, sharing the results of research cooperation policy which didn't need to add large instruments and equipments in collaboration with the School of Medicine Affiliated Hospital so that sophisticated equipment tests were carried out in the School of Medicine Affiliated Hospital.

6. Selecting optional topics at the forefront of science and didn't declare the funding from the state and only gave the Ministry, provincial and municipal department our research results.

7. The old professors can also be completed research projects at a private clinic, through shared with universities and scientific research collaboration and sharing of equipment and the results of the policy to fully use of advanced equipment conditions of institutions in conjunction with their decades of clinical experience.

After 20 years of hard work, summer and winter, we conducted a series of experimental studies and clinical validation work, finally completed 85 key national projects. All of experimental and clinical research data and conclusions of sum collection were written into more than one hundred scientific papers. There is no research funding for the paper published in the journal so that it had published two monographs. Now this monograph is the fourth publication about our new concept and a new approach to cancer therapy. All of our books are involved in tough climbing, step by step in three different research stages, the three different result levels, three different peaks, which is a series of coherent research steps and research process .

I outlined above all of my monographs background and context: from the results of a clinical follow-up and from clinical practice through review, evaluation and reflection of cases to the analysis of adjuvant chemotherapy, the drawbacks of traditional chemotherapy was found.

Looking from the natural medicine (TCM) of anti-cancer, anti-metastasis drugs in bearing tumor model in vitro, in vivo screening to find and made a XZ-C series of immune regulation medicine again into clinical validation now has committed for 16 years. More than12000 cases clinically were observed. From the experimental observation of basic research and clinical validation rising to the theoretical understanding, we put forward a series of innovative theories, some of which are original innovation and initiated a series of measures to reform the traditional therapies, and offered advice and strategies to overcome cancer, the strategic outlook. Such as the above research content and research, some of which are the first report of the international intellectual property of original and innovative research papers, which were each filled in my monographs in the form of the books published.

(C). The Social benefit assessment: cancer is a common disease of the current threat to human life, the cause of death of urban residents accounted for first, two, is self-evident, cancer is still the corpse of medical problems. Today on the occasion of the beginning of the 21st century, the main problem is the metastasis of cancer treatment, the most urgent problem to be solved is how to control metastasis, but the transfer is a phenomenon, an understanding, a research object. Invisible, intangible, how specific, how clear and detailed understanding of cancer metastasis processes, procedures and mechanisms, we proposed the transfer of anti-cancer should be research objectives, for this purpose, the target of anti-metastatic, measures must be specific, otherwise we cannot achieve the purpose of anti-metastatic. This book collected some of our papers which contained 14 new discoveries, new theories, new concepts for the process of metastasis, countermeasures specific: for example, where is the key to current cancer research, shut in where? The key is antimetastatic: 1. find and propose forms of cancer in humans three forms which this third form of cancer is shifting the way: this new understanding and new doctrine will cause a chain reaction of a series of initiatives Clinic of change and renewal, discover and proposed cancer treatment should aim for this three forms; 2. find and make the whole process of cancer development of two first-line theory that cancer treatment should not only pay attention to two things, but also more attention should be paid off line; 3.find that anti- specific measures should be focused the route to metastasis and stop them; 4. initiatives for cancer treatment discovery of new concepts, new models - the new model of immuno-chemotherapy should be carried out; 5. find and propose a new model of cancer metastasis treatment, anticancer proposed transfer therapy " trilogy ", more than some new understanding, new theoretical insights, new concepts have important academic significance and important academic value, it will have an important impact on the development of medical science tumor may be a million cancer metastasis patient benefit, out of a new road to overcome cancer. How to find measures of anti-cancer cell metastasis, where ways to explore, in the study of cancer? Chinese medicine is our advantage with this advantage to the development of anti-metastatic effect, to play our strengths and to catch up with international advanced level. XZ-C antimetastatic anticancer immune regulation medication after three years of experimental cancer-bearing animal models in vivo screening inhibition rate, but also 11 years of clinical verification applications, not only provides the benefit of millions of cancer patients with metastasis, but will also get millions of economic benefits for the country.

Part IV The Samples of the medical records and medical cases of XZ-C anticancer medication

1. Our medical records: In our clinical office all of the medical records are kept in detail such as the patients' life habits and the conditions before and after XZ-C medication and are sorted by liver, pancreas, stomach, lung, esophagus, cardia cancer, breast, bile duct, colon and rectus, etc.

The sample of XZ-C immune regulation anticancer medicine treatment(Translation):

Number	Name	Medical record	Gender	Age	Hometown	Profession	Address	Diagnosis	Test
1	Shi	6101204	Male	57	Zhaoyang	Farmer	Zhaoyang	Liver cancer	CT, MRI(06/22/1998)
2	Lan	6201222	Male	35	Dawu	Teacher	Dawu	Right lobe of huge liver cancer	CT(08/1998)
3	Lu	6201229	Male	38	Danyang	Land management personnel	Danyang	Right liver cancer	Ultrasound and CT(07/07/98)
4	Liu	6201230	Male	30	Gongen	Engineer	Gongen	Huge Liver cancer	Ultrasound and CT(07/07/98)
5	Zeng	6301242	Male	50	Zhongxiang	Farmer	Zhongxiang	Primary liver cancer	CT(08/98)
6	Ke	6301244	Male	54	Huangshi	ABC bank	Huangshi	Liver cancer	CT(08/98)
7	Song	6301257	Male	37	Yinchen	Elementary principle	Yinchen	Huge liver cancer	Ultrasound(07/01/98)
8	Yang	6401263	Male	51	Erzhong	Attending doctor	Erzhong	Liver cancer after surgery	Ultrasond(09/98)
9	Jiang	6401264	Male	57	Henan	Radio factory welders	Xiaogan	Huge liver cancer	Ultrasound(02/98)

Number	Hospital	Habbits Somking year	Habbits Somking amount	Habbits Drinking year	Habbits Drinking amount	Eating frenqently Pickle	Eating frenqently Pickles	Eating frenqently Bacon	Eating frenqently Salted fish	Eating frenqently Pickle
1	Zhaoyang hospital	30 years	1-2 package/day	30 years	3-4 oz/meal		+		+	
2	Dawu County hospital and xiehe hospital			10		+	+			
3	Xiehe hospital	6-7 year	little							
4	Gongen county erzhou city	More than 10 years	1 package/day	10 year	2-3oz/meal					
5	Zhongxiang city hospital					+	+		+	+
6	Huangshi hospital and xiehe hospital	30	1-2 package/day	More than 10 years	16oz/meal					
7	Yinchen city renmein hospital and xiehe hospital									
8	Erzhong city hospital and xiehe hospital									
9	Shanjianghangtan hospital and xiehe hospital	20year	1 package	More than 10 years	32oz/meal					
10	Railroad hospital and xiehe hospital									+

1

2

Number	Eat frequently Sausage	Eat frequently Fried food	Eat frequently Pepper	Eat frequently Garlic	Eat frequently Onion	Eat frequently Freshly vegatable	Eat frequently fruit	Eat frequently Mildew food	Drink frewunly Green tea	Drink oftern tea	Drink often others
1						+			+		
2			+			+			+		
3			+	+		+			+		
4			+	+		+			+		
5		+		+		+					
6			+	+		+			+		
7						+					
8						+			+		
9			+	+						+	
10		+				+	+				

3

Number	Drink water	Eat often Meat	Eat oftern Ribs soup	Eat often vegeteran	Work condition General	Work condition High pressure	Character Condition Cheerful	Character Condition Dull irriability	Exercise oftern
1	Well water	+						+	
2	Tap water					+	+	+	
3	Tap water							+	No
4	Tap water	+							
5	Pony water					+	+		
6	Well water	+							
7	Tap water	+				+	+	+	No
8	Well water							+	
9	Tap water	+	+	+		+	+		No
10	Tap water			+		+		+	

Number	Chronic medical history	Family medical history of three generation	Patch Pain medication disappear	Patch Pain medication reduction	Patch Pain medication effective	Patch removing swellen Bump size and site	Patch removing swellen Size change after using medication
1	1 years suffering from pleurisy, as puncture yellow liquid	No		+		06/22/1998 Check intrahepatic two placeholders ranging 1-3cm	
2	In junior high school suffering from jaundice, hepatitis, in 80 acute jaundice, hepatitis	Father passed away by esaphagus cancer				08/18/1998right abdminal and 12x10cm	
3	In 83 hepatitis B;96,97 Hepatitis B three positive	no					
4	Hepatitis B positivie and have nose bleeding	no				98.7 CTshow right liver lobe2.5x2.5x3 cm	
5	89 years was found to schistosome recurrent massive ascites,	Brother liver cancer				CT show right liver lober8x20cm	
6	Schistosome and lung T.B calification	No					
7	Hepatitis B half year	no				07/1998 right liver 8.7x7.5cm	
8	Hapetitis B two months ago	Father				09/1998 liver bump8.7x7.5cm	
9	67 had hepatitis B and hospitalization for three month. T.B, stamach ulcer	No				02/10/1998 ultrasound showed 15.4x12cm	
10	Debetis	no				9/29/1998CT showed that left liver 4.3x9.9cm	

5

Number	Treatment Operation way	Treatment intervention	Treatment Radiotherapy chemotherapy	Treatment When metastasis and where and size	Medication Time, kind and results	Comment
1	No	08/05/98 to 9/2015 two time of liver intervention			On July 14,1998 to 09/22 Taking XZ–C1,4,5,2 and XZ–C3 outside patch. After taking the medication, the pain in liver region reduce significantly and after intervention, the lesion decreased from 3.2x3.9cm2 to 2.2x2.4cm2	
2		08/98 to 11/98 three times of intervention			08/14/98 to 12/25/98 taking XZ–C1,4,5 AND C3 patch, the spirit well and appetite good and walking well and right sides of belly was softer than before and volume reduce from 10x10cm2 to 11x8cm2	After intervention the vessels were blocked and couldnt get up of the bed and the patients have great pain.
3					On 08/14/1998 to 12/25/1998 taking the medication XZ–C1,4,5 the patients spirit well and appetites well and looked like the normal person	

No.	Surgery	Intervention	Metastasis	Result after medication	Notes
4	No	Four times of intervention		After taking the medication, the patient can walk well and pain reduced	Chemotherapy mitonisyan 5Fu Heparin, The right lung has T.B bump
5				After two month taking the medication, the patient felt much better and walked well.	The brother had liver cancer remove and after the surgery passed away and the mother have liver problems.
6	Open surgery and couldn't remove the cancer	Two times of hepatic artery of intervention	Inside metastasis in liver	The patient felt much better after taking our medication	
7	Opened surgery and couldn't remve the cancer		Lung metastasis	The patient felt much better; however after the chemotherapy the patient condition got worse	The patient had great pain after once liver cancer bleeding.
8	Liver lobe and galdbladder removed a			The patient felt much better after taking XZ-C1,4,5 and spirit well	
9	NO		CT show galdbladder metastasis	After taking XZ-C4, the pain reduces and felt much better	The patient couldn't talk clear after four times of intervention
10	No		Lung metastasis	After taking our medications of XZ-C1,4,5 the patient didn't have any pain and no swellen	

2. The sample of the original medical record for each patient in Chinese: (see the pictures)

1. Typical cases of treatment of liver carcinoma

Case 1. Mr. Mao, male, 48 year-old, Taimen, officer. Medical record number: number: 100014

Diagnosis: primary liver carcinoma

Disease course and treatment: On August 1, 1994 because thepatient felt fatigued, he had ultrasound in the local hospital and found a 4.1cm x 4.5cm nodule in the left lobe of the liver. On August 26, 1994 the left lobe of the liverwas removed in the Xian Ha hospital. Pathological slides showed: liver cell carcinoma without any treatment. After operation, the patient was treated withanticancer immunological traditional medicine **XZ-C1+XZ-C4+XZ-C5** in ouroutpatient center. After taking these medicines, the patient's appetite increased, energy level increased and he was happy. He takes medicines regularly and comes to our office every month forfollow up and refillingof the medicines. He feels very well andgoes back to his work. On December 14,1996 there was another 1.3cm x 1.8cm nodule whichwas found by Bultrasound in the edge of the left liver. On December 30, 1996 he had thatnodule removed. After theoperation, he continued to take the medicine. After that, the patient tookhis medicinepersistently and regularly. InMay 2010when he cameto follow-up, his general condition was good and his face was glowing with health, his body was as strong as a healthy person's and the patient returned to work for more than 11 years. His appetite is great and his emotion is very good. He eats 600g food per day and his ultrasound is normal. **Comments**: On August 26, 1994 this patient had a 4.1cm x 4.5cm nodule removal of left liver. After the operation, the patient received XZ-C for treatment. On December 30, 1996 another 1.3cm x 1.8cm nodule was found and removed. After that, this patient continued to takeXZ-C. When hecame back for 16-year follow-up, his health condition is good and he can do labor work for many years. This patient is still alive and very well at the time of writing this book.

Implication: After the removal of the liver carcinoma the patient took XZ-C1+XZ-C4+XZ-C5 persistently, these medicines improve thymusfunction and protect bone morrow function of producing blood cells, protect liver function and improve the whole body immunology functionagainst disease. The operation and the medicine XZ-C can increase the long-term treatment of the cancer patients.

Case 2. Ms. Liu, female, 65 year-old, Jianxian in Hubei, officer. Medical record number: 110201

Diagnosis: primary huge liver carcinoma

Disease course and treatment: Because of discomfort in upper abdomen, the patient had CT in XieHe hospital which found that a 6.7 cm x 7.1 cm x 9 cm nodule in right liver, then diagnosed as primary liver carcinoma. She refused to take operation and chemotherapy. In July 11, 1995 she started to take the XZ-C1+XZ-C5. After 2 months, her emotion and appetite get better and her weight increased. In September 20, 1995 on follow-up ultrasound, the nodule was reduced. In November 1995 she had a chemoembolization and didn't have any other therapy. She continues to take the XZ-C for more than 6 years and continues to follow-up more than 10 years. This patient's condition is good. In May 2005 this patient is as healthy as a normal person.

July 4,1995 July 11, 1995 November
1995 1996 1997 1998 1999 2000 2001 2002 2003 2004 2005
CT XZ-C chemotherapy XZ-C XZ-C XZ-C XZ-C XZ-C XZ-C XZ-C XZ-C XZ-C XZ-C (we wrote this book day)

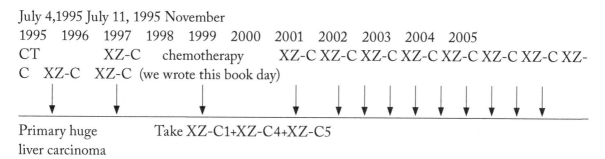

Primary huge   Take XZ-C1+XZ-C4+XZ-C5
liver carcinoma

Comments: On July 4, 1995 this patient was diagnosed with primary liver carcinoma by CT and then took XZ-C after 1 week. After 2 month, the CT scan showed that the nodule become smaller. On November 21 the chemotherapy procedure was conducted, and then she continued to take XZ-C regularly and persistently for 10 years. Now this patient is as healthy as a normal individual.

Implication: The chemotherapy+XZ-C have good results on liver carcinoma treatment. The chemotherapy can stop the blood supply to the cancernodule and chemotherapy can kill some of the cancercells. There are living cancer cellsinside and under the tumor nodulemembrane after chemotherapy; the tumor cellsdidn'tdie completely and then grew fast after circulation built up. XZ-C can protect thymus and improve the immune ability, protect the bone morrowfunction and improve the body immune function. In addition, 85% hepatic canceroccurredinthe cirrhosis patients so chemotherapy will damage the liver function. XZ-C will protect the liver.The combination of chemotherapy+XZ-C willinhibit the tumor and protect the host to improve thelong-term treatment. This is called"take out the bad and keep thegood" inChinese.

Case 3. Mr. Kei, male, 54 year-old, Yanxi in Hubei, officer. Medical record number: number: 6301244.

Diagnosis: primary liver carcinoma

Disease course and treatment: The patient had pain on the upper right abdomen for half of a month and his appetites decreased. CT inYanxia showed nodules in the right front and back lobe and left lobe. The patient was diagnosed with primary liver carcinoma. On August 20, 1998 the patient had opening surgery which revealed thatthemain tumors were in the entrance of the common duct and there were metastasis in both of left and right liver, which could not be removed. Therefor a tube for the chemotherapy was placedthrough thehepatic artery.After theoperation,the chemotherapy was used once. In October 1998 the second chemotherapy was used. Because the tube was blocked, the patient stopped using the tube. On September 8, 1998 he started taking XZ-C1+XZ-C4+XZ-C5. After taking this medicine one month, the patient's emotion and appetite were good and his body weight increased and his face was glowing with health. On his physical exam the abdomen was soft and flat and the spleen and liver could notbe felt;his general condition was good. He could support himself very well and picked up his medication by himself. On June 4, 2002 when he came back for his follow-up, his healthy condition was good; his face was glowing with health, his walking, acting and smiling were like a normal, healthy person. On the physical exam there was no abnormality found.

Comments: On August 20, 1998 liver carcinoma was found in the right and left liver and could not be removed, and a chemotherapy tube was placed, through which the chemotherapy was twice given after CT scan showed many lesions in the left lobe, right front and right back lobe. On September 8 the patient started to take XZ-C1+XZ-C4+XZ-C5. Until 2002 this patient's condition was good and didn't have metastasis.

Implication: When liver cancer could not be removed, the liver artery tube could be placed,then XZ-C1+XZ-C4+XZ-C5 was used to protect Thymus, bone morrow, liver to improve the host immune system function and induce the host to produce more anticancer factors to control the tumors and to control the development of the cancers.

Case 4. Mr. Pu, male, 51 year-old, Yin Zheng, officer. Medical record number: number: 500989

Diagnosis: primary liver cancer

Disease course and treatment: There is a 4.6cm x 3.6cm nodule in left liver and a 1.6cm x 1.6cm nodule in right liver after the patient had CT on October 30, 1997. Diagnosis was liver carcinoma. There is a 5.9cm x 4.0cm x 5.4cm nodule in the left liver lobe and a 2.1cm x 1.8cm lesion in the right liver lobe when the patienthad Ultrasound in theXieHehospital.Liver angiography showedthat the patient had liver cancer. HBsAg(+), AFP(-).Because this patient's liver functionwas poor, he couldn't stand the operation and put on the tube for chemotherapy. This patient is alcohol drinker for 40 years (250ml/per meal average). In 1996 he had Hepatitis B. In 1966 he had blood fluke. On November 25 the patient starts to take XZ-C1+XZ-C4+XZ-C5. In 1998 and 1999 the patient continued to take the medicine. The patient's condition is good, and his face is red and smiles. On November 2, 1999 he came to follow-up and the ultrasound showed the lesion was reduced. He can do light work and feels very well. For more than 2 years, he continues to take XZ-C1+XZ-C4+XZ-C5. After these medicines the patient's energy level is improving and appetite is improving. In June 2002 he went to Beijing for treatment (before he went toBeijing,he was good and walking as the normal person).During the operationthere is a 5cm x 6cm nodule in the liver which isthe same as 5 years ago and there are cancer cells in the common duct and now metastasis, and no fluid in the abdominal cavity. There is no metastasis in the liver, however because the nodule is close to the hepatic artery entrance, it is very difficult to remove the cancer nodule and then place the drainage tube. After surgery, this patient didn't have urine and had acute renal failure. He passed away on day 6.

Comments: On October 30, 1997 CT showed a4.6cm x 3.6cm nodule in left liver and in November 1997 there is a 1.6cm x 1.6cm nodule in right liver. Because the liver function was poor, the patient didn't have operation and tube placement and other treatment. On November 25 he started to takeXZ-C1+XZ-C4+XZ-C5 and continued for 5 years. His health condition was fine.

Implication: XZ-C can improve thehost immunesystem ability (including the cell and antibody immune function) to protect the central and peripheral immuneorgans, to protect the liver and kidney, andto produce anticancer factorsan dprevent cancer cells metastasis and spread.XZ-C is a medication with no side effects which helps the patient in "fight with bad and help the right". In addition the patient's disease condition was under very good control without metastasis so thattherapeutic effectwas very good. This patient tookXZ-C for 5 years, during which time his condition wasstable and theliver cancer lesionwas not increasing and there were no metastasis. Hisgeneral condition was good and not uncomfortable and the patient walked as a normal person. He went to Beijing and was diagnosed as liver cells carcinoma whichwas in theentrance of the liver andcouldn't beremoved becauseof the cancercells in the common duct. The patient underwent surgery for the placement of the T-tube for chemotherapy. After the operation, this patient didn't have urineand died of acute renal failure. If he had not had the operation which destroyed the liver and kidney function,hemight have survived to the present day.

Case 5. Mr. Huang, male, 53 year-old, Wuhan. Medical record number: number: 11202225

Diagnosis: primary huge liver cancer, liver cirrhosis after hepatitis,the later stage ofJapanese blood fluke,Portal hypertension.

Disease course and treatment: Patient's appetite decreased and he felt uncomfortable in his abdomen. InSeptember 2000CT showed a 13.6cm x 11.8cm lesion in the right liver lobe. In September 7, 2000MRI showed a huge 13.1cm x 11.4cm x 12.5cm lesion in right lobe, diagnosed as huge liver cancer in rightlobe. The patient hadhepatic arterial chemoembolization (HACE) and embolization (HAE) and the chemoembolization medicinewere hydroxycamptothecine 25mg +5-Fu 1000g and Iodized 10ml +Mitomycin 10mg. Currently his general condition is good. The change of hisliver lesions are the following which are stable andgetting small: CT showeda 11.1cm x 11.8cm lesionin the right liver lobe onOctober 12, 2000, a10.8cm x 9.8cm lesion in theright liverlobe on December 14, 2000, a 10.5cm x 9.5cm lesion on Feb 2001 and a 9.8cm x 8.9cm lesion on September 3, 2001in the right liverlobe. This patient started to take XZ-C1+XZ-C4+XZ-C5 on January 9,2002and hisgeneral condition is good, just as his emotion, appetite and sleep are very good. Hecomes back for check-upevery month and takes his medicine regularly. OnOctober 21, 2002 during his follow-up, his general condition is good, emotion isstable, andappetite is good and bowel movement is good andhis routine is regularand he exercises regularly. He reports not having had a cold during the last four years. He lived as a normal healthy person.

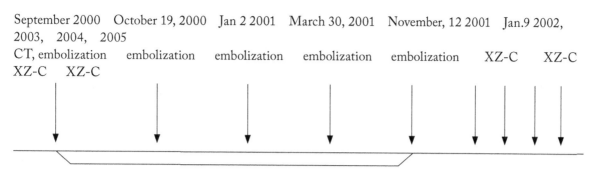

September 2000   October 19, 2000   Jan 2 2001   March 30, 2001   November, 12 2001   Jan.9 2002, 2003,   2004,   2005

CT, embolization   embolization   embolization   embolization   embolization   XZ-C   XZ-C
XZ-C   XZ-C

Lesion in the right liver   embolization
13.6cmx11.8cm

Comments: This case is primary huge liver carcinoma which had five times embolization and the lesion was getting smaller and had very good response. Last embolization is on November 12, 2001 and the lesion is 9.8cm x 8.9cm. He started to take XZ-C1+XZ-C4+XZ-C5 on Jan 9, 2002. The XZ-C1 can kill the cancer cells and not kill the normal cells; XZ-C4 protects thymus and inhibits thymus shrinkage; XZ-C5 protects liver function. This patient continues to take this medicine for more than 3 years, however when he came back for follow-up in the fourth year, his health condition is general, disease is stable and there is no metastasis and no further development. His emotion is stable, his appetite is good, and he walks as a normal healthy person. The experience from this case is for primary huge liver cancer, first embolization treatment are given to make this lesion smaller and stable, later use XZ-C to support the long-term therapy and to protect the liver function and to improve the immune system and to control the metastasis.

Case 6. Mr. Lee, male, 53 year-old, Wuhan, farmer. Medical record number: number: 9901979

Diagnosis: primary huge liver carcinoma, late stage Japanese blood fluke hepatic cirrhosis.

Disease course and treatment: On January 22, 2001 the patient felt pain in the right back. In Feb 26, 2001 ultrasound showed a nodule in the liver. On January 31, 2001 CT showed a 14cm x 1cm lesion in the right liver lobe diagnosed as primary huge liver cancer in the right liver. On March 1, 2001 the open abdomen surgery was done in Tongjin Hospital and the pump implantation in the portal vein because the lesion was huge and couldn't be removed. After the surgery the patient received chemotherapy once. This patient had 30 years Japanese blood fluke. On March 9, 2001 this patient started to take XZ-C medicine. He used XZ-C1+XZ-C4+XZ-C5, LMS, MDZ, and XZ-C3 placed on a fist-size lump in the right rib edge area. After one month of taking this medicine, the patient's condition is getting better and his emotion is stable and happy. His appetite is increasing. The lump in the right rib edge area is getting smaller and softer than before. After he continued to take this medicine for three months, his general condition is good and his appetite and sleep are good. His energy level is recovering and he is walking as a normal person. On October 22, 2001 Ultrasound showed a 6cm x 7.8cm lesion in the right lobe liver and he continues taking XZ-C1+XZ-C4+XZ-C5 and using XZ-C3 on the lump. On November 19, 2003 during his follow-up, ultrasound showed this lesion size the same as before, kidney function is normal and CXR didn't show abnormality, there is no positive lymph node and the lump on the right rib edge is soft and getting smaller and the boundry is clear and not painful. This patient continued to use XZ-C1+XZ-C4+XZ-C5.

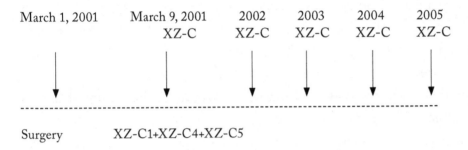

| March 1, 2001 | March 9, 2001 | 2002 | 2003 | 2004 | 2005 |
| | XZ-C | XZ-C | XZ-C | XZ-C | XZ-C |

Surgery   XZ-C1+XZ-C4+XZ-C5

Comments: This case is diagnosed as primary huge liver cancer and the lesion can not be removed so that the portal vein pump was placed for chemotherapy once. In March 2001, he started to use the XZ-C1+XZ-C4+XZ-C5 and topical XZ-C3 for 4 years. His general condition is stable and didn't develop further and didn't metastasize.

Case 7. Mr. Wang, male, 40 year-old, Shangdou, teacher. Medical record number: 900164

Diagnosis: primary liver cancer

Disease course and treatment: The tumor was removed in the mediastinum on June 28, 1989. The pathology showed the thymoma with lymphocyte type and high malignant tumor and without treatment. In Feb 1995 ultrasound showed a lesion in liver. On Feb 23, 1995 CT showed a 8.2cm x 8.7cm lesion in right posterior lobe and many nodes mixed together. On June 5, 1995 the hepatic artery graph embolization was done. The chemotherapy was injected in the lesion and on November 10, 1995 this right liver lesion was removed and the pathology showed liver cell cancer. On December 21, 1995 ultrasound showed a 3.8cm x 3.2cm lesion in the right liver lobe which was the recurrent lesion after the surgery and there was fluid in the right chest cavity and the right low lung is not distended and CXR showed right low lung metastasis. On

December 23, 1995 this patient took the XZ-C1+XZ-C4+XZ-C5 for more than two years and follow-up more than five years. His general condition is good and he continued to teach and work normally without other treatment.

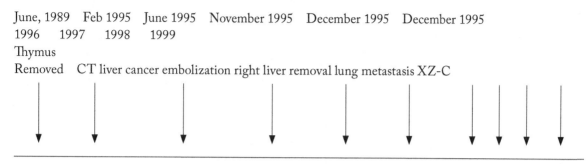

June, 1989   Feb 1995   June 1995   November 1995   December 1995   December 1995
1996   1997   1998   1999
Thymus
Removed   CT liver cancer embolization right liver removal lung metastasis XZ-C

taking XZ-C1+XZ-C4+XZ-C5

Comments: In May 1995 CT showed a 7.1cm x 6.6cm lesion in the right liver lobe. In 1995 the embolization was done once. On November 10, 1995 this right liver lesion was removed and diagnosed as liver cancer. On December 21, 1995 ultrasound showed a 3.8cm x 3.2cm lesion in the right liver lobe which was the recurrent lesion. On December 23, 1995 this patient took the XZ-C1+XZ-C4+XZ-C5 and his condition is good for more than four years.

Implication: there is very good result for liver cancer while using the combination of embolization +operation removal+XZ-C immune anticancer medicine.

Case 8. Mr. Zhao, 34 year-old, JinZhou, accountant. Medical record number: 380742

Diagnosis: primary huge liver cancer

Disease course and treatment: On Feb 26, 1997 there was a 13cm x 10.4cm lesion between the liver quadrate lobe and left lobe because the patient feel uncomfortable about her stomach and had ultrasound test, then MRI showed a 7.9cm x 11.2 cm x 11.0cm lesion and portal vein had the cancer thrombus. On March 1, the patient had fever of 39°C. On March 2, the patient was transferred to the XieHe hospital because of high fever and there is a 5cm x 6cm hard lump under sternum. On March 10 the embolization was performed and the patient had great reaction to this. This patient had embolization on April 30, on July 9, and on September 18. Then lump decreased significantly. On March 4 the patient started to take XZ-C1+XZ-C4+XZ-C5 to stabilize the lesion and to control the spread and to prevent the metastasis. After taking the medicine, the patient's emotion and appetite are getting better and the general condition is getting better and life quality is getting better. The lump under the sternum couldn't be palpated.

Feb 26 , 1997	March 3, 1997	March 10,1997	April 30,1997	July 9, 1997	Sept 18, 1997,	1998	1999	2000
XZ-C	Embolization	Embolization	Embolization	Embolization	XZ-C	XZ-C	XZ-C	
CT								
MRK								

Taking   the XZ-C1+XZ-C4+XZ-C5

Comments: For this primary huge liver carcinoma, four times embolization were performed and the patient took XZ-C persistently so that the combination of embolization and XZ-C had good treatment result and life quality increased. The lump under sternum went away. In the past three years the patient's general condition is good.

Implication: The combination of embolization and XZ-C had good results and supported the long-term results. Embolization can kill the parts of cancer cells and decrease lump size, however there are residual alive cancer cells and continued growth so that after embolization the patient took the XZ-C1+XZ-C4+XZ-C5, which can kill 10^5 cancer cells. Taking XZ-C for long-term can control tumors and stablize the lesions, preventing metastasis. An important problem with embolization chemotherapy is that cancer cell division continues while chemotherapy can only be used periodically due to the toxic side effects. The cancer cells can grow back during the intervening period. The embolization can damage most of the cancer cells and XZ-C can support our immune ability to kill the residual cancer cells.

Case 9. Mr. Zheng, male, 48 year-old, Enshi, officer. Medical record number: 500987

Diagnosis: primary liver carcinoma

Disease course and treatment: In January 1996 a thumb-sized lesion was found in the right liver lobe and was treated with protection of liver treatment. In October 1997 a 5.7cm x 5.7cm lesion was found by ultrasound. In October 1997 the patient had open abdominal surgery and the lesion couldn't be removed so a hepatic tube was placed for pump chemotherapy. Pathological diagnosis is liver cells carcinoma.

In December 23, 1997 chemotherapy was given for the second time; however the reaction is great so that the patient didn't have chemotherapy again. In December 25, 1997 the patient started to take the XZ-C. At follow-up, his condition is stable and healthy and he is happy. His appetite is good and energy level is up and he walks and performs other activities as the normal individual. In November 1998 the patient returns to regular work as teacher and his energy level is great.

Jan   Oct   Dec   Dec 25   April   May   July   Aug   1998   Oct   1998   Dec   1998   Jun1999
1996 1997 1997 1997   1998   1998 1998

CT   CT lesion operation,

    Increase   XZ-C --

                Taking XZ-C1+XZ-C4+XZ-C5

Comments: In January 1996 a lesion was found in the right liver and in November 7, 1997 the chemotherapy pump was placed during surgery following which chemotherapy was used twice. After the second time in Dec 23, 1997, the patient only received XZ-C1+XZ-C4+XZ-C5 for three years. His condition is good.

Implication: The hepatic arterial chemoembolization and XZ-C1+XZ-C4+XZ-C5 had good result because the chemotherapy can kill most of cancer cells and XZ-C1+XZ-C4+XZ-C5 can kill cancer cells and protect hosts as well as improve the host immune function and get rid of the rest of the cancer cells.

Case 10. Ms. Wei, female, 36 year-old, Chibi in Hubei. Medical record number: 15603095

Diagnosis: Liver cell cancer

Disease course and treatment: The patient had pain in upper abdomen and her appetite decreased and she was tired for more than half month so that she had CT which showed a lesion in left liver and AFP is more than 400ug/L. On June 6, 2004 the left half of the liver was removed and a portal vein chemotherapy pump was placed in Chibi hospital. During the operation, a lesion was found in most of the left liver so that the pump was placed after the removal of the left liver lobe (the end into hepatic portal vein). After operation, the chemotherapy was used twice through the pump and ultrasound showed a 1.7cm x 1.8cm lesion in right liver. Pathology shows: liver cells cancer. On Sept 27, 2004 the patient started to take XZ-C1+XZ-C4+XZ-C5, LMS and MDZ and follow-up every month to fill up the medicine. On April 2008 ultrasound showed no lesion in the liver and AFP is normal. The patient's general condition is good. Her emotion is stable and her appetite is good. Her body weight is increased and her energy lever is good and she works in other city. She continued taking the medicine for more than 7 years and she is healthy.

Comments: After left liver removal and pump chemotherapy which was used twice with right liver lesion, the patient still continued to take XZ-C to protect thymus and bone morrow for more than seven years and her health condition is good. Recently she works in another city and fills up her medicine every month.

Case11. Mr. Huang, male, 38 year-old, Hubei, worker. Medical record number: 13402661

Diagnosis: primary liver carcinoma

Disease course and treatment: In Feb 16, 2003 during physical exam, the ultrasound found a liver tumor and CT showed a 9.8cm x 5.8cm lesion in positive right lobe for which boundary line is not separate, clear. Diagnosis was liver cell carcinoma. AFP is 91.875ug/l. In March 8, 2003 the right half liver was removed, for which Pathology diagnosis is liver cell carcinoma. The patient only takes XZ-C after operation. He takes XZ-C regularly and persistently for more than 8 years, during which he follows-up every 2 months. His general condition is good. He returns to work for more than four years and energy level is great. On December 10, 2009 he comes back to follow-up and fills his medicine and his general medical control was great and appetite is good and no other complaints. This year he works in another city and he is healthy.

This is the case which after operation the patient survives more than eight years through only taking XZ-C medicine.

March 8, 2003	April 2003	2004	2005	2006	2007	2008	2009	2010
Right half liver removal	XZ-C	XZ-C	XZ-C	XZ-C	XZ-C	XZ-C	XZ-C	XZ-C

Liver cell cancers taking XZ-C1+XZ-C4+XZ-C5

Comments: This is a case in which, after right half liver removal and the patient only taking XZ-C medicine to improve thymus function and to improve the immune function, the patient survives more than eight years. He comes to work four years now.

Implication: XZ-C medicine can work as an assistant therapy for the surgery to improve the host immune function and to prevent recurrence and metastasis.

Case 12 Mr. Lee, male, 60 year-old, Wuhan, officer. Medical record number: 270003392

Diagnosis: liver cells cancer

Disease course and treatment: In November 2005 during the physical exam B showed a 5.4cm x 4.0cm lesion in right liver lobe. In the same month the patient had right half liver removal. Pathology diagnosed as liver cell carcinoma. After the operation, on November 28, 2005 he started to take XZ-C1+XZ-C4+XZ-C5, LMS and MDZ to protect thymus and bone morrow. He takes the medicine regularly for more than five years and his general condition is good and his appetite is great and he is healthy.

November 2005	November 28 2005	2006	2007	2008	2009	2010
Right half liver removal	XZ-C	XZ-C	XZ-C	XZ-C	XZ-C	XZ-C
Liver cell cancer	taking XZ-C1+XZ-C4+XZ-C5, LMS and MDZ					

Comments: The patient had a lesion in the right liver, which had right half liver removed. After operation, the patient only takes XZ-C1+XZ-C4+XZ-C5, LMS and MDZ for more than five years and his health condition is good.

2. Typical cases of assistant treatment after operation in pancreatic carcinoma

Case13. Ms. Yao, female, 73 year-old, Wuhan. Medical record number: 240469

Diagnosis: gallbladder adenocarcinoma

Disease course and treatment: In Dec 1995 the patient felt pain in right upper quadrant getting worse, then admitted to hospital in Feb 1996. On March 26 1996 the patient was diagnosed as gallbladder cancer during operation, then removed of the gallbladder and put T-tube placement to have bile drainage. Pathological diagnosis is papillary adenocarcinoma involved in muscle layers with gallbladder stones. On April 26, 1996 the tube was removed and the patient started to take XZ-C1+XZ-C4. On Jan 23, 1997 the patient had severe pain and was diagnosed as common duct blockage and jaundice by ultrasound. Common duct dilated into 1.5cm. After taking the medicine for 2 months, the jaundice went away, appetite increased, energy level increased. She took the medicine regularly for 15 months. In July 1997 the patient recovered completely, walked normally, activities are the same as a normal individual. She did the chores every day. On December 4, 1999 her son come to office for follow-up: after taking this traditional medicine for one and half years, the patient is doing fine; she is happy and has recovered her energy level and does chores, plays cards and goes to shop. Her activities are the same as other women.

Comments: On March 26, 1996 the patient was diagnosed as gallbladder cancer and the gallbladder was removed. The patient didn't' take any other treatment because of her age and weakness. On April 26, 1996 she start to take XZ-C1+XZ-C4. On Jun 1997 jaundice came after blockage of common duct. She continues to take XZ-C for 2 month and the jaundice went away. She took XZ-C regularly and persistently. Follow-up the patient for four years, she is fine.

Implication: Taking XZ-C1+XZ-C4 for long term treatment can improve quality of life and prevent metastasis and improve the patient's survival rate.

Case 14. Mr. Zhou, male, 53 year-old, XiaoGan, officer. Medical record number: 950004284

Diagnosis: Pancreatic adenocarcinoma

Disease course and treatment: In August 15, 2007 the patient was diagnosed as hepatitis and had CT which showed tumor on the pancreas and blockage of the common duct. The patient had operation for removal of the pancreas and duodenum. Pathology showed malignant pancreas adenocarcinoma and metastasis of the common duct and duodenal wall and the membranes of the pancreas. There are no lymph node metastases around the pancreas. After four weeks chemotherapy the wbc and platelet, and other side effects were significant. On June 16, 2008 the patient started to take XZ-C1+XZ-C4+XZ-C5+LMS+MDZ. This patient's general medication is fine and his appetite is great. He takes his medication regularly and fills his medication regularly for more than four years. In Sept 2010 when he came back to follow up, his medical condition was good and there was no lymph node enlargement and his abdomen is soft and there is no lump palpation. Now the patient is back at work for one year and he is healthy.

August 21, 2007	June 2008 2009 2010
Removal of pancreas and duodenal chemoth chemoth chemo chemo	XZ-C
Pancreas cancer	Taking the XZ-C1+XZ-C4+XZ-C5

Comments: This patient had removal of the pancreas and duodenum and after four times chemotherapy, the side effects were significant and then started to take XZ-C for more than four years and now goes back work.

Implication: After the pancreas adenocarcinoma operation, the XZ-C can protect the thymus and protect the bone marrow to control the metastasis and to improve survival rates.

Case 15. Mr. Fong, male, 50 year-old, Hubei Lou Tang, peasant. Medical record number: 330651

Diagnosis: Pancreas cancer

Disease course and treatment: Because of discomfort in upper abdomen for more than three months, he had jaundice and had opening abdomen surgery showing: No stones in the bile system and enlargement of the pancreas. The tumor couldn't be removed and Pathology showed pancreatic cancer. CT showed enlargement of pancreas head and dilation of the bile duct in liver. After the operation the jaundice extended persistently. On December 11, 1996 he started to take the XZ-C and after one month his medical condition got better and his appetite increased, however he still had little jaundice and weakness and sweating. After taking XZ-C and soup two months the jaundice and pain reduced and got better. After four months, the jaundice was gone completely and his appetite and energy level were good. His pain in abdomen was mild. In July 1998 he returned to work and did mild labor work and his face looks red. He continues to take his medicine for many years. On April 6, 2004 his family introduced a new patient to us and told us that this patient is fine and his activities are as a normal person's and he does his chores very well.

omments: This patient has pancreas head cancer and jaundice. On November 28 1996 during the operation, this tumor cannot be removed and the Pathology is pancreas cancer with the dilation of the bile duct system in the livers. On December 11, 1996 this patient took ZX-C and soup. After seven months his jaundice is reduced and he continues to take medicine to improve his immune system. Until July 1998 his condition is completely normal. He continues to take his medicine for more than four years and later changed to taking the medicine periodically to support his healthy condition. This patient has followed up for more than nine years and his condition is very good.

3. Typical cases of assistant treatment after operation in stomach carcinoma

Case 16. Mr. Chan, male, 65 year-old, Wuhan, retired officer. Medical record number: 280555

Diagnosis: Adenocarcinoma in the pyloric area of the stomach and recurrence after surgery in the remaining stomach

Disease course and treatment: This patient had pain in the upper abdomen for more than one year and in June 1993 he was diagnosed as stomach cancer and had removal of the great curvature in the stomach. After the operation, he had FM chemotherapy once which caused anemia and weakness and wbc is 1900. 8 months after operation, the patient had abdomen pain with vomiting and had left upper abdominal pain for half year. On March 25, 1994 the Barium showed: there was no filled on the upper area of the stomach and part damage of the membranes and the narrow change in the cutting parts. A barium swallow showed recurrence of the stomach cancer. On May 3, 1996 ultrasound showed that there is no lesion inside the liver. Because this patient couldn't eat rice and just eats noodles and liquid food so that he had fatigue and no energy, he didn't want to have operation. In June 1996 he started to take XZ-C. After that he is fine and his appetite is increased and he takes this medicine regularly for more than four years. On May 6, 2000 when he came back to follow-up, his general condition is great and his face looks red and healthy. Walking and activities are normal as the others and he eats rice soup and banana often as his meal.

June 1993	March 1994	June 1996	June 1997	June 1998	June 1999	Dec 1999	May 2000
Stomach operation							

taking XZ-C

Comments: In June 1993 the patient had stomach removal. In March 1994 the cancer recurred and the junction part turned narrow. After taking XZ-C+XZ-C4 only, for more than six years his health condition is great.

Implication: For the recurrence of the stomach cancers, the junction of the surgery was not closed completely and the patient could still eat food. After taking the medicines to improve thymus function to control the tumor growth and prevent the tumor growth and metastasis. The patient's medical condition is stable and he is still alive.

Case 17. Mr. Liu, 65 year-old, Wuhan, economist, Medical record number: 2200421

Diagnosis: fundus and cardia stomach carcinoma

Disease course and treatment: In Jan 1995 the patient had stomach pain for six months and had endoscopy which showed stomach pyloric adenocarcinoma and had surgery for primary stomach removal and to connect the esophagus with stomach body. After the operation the patient was weak and thin so he didn't have chemotherapy. On March 16, 1996 he started to take the XZ-C1+XZ-C4 for more than five years persistently, and then changed to periodically taking the medicine.

Jan 1995	March 1996	1997	1998	1999	2000	2001	2002	2003
Operation	XZ-C	XZ-C						

Taking the XZ-C1+XZ-C4

Comments: In Jan 1995 this patient had the removal of the cardia and fundus of the stomach which connected the esophagus with the stomach body. Because of his weakness, he didn't take chemotherapy and takes the XZ-C1+XZ-C4 only for more than ten years and his medical condition is fine.

Implication: After the operation, the medicine XZ-C can control the cancer, preventing recurrence and metastases and has very good curvature results.

Case 18. Mr. Cheng, male, 65year-old, worker. Medical record number: 260518

Diagnosis: Recurrence and metastasis of stomach cancer

Disease course and treatment: On June 1, 1994 the endoscope showed a 3cm x 3cm ulcer in the stomach pyloric area for which the Pathology was adenocarcinoma in the pylorus. In June 1994 the patient had surgery to remove the cancer. Pathology showed cancer cell in the muscular layer and not the lesser curvature and mucous adenocarcinoma. In May 1996 the patient felt pain in the upper abdominal area and decreased appetite and fatigue. On May 14, 1996 he was admitted into the hospital and had fever, pain in the abdomen, low protein and ascites and fluid in the chest. There were many cancer cells in the ascetic fluid. Because of the heavy ascites the patient came to our office and started to take our medicine. After taking this medicine the patient's general medication condition is very well and appetite was great and his ascites is reduced and his energy level is increased. He came back to follow-up regularly. After the surgery six years and recurrence for four years the patient's condition is great and appetite is great and activities are as the normal persons.

Comments: This patient had surgery in June 1994. After that he didn't have any treatment. In May 1996 he had fluid in his chest and his abdominal cavity. Because the ascites is heavy, he started to take the XZ-C and his general medical condition is good and follow-up with us for more than four years.

Implication: One year after surgery this patient had fluid and cancer cells in his chest and abdominal cavity. He takes the medicine persistently and his medical condition was controlled and his life qualities are improved and he survives very well with his cancer.

Case 19. Mr. Wang, male, 53 year-old, Xinzhou, peasant. Medical record number: 800157

Diagnosis: Recurrence of stomach carcinoma

Disease courses and treatment: In February 1994 the patient felt uncomfortable and endoscopy showed stomach carcinoma. In June 1994 he had stomach removal and followed with chemotherapy for two courses of treatment with 5-Fu+MMC. On May 30, 1995 a barium scan showed damage of the junction sides and narrow area for more than five cm and partially obstructed and there is a 5 cm diameter mass in the junction area. On June 2, 1995 he started to take XZ-C1+XZ-C4. After taking his medicine his general medical condition is great and appetite is increased and can eat the rice and bananas. He comes back to follow up regularly for more than two and half years. His health condition is great.

June,1994	July, 1994	August, 1994	May 30, 1995	June 2,1996	1996	1997
Operation	215soph.	Chem.	GI recurrence	XZ-C	XZ-C	XZ-C

Taking the medicine

Comments: The patient had recurrence of stomach cancer after the partial removal of the conjuction of the stomach. In June 1995 he started to take the XZ-C and follow up with us for more than two and half years. His condition is great.

Implications: XZ-C can stable the recurrence of the cancinoma and improve the patient's condition well and had very good results.

Case 20 Ms. Zhang, female,39 year-old, Wuhan, account, Medical record number::
1700321

Diagnosis: the stomach cancer from the stomach ulcer, low differential adenocarcinoma

Disease courses and treatment: in March 1994 because of the uncomfortable in the
upper abdomen for one month and getting worse for one week so that the endoscopy
showed the stomach ulceration. On April 20 1994 the major stomach was removed and
had chemotherapy for six courses of the treatment after the operation with xxxxx+xxxxx
to protect the livers. Pathology showed the low differential stomach canciroma and
had lymph nodes metastasis. On November 22 1995 he started to take XZ-C1+XZ-
C4+XZ-C8 only to protect the bone marrow and follow up with us for more than ten
years. He doesn't have metastasis and recurrence and his condition is great.

April 20, 1994	Chem 6 times	November 22, 1995	1996	1997	1998	1999	2000	2005
Operation		XZ-C	XZ-C	XZ-C				

Taking XZ-C1+XZ-C4+XZ-C8

Comments: this patient had low degree adenocarcinoma in the stomach and lymph
node metastasis. On April 20 1994 he had the removal of his major stomach, then
he had six courses of the chemotherapy. On November 22 1995 he took the medicine
only and followed up with us for more than ten years. His medical condition is great.

Suggustions: After the operation the combination of the chemotherapy and XZ-C
medicine can improve the long-term treatment. XZ-C can prevent the cancer recurrence
and metastasis.

Case 21 MR.Zhou, male, 57 year-old, officer, Medical record number::1900368

Diagnosis: pyloric and greater curvature of the stomach carcinoma from the ulceration

Disease courses and treatment: In September 1995 after the removal of the stomach
caner, he had two courses of the chemotherapy and the side effects were significant
and his hair lost. Pathology: medium differential adenocarcinoma without the lymph
nodes metastasis. On January 5 1996 he started to take the medicine and his medical
condition is getting better and his appetite is good. He persistenly takes his medicine
for more than four years and his medical condition is stable.

September 1995	1995	1995	Jan 5 1996	1997	1998	1999
The removal of His stomach	Chem(1)	216 soph.(2)	XZ-C	XZ-C	XZ-C	XZ-C

Comments: the patient had the cancinoma from the stomach ulceration, with medium differential. On September 25 he had the operation and took two period of the chemotherapy after the operation, however the reaction was strong so that he took the XZ-C only since then to prevent the recurrence and metastasis of the cancinoma. He took this medicince for more than four year and his medical condition is great.

Sugguest: After his opeariton his immune system function is decreasing so that the chemotherapy was used for short-term and XZ-C1+XZ-C4 for long-term to protect thymus and to prevent the recurrence and metastasis.

Case 22 MR.Yi, male, 58year-old, Shanxing, Medical record number::8801750

Diagnosis: stomach carcinoma

Disease courses and treatment: after the pain in the stomach two years, on April 27,2000 he had the endoscope which showed the stomach cancer which low-grade adenocarcinoma in the body of the stomach so that he had radical removel. After five days of his surgery, he had a chemotherapy. On June 19 2000 he started to use XZ-C1+XZ-C4 to protect his thymus and the patients took the medication persistently. So far he takes this medication for more than eleven years and continues to follow up with us. On Jan eight 2010 when he came back to follow up, his general medical condition was very well.

April 27 2000
Operation　　Chemotherapy once　June 19 2000　2001　2002　2003　2004　2005　2006　2010

Comments: after the radical operation, there is once chemotherapy. Because of the reaction, he kept using the XZ-C to protect his thymus and bone marrow to prevent the immune system and protect the metastasis and recurrence. He kept using the small amount medication to get good health.

Case23 Ms. Zheng, female, 54year-old, worker Medical record number::12602507

Diagnosis: the stomach adenocarcinoma

Disease courses and treatment: in September 2002 the endoscope showed that stomach cancer. On Octocber 14 2002 he had radical operation. Pathology showed I-II stages and in the deep muscular layer and 2/3 lymph nodes metastasis and once chemotherapy after the operation. WBC decreases and then stop. On Octocber 25 2002 he started to take XZ-C1+XZ-C4. After that he is llively and his appetite is good and his physical strengthen gradually increase and have continues to take this medicine for more than eight year-old. On September 4 2010 when he follow up to us, his healthy condition was great.

Octocber 14, 2002	chemotherapy Octocber, 25 2002	2003	2005	2006,	2007	2008	2009	2010
Radical	once	XZ-C			⟶			

Comments: after this patient had operation and once chemotherapy, his reaction is strong so that he started to take XZ-C to protect his thymus and to prevent his bone marrow to inhibit the recurrence and metastasis. For eight years he takes this medication persistently and his medical condition is healthy.

Case 24 Mr. Liao, male, 60 year-oldu, Wuhanjiongxia, Medical record number::7101403

Diagnosis: the pyloric carcinoma

Disease course and treatment: Because he had pain in the upper back and under stern for more than four months, he had endoscopy and bisopy done which showed the low grade pyloric adenocarcinoma. In December 1998 he had the radical removal of the total stomach the xian hei which the Pathology showed the same results as before and had the metastasis of the lymph nodes in the lesser and greater curvative. He had once chemotherapy and on Jan 31 1999 he started to take XZ-C1+XZ-C4 and he is spirited and his appetite is good and his physical lever is great. He followed up with us for more than twelve years and his general medical condition is great.

December 1998
Stomach removal   Jan 31 1999
                     XZ-C

Comments: this patient had the stomach removal and chemotherapy. After one month later he started to take the XZ-C to protect the thymus and bone marrow. For 12 years his healthy condition is good.

4. Typical cases of assistant treatment after operation in lung carcinoma:

Case 25 Mr. Liu, male, 68year-old, Changzhou, officer, Medical record number::8701735

Diagnosis: the central lung cancer on the right upper of the lung with the metastasis

Disease courses and treatment: in Octocber 1998 he coughed two weeks with the pain in the right shoulder and was treated with inflammation. In Jan 1999 his cough is getting worse and this appetite is decreased and fatigure and getting weak. On CT there is mass on the right upper lung showing the central lung. He had endoscope and biopsy which showed that lung adenocarcinoma in the xxxxxx. He and his family member don't want to have operation. In Feb 1999 after chemotherapy for one course, his reaction to the chemotherapy was strong and stopped to use it. This patient had metastasis in the left lung which showed there are two lesions and he coughed with mucous and blood sputdu and difficult walking. On April 23 2000 he started to take the XZ-C1+XZ-C4+XZ-C7, LMS+MDZ for three months and his general condition is good and he is lively and his appetite is great. In December 2000 his medical condition is stable, and he is lively. His appetite is good and his breath is smooth and his face is red. He walked as the normal person and sometimes he coughs. He persistently takes this medication for more than four years and when he comes back to follow up during the five years, his general condition is great and he walked as the normal healthy person.

Comments: this patient has the central lung cancer in the right upper lung. In April 2000 he started to use XZ-C1+XZ-C4+XZ-C7. XZ-C1 is used to kill the cancer cells only without kill the normal cells; XC-C4 protect the thymus and increase the thymus weight and to protect the bone marrow, XZ-C7 inhibit the lung cancer cells and protect the lung and solve the suptid. After short-term chemotherapy he started to take the XZ-C to strengthen his long-term therapy. XZ-C improve the whole body immune system and he is lively and his appetite is good and his spleen is great and help the patients against the diseases and help the patient's organ functions and the nutrition condition and metabliztion recover so that the patients' healthy condition is recovery.

This patient didn't have the operation. In Feb 1999 he had chemeotherapy, however there is left lung metastasis after chemotherapy. Afterh that, he only took the XZ-C to control the metastasis. He persistently took the medicine for more than four years and his medical condition is great without any complaints. He followed up with us for more than seven years. In May 2005 when he came back to follow up, his general medical condition is great and his appepital is good without other symptoms. His walking and activities and he talks cheerfully and humorously.

Case26 Mr. Zhou, male, 49year-old, Wuhan, officer, Medical record number:s: 410804

Diagnosis: lung cancer in the right low labor

Disease courses and treatment: In 1996 the patient started to have cough and chest tightness and low fever and difficult breath and was treated as the Cold. In April 1997 he suddenly started to cough blood and X-ray and CT showed the right lung cancer in low lobe. And at the same month he had right low lobe lung removal and Pathology showed that lung low grade adenocarcinoma. After the operation, his condition is stable and didn't have chemotherapy and radioactive therapy. On May 15 1997 he started to take XZ-C:1, 4, 7, vitamin C, B6 E, A. After he took these medicine his energy level is increase and appetite was great and his face is red and there were no recuurence and metastasis and no complaints. In June 2004, the patient came back to follow up with us he continues to take these medicine more than three years. Everything is stable. So far his condition is stable as the normal healthy person after he took his medication more than eight years.

Comments: this patient has right low lobe low grade adenocarcinoma. After the operation, he didn't have radioactive and chemotherapy treatment and he only takes the XZ-C medication XZ-C1+C4+C7. After taking these medicine more than eight years, his energy level is high and appetite is good and his healthy condition is great.

Case 27 Mr. Zheng, male, 52 year-old, Wuhan, driver, Medical record number::11302254

Diagnosis: right lung low grade adenocarcinoma with lymph node metastasis

Disease courses and treatment: because of bloody cough he had the CTscan which showed that right low lung tumor and the bronchoscopy didn't show abnormal. On December 12 2001 he had the removal of the right middle and lower lobe and one lymph node between lobe and two lymph node in the entrance were found. Pathology showed that low grade adenocarcinoma with lymph node mestastasis. After the operation he has once chemotherapy. In 2002 he started to take XZ-C to prevent the tumor recurrence and metastasis. He continues to take the XZ-C1+C4+C7+LMS+MDZ for more than three year and his condition is stable and he is energetic and his appetite is great.

Comments: this patient has the right low lobe adenocarcinoma with lymph node metastasis. After the chemotherapy once, then using the XZ-C1+C4+C7 as the supplement treatment. XZ-C1 kills the cancer cells without killing the normal cells. XZ-C4 protects the thymus and bone marrow; XZ-C7 to protect the lung function. He continues to take his medication for more than three years and there was not metatastasis. When he came back to follow up for his fourth year treatment, his condition is stable and his appetite is great and walked as the normal healthy person.

Case 28 Mr. Long, male, 60 year-old, Huangguang, officer, Medical record number: 521028

Diagnosis: Right lung middle and low lobe adenocarcinoma with diaphragm lymph node metastasis

Disease courses and treatment: In January 1997 he started to cough and fever and was treated as pneumonia. In December 1997 CT showed right lung cancer. The bronchoscopy showed that right side central low grade adenocarcinoma with diaphragm lymph node metastasis and then he was treated as intervation treatment and XZ-C treatment. He had his first chemotherapy through the brochial artery on Dec 31 1997 and the second chem. On Jan 20 1998, The third chemotherapy in March 1998. On July 8 1998 he received the 35th radioactive therapy. In September 1998 after the radioactive therapy, the twice chemotherapy were given(one months). From February 14 1998 to March 14 1998, May 9 1998 to June 9 1998, July 1 1998 to August 1 1998 the patients took ZX-C1 +XZ-C4+XZ-C7 by oral. After that the cough decreased an general conditions well, the vital energy and appetites are good, the energy level come back, he walked and acted as the normal person, dry cough. On Auguest 9 1998 because of the radioactive esophagitis which cause the swellon, congestion and difficulty swallowing, horse voice, then XXXX the XZ-C2 and inhaling the Chinese herbs, continue to take XZ-C medicine, his vital viguour and appetites are very well and can take the food.

Common: This patient have the right low lobe lung cancer with diaphragm lymph nodes mestatasits which was treated with intervation+XZ-C, after the long-term usage of the XZ-C regulation and control medicine, his general medical condition is good and appetite is good. Follow-up with us more two years and eight month, the condition is stable.

Suggestion: Left lung cancer with diagraph lymph node metastasis cannot be operated so that he was treated with chemotheray+Radiavtive+Chinese medicine, first radi+chem to kill the tumor cells, then continue to use the XZ-C immune medicine to protect thymus and improve th whole body immune level, so that to strength the curative therapy and protect the recurrence which has the effective effects.

Case 29 Mr. Xie, male, 55 year-old, Xiang Fen, Medical record number::340663

Diagnosis: Right upper lung adenocarcinoma

The disease courses and treatment: The activities of the right shoulder and right hands decreased about half of years and two months cough and little XXX without blood. On November 26, 1996 Chest X-ray showed that there is round lump on the right upper lung, which was confirmed by CT. On December 16 1996 he had the removal of the right upper lung and the pathology showed that right upper lung adenocarcinoma. On December 23 1996 he started to take XZ-C to prevent the recurrence, metastasis and he didn't take any other therapy. After taking XZ-C for a long-term, the patient is stable and his appetite is good and the vigour is very well and the energy level recovered and didn't have any other symptoms. His face glow with health so far it has been three and half years and everything is good as the normal healthy persons. He had many times of Chest X-ray which showed the normal. Ultrosound is normal.

Commens: this patient took XZ-C1+XZ-C4+CX-C7 for three years after the operation, so far he still used the XZ-C without other therapy. He is healthy as the normal persons.

Suggestions: After the lung operation, to take XZ-C for a long term can prevent the reccurence and metastasis for longterm. Because XZ-C protect thymus and bone marrow and can improve the immune function, the immune function of the patients can keep the high level without using radioactive and chemotherapy. Only treated by XZ-C for more than three years, he is well and as healthy as the normal persons.

Case 30 Mr. Huang, male, 54year olds, Xiaogan, the officer, Medical record number:: 4600907

Diagnosis: Lung cancer

Diseases courses and treatment conditions: In September 1996 cough blood and recovered with the antiinfection. In Aprle 1997 coughed again the symptoms can not be treated in the local hospital. On August 15 1997 the bronchoscopy and biopsy showed that lung squamous carcinoma. On August 31 1997 he have the left low lung removal and the pathology showed that left low lung squamous carcinoma with the lymph nodes of the lung entrance metastasis(1/3). Since September 1997 he took XZ-C to prevent the recurrence and matastasis. After taking the medicine, he is vagorous and his appetite is good. Every month he came back to get the medicine. In April 1999 when he came back to follow-up, he is healthy and his face is glowing with health, walking and acting and talk cheerfully and humorously, the superclavica, xxx, xxxxl lymph nodes and liver and spleens have no lesions, his body weight is 63kg. Chest X-ray and CT have changed sincere the surgery. After the surgery he started to take the medicince XZ-C1+XZ-C4+XZ-C7 for more than two and half years without other therapy. He is healthy.

Comments: This patient had the removal of the left low lung on Auguest 31 1997 and the pathology showed that left lung squamous carcinoma with the lymph nodes in the lung entrance metastasis(1/3). On September 19 1997 he started to XZ-C1+XZ-C4+XZ-C7 without other therapy for more than three years and he is healthy.

Suggestions: after the lung removal, to take XZ-C can improve the immune function and strengthen the body and maintain the curative therapy which can form the environment of no benefits for the tumor growth to prevent the tumor recurrence.

Case 31 Mr. Wang, male, 61year-old, Machen, officer.

Diagnosis: the central left lung cancer.

Disease courses and the treatment condition: On July 29 2006 the left lung cancer was found during the physical examinatoion. On August 21 2006 the total lungs in Tongjin hospital and cleaned the lymph nodes and part of the heart capsule+left part of artrium+ the xxx nerve removal. After seven days the left chest cavity had pneumothorax and induced by the tube. After the operation the patient was weak without the chemotherapy and radioactive. On October 10 2006 he started to take XZ-C and he is energetic and his appetite is good. He persistently took his medicince for more than five years. On Octocboer 8 2010 he came back to followup and his health condition is good.

Comments: this patient has the left central lung carcinoma which the surgery is very difficult and have the removal of the total parts of the lung in the heart cavity+ lymph nodes in the digraph+parts of the heart capsule+parts of the left antrium+ xxx nervous. After the operation, the tube was used to induce the fluid. Because of the age he didn't receive any therapy. On November 11 2006 he started to take XZ-C and he took them regularly and he is vagour and his appetite is good formore than five years.

Suggestions: Left central lung cancer, the surgery removal is a difficult procedure. After the operation, the immune function decreases and the patient was weak. After taking

XZ-C to protect the thymus and bone marrow, the therapy is excellent. This patient medical condition is stable.

Case 32 Mr. Guang, male, 64 year-old, Fushan in Guangdou, business man, Medical record number::220003302

Diagnosis: right lung adenocarcinoma

Disease course and treatment: in May 2005 CT in the southern hospital showed tha the right lung cancer in the peripheral. On May 16 2005 he had the removal of the right upper lobe lung and Pathology showed that peripheral lung adenocarcinoma in the right lung with XXXXX and no lymph node metastasis. After the surgery once chemotherapy. On July 13 2005 he came to our office for XZ-C1+XZ-C4+XZ-C7+LMS+MDZ, and continued to take them for more than five years without other therapy. His condition is stable

Comments: this patient had the right upper lobe lung cancer with the removal. After the chemotherapy, he had great reaction so that he stoped. In July 2005 he started to take XZ-C which he refilled every three months. He persistently took his medicine for more than five years and his medical condition is good.

Case 33 Mrs Ling, female, 64year-old, Danan, Medical record number::670003868

Diagnosis: after the removal of the right lung cancer, with both of the sizes metastasis and bone metastasis

Disease course and treatment condition: in March 2006 the patient coughed without the reasons. In May 2006 CT showed the right upper lung cancer and In June he had the removal of the right upper lobe + lymph node in the secondary hospital in the Daniang. The pathology showed that small cell lung cancer. In July 2006 after chemotherapy, CE xxx for two weeks the bone marrow were inhibited for the three degree. In September after the operation CT showed that both lung had metastasis nodules. Because of read my book<< the new ways and new concepts of the cancer treatment>>, he started to take XZ-C1+XZ-C4+XZ-C7+LMS+Vit. He took the medicine persistently for more than four years. His healthy condition is fine and he is energetic and his appetite is good and walking as the normal healthy persons.

Comments: this patient had right upper lobe small cancinoma. After the operation, he had twice chemotherapy and the bone marrow were inhibited to three degree so that he started to use XZ-C medicine to protect his thymus and bone marrow as the supplemental therapy to prevent the recurrence and metastasis.

Suggestions: XZ-C can be used as the assistant therapy after the surgery to improve the immunce function and to prevent the recurrence and metastasis.

5. Typical cases of assistant treatment after operation in sophagi carcinoma

Case34 Mr. Ding, male, 63year-old, Wuhan, officer, Medical record number:s: 600106

Diagnosis: the middle esophagus cancinoma

Disease course and treatment: in January 1994 the patient had the xxx difficulty of the swallow and after the barium swallow tests the diagnosis was confirmed. On Feb 3, he had the removal of the cancer with the reconixxxxx of the esophague and stomach. After one month of the radioavitvotherapy, because of the heart problems, he didn't use the chemotherapy, On April 5 1995 he started to take XZ-C and then he is energetic and appetite is good. From 1996 to 1999, he refilled his medicine every month and take the medicine persistently. In July 2005 his hair was gray. Recently one year his hair started to turn black and currently his black hair is full of his head and his facial skin is mor tenderer than before, his face is glowing of the health. He is the same as the normal persons. So far he has taken the medicine more than 16years and will continue to take his medicine.

Comments: The patient had the removal of the esophageus on Feb 3 1994. After 40 days of the operation he had radioactive and immune therapy and continued to take the medicine more than 16 years and his healthy condition is good.

The experience of this treatment: During the fourty days after the surgery, he received the radioactive and immune therapy. After that he took the immune therapy persistently to protect his bone marrow and thymus. XZ-C1 can inhibit the cancer mutation and XZ-C4 can improve the immune functions and induced the anticancer factors to protect the immune organs and stop the rest cells into the proliferation stages. If persistently using, the body will be the high immune function level and to prevent the recurrence and the health will recover.

Case 35 Mrs. Huang, femal,66 year-old, Wuhan han yan, Medical record number::10102008

Diagnosis: the squamous carcinoma of the low esophagus

Disease courses and treatment: in December 2000 the patients started to vomit and to have progressively swallow difficultly and only swallow the half of xxxx food. EGD showed that there was narrow in the low esophagus, congestion, ulcer and xxx. Pathology showed squamous carcinoma in the lower esophagus. According to his medical condition he should be treated for a surgery, however because he could afford to the medical cost, he started to take XZ-C. After one month, he is energetic and his appetite is getting better and can eat the soft food, noodle and rice soup. After she continued to take these medicine for six months, he is vagour and his appetite is good and can eat the soft food and noodle and rice soup. Until June 2003 she took the medicine more than two and half years and his health condition is good and can eat the regular rice and felt fine as the normal healthy persons. However she stopped to taking the medicine for more than four and half months. Until Octocber 16 2003 he suddenly had the difficulties to swallow the food and vomit the brown food. She could not eat for more than three days. After adding her some fluids and continued to take XZ-C until Octocber 31 2003 she can eat the food again. After that, she never stopped taking the medicine again. Now she is 70 year-old and healthy the same as the normal persons. She is energetic and her appetite is good and can eat regular food. She lived in the seventh floor and everyday she will come down the first floor and sometimes she help others to fill the bicycle wheels.

Comments: This patient had the low grade squamous carcinoma in the low esophagaus which was diagnosed by EGC and pathology. At that time he could only eat the liquid food and half of XXXX food. She makes her living by filling the bicycle wheels and didn't have money for her surgery so that she started to take XZ-C medicine. After taking the medicine half of year her symptoms turned good. Aftertaking the medicine two andhalf years she recovered as the normal person and didn't have any complain. Because of her incoming condition, she didn't get any other tests and treatment. When she came back to followup, she had taken the medicine more than five years and her condition is good.

To take XZ-C for longterm can improve the patients immune function and the pateitns energy level will increase and the appetites will increase and the sleep will be good. XZ-C4 can protect the bone marrow and thymus to improve the nutrition and the metabolism will turn good and will get rid of the free bases to control and to repair the diseases.

Case 36Mrs Hang, female, 65year-old, Huangpi in Hubei, Medical record number::10402074

Diagnosis: the middle esophogus carcinoma

Disease courses and treatment condition: In April 2001 the patient had difficulty swallowing and chest and back pain and gradually increased. Until June only can eat the liquid food and vomit the mucous staffs. On June 6 2001 the barium swallow tests in the xxx showed under the aorta branch xxxx 2cm there is a 10cm lenghth narrow and 6cm xxxxxlump in the left wall and the muscous stop. Because of the cost, she didn't have the operation, radioactive and chemotherapy. On June 25 she started to take XZ-C. After three months, her general condition is better and her appetite is getting better and the difficultying swallowing is getting better and can eat the rice soup, noodle. She continued taking the medicine until March 2002 then can take the rice and regular food. In July 2003 she just took XZ-C4+XZ-C2. In April 2005 when she followed up with us, she is energetic and her appetites was great at that time she had been taking XZ-C for more than five year. He condition is stable and can eat the regular food and can do light house work.

Comments: This patient had esophageal cancer which she only took XZ-C to control her condition without the operation, radiactiv therapy and chemotherapy. For more than four years, there was no metastasis and her condition had been controlled and can eat the regular food and rice. She is as healthy as other old persons and can do some choresevery day.

She kept taking her medicine regularly.

Case 37 Mr.Huang male, 66year-old, Huanpi, officer, Medical record number::300584

Diagnosis: the middle and low esophagous carcinoma

Disease courses and treatment: in March, he had the difficulty to swallow and the barium swallow test showed that the middle and low esophagum cancer. In May 1996 he had the removal of his cancer without other therapy. On June 19 1996 he started to use the XZ-C as the supplemental therapy to prevent the reccurrence and metastasis. He only takes XZ-C to protect his thymus and bone marrow for more than three years, then he changed into periodly taking the medicine. He is energetic and his appetite is good and walking and other activities are the same as the normal persons. In April 2005 when he came back to follow up with us, his condition is stable.

Comments: after the operation of his esophague, this patient only took XZ-C to assisting his therapymore than nine years, his condition is stable.

6. Typical cases of assistant treatment after operation in breast carcinoma

Case 38 Mr. Zhen, female, 44 year-old, Wuhan, Medical record number:s: 700121

Diagnosis: Breast adenocarcinoma

Disease courses and treatment: right breast lump was found for three months which the needle biopsy showed breast cancer. On February 20 1995 she had the removal of the breast cancer and once radioactive therapy after the operation. Because of the weakness, she couldn't tolerate it. On May 11 1995 she started to take XZ-C1+XZ-C4 and continued to take them for more than three years. After she took the medicine, her energy level was improving and her appetite was increasing and her weight is increasing. Following up with us every month and her medical condition is stable.

Comments: this patient had the removal of the breast on Feb 20 1995 and once radioactive therapy after the operation. Because of the weakness the radiative therapy was stopped. In May 1995 she started to take the XZ-C1+XZ-C4. After three years her condition is stable. When she came back for her five year follow-up, she is healthy.

Case 39 Mrs Pan, female,68year-old, Shengyang

Diagnosis: multiple bone metastasis after the removal of the breast cancer.

Disease courses and treatment: in 1984 the patient had the removal of the right breast cancer I stage, the pathology showed that simple breast cancer without lymph node metastasis. After the xxx +xxxx chemotherapy for two years, she started to use some immune enhancing drug. In January 2001 she felt the right shoulder pain and ECT showed that multiple bone metastasis and the supericlavical lymph nodes enlargement. Since March 27 she had 25 times radicacto therapy on the sites of the right superoclaviceal lymph nodes and the whole blood counts decreases and the white cell counts decrease into 2.9x109/L. After the radiactherapy, her condition stable.

On June 15 2001 he started to take XZ-C such XZ-C1+XZ-C2+XZ-C4+LMS+MDZ+VS for two months and her symptom significantly increased. After six months ECT was normal and she is stable. On September 2 2002 on the phone she told us that she is stable and takes her medicine regularly for more than four years. In

April 2005 She called us that she is energetic and her appetites is great and walking as the normal healthy persons. On her physical examination, Ultrasound of her liver and gallbladder, Chest X-ray, ECT etc she is normal.

Comments: this patient had right breast cancer after the operation for more than 17 years with bone metastasis and right shoulder pain. After the radiactiv therapy her medical condition is getting better. After taking XZ-C for a long period to protect thymus and bone marrow function, her metastasis was controlled well.

Case 40 Ms. Liu, female, 49year-old, Wuhan, account, Medical record number:: 4500884

Diagnosis: Left breast ductal adenocarcinoma

Disease courses and treatment: on May 19 1997 left breast had a lump 3cmx3cm. after the removal, the Pathology showed that left ductal infiltrated cancinoma. On June 3 1997 the second operation of the radiactie left breast cancer was done, which showed that there is no lymph node metastasis. Twice chemotherapy by taking XXXX were used after the operation. Because of the strong reaction to the chemotherapy, she started to take the XZ-C on August 24 1997. After that she is energetic and her appetite is increasing. After three months, she can go back to her work. After four months, the 3cmz3cm of the two lumps were found and the adjecxxxx is not clear, which the biopsy is breast proliferatin. After using the XZ-C1+XZ-C4 the lumps went away. For three years, she only takes the XZ-C medicine and her medical condition is stable and worked as the normal persons.

Comments: this patient had the removal of the breast cancer with twice chemotherapy. On August 24 1997 she only takes XZ-C to protect her thymus and bone marrow. For more than eight years, she is stable.

Suggestions: after the surgery she used twice chemotherapy for short time which the reaction is great so that she only used xz-c to induce the production of the anticancer factors to improve the immune function and to protect the host immune functions.

Case 41 Ms. Lee, female,33 year-old, Changda in Hunan, worker, Medical record number::3400667

Diagnosis: Left simple breast cancer.

Disease courses and treatment: On November 29 1996 she had the removal of the breast cancer in Changda which showed the right armpit lymph node metastasis(3/5). After one month, CMF was done which she used once/week, for more than four weeks.

On December 25 1996 she started to use XZ-C to protect her bone marrow. After taking the medicine, her whole blood went back to the normal level. From April 2 1997 to May 14 1997 she had radioactive 15 times in right breast inner line, 15 times under the armpit right and 25 times in the right breast outside lines. XZ-C were taken as the supplement therapy without the side effects. The patients is stable and reaction small and even no side effects when she took XZ-C with radiactherapy and chemotherapy. In June 2004 she only took XZ-C. Every three months she came to Wuhan to refill her medicines. Her condition is stable. In Dec 2004 when she came back to follow up with us, she is energetic and appetite is good and her face is glowing of the health. Acting is as the normal healthy persons. She came to refill her medicine from XXXX to WuHAN.

Comments: the curative experience of the treatment: 1). During the radiacti and chemotherapy the XZ-C4 can reduce the reaction, during the interval time between the radiac and chemotherapy and after them XZ-C can strengthen longterm curative effects to protect the recurrency. 2) after the surgery about six months the radia+chemotherapy +XZ-C can kill the remaining tumor cells or the small tumor lesions, meanwhile to protect the host immune organs. After taking the medicine for six months, the patient's general condition is good so that XZ-C can get rid of the wrong and strengthen the long-time curative effects. After 9 years of the operation, XZ-C can strengthen the long-term therapy.

Case 42 Ms Zhang, female, 65year-old, officer, Medical record number::13502682

Diagnosis: Breast ductal adenocarcinoma

Disease courses and treatment conditions: in 2002 on PE, a small lump was found in the breast, which is considered as breast cancer. In 2003 she had breast radiacal removal in Wuhan center hospital, which the Pathology showed that breast ductal adenocarcinoma without metastasis. She has the Diatebite and chronic renal inflammation. On April 2003 she started to take XZ-C1+XZ-C4 and has been taking the medicine for more than eight years. Every month she come back to refill the medicine and her healthy condition is well.

Comments: This case is the removal of the breast cancer, after the operation due to the chronic renal inflammation so that she started to take XZ-C and XXX soup to protect the thymus and bone marrow for more than eight years to prevent the reccurrency and metastasis. In addition, her kidney inflammation was getteing better and never recurrent. She come back to refill her medicine every two weeks. She is healthy and stable.

Case 43 Ms Liu, female, 49 year-old, Changsha in Hunan, teacher, Medical record number::260003372

Diangosis: breast infiltrating ductal cancer.

Disease courses and treatment condition: in February 2005 a left breast lump was found which is 2cmx1.5cm, biopsy showed that high degree mutation. On March 8 2005 she had CAF. On May 30 2005 the breast cancer was removed partially, pathology showed the breast cancer so that the breast cancer radiact removal was performed Pathologyshowed that left breast cancer infiltrated ductal cancer. LN0/20 with the C-erB2(++), P53(+), PR(-), ER(-), nm23(+). After the surgery the chemotherapy was used for six cycles. On Octocber 22 2005 she started to take XZ-C to strengthen the curative effects and to prevent the recurrence and metastasis.

Comments: in this case before the operation the lymph nodes under armpit were palpatited. Chemotherapy for six cycle was used before the operation and after the operations to strengthen the long time curative effect. She persistently takes these medicine more than six years and her healthy condition is stable.

7. Typical cases of assistant treatment after operation in colon and rectal carcinoma

Case 44 Mr. Yan, female, 71 year-old, Wuhan, teacher, Medical record number:s:100188

Diagnosis: ascending colon carcinoma

Disease courses and treatment: Because of abdomen pain and bloody stool, the patient was diagnosed as colon cancer by colonoscopy with biopsy. On December 19 1994 he had half of the right colon removal. Pathology showed the medium grade of colon adenocarcinoma involved in serosa. After the operation, he didn't accept other therapy.

On July 4 1995 he started to take XZ-C1+XZ-C4 as assistant therapy to prevent the recurrence and metastasis. He only takes XZ-C more than ten years and his healthy condition is very good. In April 2005 when he was 81 years old and came back to follow up with us, he was healthy and played the card every day in the afternoon.

Comments: this case is that after the removal of the ascending colon, the patient just takes XZ-C medicine as the assistant therapy to protect recurrence more than 10 years and his condition is stable.

Case 45 Mr. Yin, female, 60 yr, Huangpu, Medical record number::8301655

Diagnosis: sigmoid colon cancer and the removal of half of the left colon.

Disease courses and treatment: In August 1998 the patient had bloody stool and was treated as hemorrhoid. In Octocber 1999 when he had the colonoscopy in Xiehu hospital which there is narrow in the 32cm from the anus. On December 3 1999 he had the removal of half of the left-colon. Pathology showed: sigmoid xxxx adenocarcinoma involved in the whole layers of the colon and the metastasis of the nearby lymph nodules(6/8). On Jan 12 2000 he started to take XZ-C: XZ-C1+XZ-C4+LMS+MDA+VT to protect recurrence and metastasis. After he continues to take the XZ-C more than three years and eight months, his son came to refill the medicine on August 4 2003 and told us that his medical condition was good and did the chores every day and planted a lot of different kinds of flowers and vegatables watering them with ten buckles of water. The patient has been in the good condition and happy and has good energy. After his operation, he continues to take the XZ-C medicines only everyday without other chemotherapy. When he followed up with us, he already took the medicine more than five and half years.

Comments: the case is that sigmoid colon carcinoma with metastasis of the nearby lymph nodes. After the removal of the operation the patient didn't have chemotherapy because of the decrease of the white blood cells so that he took the XZ-C as the assistant therapy to protect the bone morrow and thymus to improve the body immune system to protect the reccurrence and the metastasis. After five and half years, his condition was good.

Case 46 Ms. Yun, female, 63year-old, Jiling, officer, Medical record number::8601705

Diagnosis: the rectal adenocarcinoma

Disease courses and treatment: in Octocbor 1999 the patient has the bloody stool and the the rectaoscopy showed there is a flower-like tumor in the 10cm distance from the ana and Pathology showed the rectal cancer. On November 22 1999 the rectal radioactive surgery was done in the affliatite hospital with Dixon ways. After the operation the patient's condition is stable. On December 2 the chemotherapy was done(urine xxxx 1.0g/day, for five days, xxx 100mg/day for three days). On December 9 the white blood cell counts decrease into 0.09x109/L, on December 10 the white blood cells decrease into 0.06x109/L, injection of the medicine of increasing the white blood cells for five days, the white blood cells into1.1x109/l and had the pneumonia and fever with 40C. On January 2 xxxx after treatment with xxxx+xxxx, the patient still has fever and had the throat infection with three bacteria and can not eat and drink anything. After using XXX for five days, the temperature dropped into 38C. Because this patient had hypertension, diabetes and lung diseases, her medical condition is weak and severe and had twice warrancy from the hospitals. After two months of the treatment, she is stable. On March 20 2000 she started to take XZ-C for half of the years and her medical condition is stable and can do a little chores and can support her daily life by her own. On September 2000 she recurred very well and can shop in the nearby market and do little chores. She has been taken the medicine for more than five years consistently. In May 2005 her daughter come to refill the medicine and told us that she is totally fine and still do some house chores as healthy as other normal healthy individuals.

Comments: this case is the radial rectal cancer removal and the chemotherapy. After these her immune function and bone morrow function were inhibited so that she had throat and both the lung infections, which later are two fungus infections. After the treatment her condition started to get better and started to take the XZ-C which XZ-C1 only inhibited the tumor cells without affecting the normal cells and improve the immune fucntions, XZ-C4 to protect thymus and bone marrow to improve the immune function. The chemotherapy can inhibit the bone marrow so as to lead the bone marrow inhibition to some degrees which can affect the patients for more than 2 to 3 years so that XZ-C which have protect thymus and bone marrow function need to be taken for several years to benefit the bone marrow and immune functions

Case 47. Mr. Qian, male, 66year-old, Wuhan, accounting, Medical record number::5401066

Diangosis: rectal carcinoma

Disease courses and treatment conditions: occasionally diarria and constipation with bloody stool for two years. The rectal examination showed that there was a 3cmx3cm lump at the 6 clock point in the xxxx position. On January 20 1998 the colonoscopy showed the polypoid mutation of the rectal colon. On January 24 1998 Dixon which the 40cm of the colon were cut off was done in the xiehae hospital, Pathology showed that rectal cancer with middle division and invade into the muscular layer without lymph nodes metastasis and the margin clear. After thesurgery, on March 3 1998 he started to use the XZ-C and took this medicine persistenly for more than eight years and he come back to work for more than five years He is stable and still continued to use these medicine.

Comments: this case is rectal adenocarcinoma. In January 1998 Dixon was done and Pathology showed that rectal adenocarcinoma, middle-degree. After the operation he only took the XZ-C1+XZ-C4 for more tha eight years. His medical condition is stable.

Suggestions: After the rectal Dixon without the chemotherapy, he only took the immune regulation medicine XZ-C to protect his thymus and bone marrow to improve his immune functions to improve the life quality and prevent the recurrence and metasatasis. He was stable.

Case 48. Ms Year-oldng, female, 32year-old, Zhaoyang, accounting, Medical record number::500993

Diagnosis: rectal villious adenocarcinoma

Disease courses and treatment condition: the patient had bleedy stool. In September 1997 the Colonoscopy and biopsy showed the rectal cancer. On September 17 1997 she had the rectal radial operation which showed that the lump was 1.0cmx1.0cm on the bases and was 4cm distance from the ana. Pathology reported the rectal villious adenocarcinoma and invaded into the all of the wall of the intestines with the menstema lymph node metastasis. After the operation she had chemotherapy once. Because of the decrease of the white blood cells she stop chemotherapy and started to use XZ-C1+XZ-C4. Her medical condition is well and stable. She continued to take the medicine for more than eight years only without chemotherapy and other therapy. She did her chores as the normal persons.

Comments: this case is the rectal radial removal on September 17 1997, during the operation, the metastasis were found in the mestaen membrane lymph nodes and invades the whole wall of the intestines. After the operation she had the chemotherapy once which had been stopped because the side effects were severe. Since December 3 1997 she started to take XZ-C only for more than eight years to prevent the reccurrence and metastasis after the surgery. Her medical condition is well.

Case 49. Ms. Cheng, female,68year-old, physician, Medical record number:: 15403059

Diagnosis: Colon cancer

Disease coursed and treatment condition: Because the treatment for the obstracle didn't improve, the operation was done in XinHua hospital on April 30 2004 and found the colon cancer, then the right half of the colon was removed. Pathology showed: the colon capillary adenocarcinoma and the obstracle. After the operation, she received once chemotherapy which she can not tolerate. She started to take XZ-C. After that she is energetic and her appetite is good. She took the medicine persistently for more than six years and she is healthy.

Comments: this patient have obstracle from the Colon cancer and had surgery to remove the right half of the colon. After once chemotherapy she couldn't tolerate and then she started to take the XZ-C for more than six year. Her medical condition is well and she is healthy.

Case 50. Ms Zhang, female, 38year-old, Hanchuan, Medical record number::400003595

Diangosis: colon cancer

Disease courses and treatment conditions: the patients had occasionally abdominal pain for more than five months and the Colonoscopy showed the colon lump in the descending colon. On Octocber 4 2005 the left half of the colon and right overian were removed and Pathology showed that the low grade adenocarcinoma and the metastasis to mesentery and right overain. After the operation six cycle of the chemotherapy were done. On August 18 2006 she started to take the XZ-C medicine such as XZ-C1+XZ-C4+LMS+MDZ persistently for more than five years. She is healthy and refilled the medicine every month.

Comments: this case is left half of the colon and right overian removal. After the operation, the six cycle of the chemotherapy was used, then take XZ-C to strengthen his immune systems. She is healthy after she takes the medicine persistently for more than five years.

Case 51 Mr.Luong, male,60year-old, Shichuang, professor Medical record number::8801759

Diagnosis: rectal carcinoma

Disease courses and treatment: in November 1999 there was blood in the stool and he was treated as hemorriod. In Febrary 2000 he was diagnosed as rectal cancer by the colonoscopy with biopsy. On March 2 2000 he had radical rectal cancer removal in Tongjing University, which is Mile models, Pathology: medium grade rectal adenocarcinoma. After the surgery, he had 12 radiactive therapy and once chemotherapy. On May 30 2000 he began to take XZ-C1+XZ-C4+LMS+MDZ. After he took this medicine, his appetite is good and persistently takes small amount medicine to protect thymus and to protect the bone morrow and follow-up with us monthly for more than ten years and his healthy condition is good and every test is normal.

Comments: this patient had the Mile surgery. After theoperation, he had 13 radiactive and one chemeotherapy, then only take the XZ-C to protect thymus and bone marrow. He persistently takes his medicine and every month he refilled his medicine. So far he has been taking his medicine more than ten years and his medical condition is stable.

8. Typical cases of assistant treatment after operation in galdbladder carcinoma

Case 52 Mr. Shong, male, 51 year-old, Tianmen, officer, Medical record number::14302843

Diagnosis: adenocarcinoma in the distant common ducts

Disease courses and treatment: After one week painless jaundice, the CT showed the tumor of ampulla of vater. On September 7 2003 he had pancreas and duodenum removal in Zhanjiang xxxx central hospital and the operation was done very well and the size of the tumor is the same as the thumb. Pathology: high-grade adenocarcinoma involved in the whole lumon layer and the head of the pancreas. After twice chemotherapy he came to our outpatient center to take XZ-C: XZ-C1+XZ-C4+XZ-C5+LMS+MDZ+Vit. He continued to finish Chemotherapy so that he had chemotherapy and immune regulation medicine. After finished six periods and continued to take XZ-C4+XZ-C5 to protect thymus and to protect his bone morrow. After taking the medicine, his general medical condition is good and his appetite is increasing. So far he had taken

XZ-C for 7 years and his general medical is good and his healthy condition is good and healthy condition is good. He comes back to work more than three years and he is physical strength and he look a regular heathy person.

Case 53 Ms. Dai, female, 59year-old, Wuhan, Medical record number::790003988

Diagnosis: Gallbladder adenocarcinoma

Disease courses and treatment condition: because of the gallbladder stone found in PE, the gallbladder was removed on March 22 2007 in Zhengshun Hospital. After the operation the sample was grossed as 1.8cm in the base of the gallbladder ranges from 2.5cmx3cm. Pathology showed that high division of the adenocarcinoma and IHC showed CK(++), CEA(+). EGD showed that the chronic ulcerative gastritis with bile gastritis. H.pyloric (+), after the operation she took the xxxx. She started to take XZ-C such as XZ-C1+XZ-C4+XZ-C5+ LMS+MDZ and treatment of H. Pyloric bacteria. After one month of the XZ-C he is stable and his appetite is good. She have been taken the XZ-C for more than four years and her medical condition is stable.

Comments: This case is gallbladder cancer. Before the operation the diagnosis is gallbladder stone. After the gallbladder removal through laparoscopy, the Pathology showed that high division of the adenocarcinoma. He took XXX for two cycles of the chemotherapy and took XZ-C to assisting the therapy. For more than four years he has been taken XZ-C and his appetite is good and his energy level is good.

Case 54 Mr. Guong, male, 57year-old, Wuhan, Medical record number::260003376

Diagnosis: middle degree of adenocarcinoma in the gallbladder.

Disease courses and the treatment condition: Because of the abdominal pain in September 2005, the test was done and showed polyp in the gallbladder. The gallbladder was removed with laparoscopy on October 18 2009 in Wuhan first hospital. Pathology showed that middle degree gallbladder cancer without the liver metastasis. After the operation, he didn't have the chemotherapy and radioactive therapy. On Octocber 31 2005 he came to our outpatient center and started to take XZ-C1+XZ-C4+XZ-C5+LMS+MDZ to assisting his therapy. After he took his medicine for more than five years, his medical condition is stable.

Comments: this case is gallbladder carcinoma was diagnosed as the polyp of the gallbladder and the removal of the gallbladder through the laparoscopy. Pathology showed that gallbladder carcinoma. Because of the early stage of the carcinomam, he didn't receive other therapy. He only takes XZ-C to assisting his surgery for more than five years. He is healthy as the normal persons.

9. Typical cases of assistant treatment after operation in kidney and bladder carcinoma

Case 55: Mr. Cheng, male, 62year-old, Wuhan, engineer, Medical record number:s: 210412

Diagnosis: Renal pelvis carcinoma in the right kidney and the recurrence after the bladder carcinoma operation.

Diseases courses and treatment: the patient had cytoscopy which showed the bladder carcinoma in November 4 1995 afterthe bloody urine for two years. On November 21 1995 CT showed that rght renal pelvis tumor. On December 6 1995 the right kidney and urother were removed and his bladder was removed by the xxx and after the operation the local xxxx chemotherapy was used for seven times. On March 8 1996 the cystoscopy showed there was the hard lump in the left wall of the bladder in order to prevent the reccurrence of the tumor, he started to take XZ-C1+XZ-C4+XZ-C6. After taking this medicine he is well and his appetite is getting better.. On June 24 1996 the cytoscopy showed that the bladder walls are smooth and the surface is smooth and the new things were gone. He continued to take XZ-C medicine to prevent the recerence and metastasis. Until June 11 1997 the cystoscopy showed the bladder is normal. On December 28 1998 the cystoscopy is normal. On June 26 1999 when he came back to follow up, his condition is stable and he continues to take the XZ-C1+XZ-C4+XZ-C6 for more than ten years to prevent the recurrence and metastasis. On May 6 2005 when he follow-up, he is stable and his condition is good and is the same as the normal individuals.

Comments: this case is the recurrence of the bladder cancinoma after the operation. After taking this medicine more than ten years to prevent the recurrence and metastasis, his medical condition is good and after many cystoscopy, the bladder is normal.

Suggestion: XZ-C can improve the patients immune function and prevent the tumor recurrence and metastasis and control the primary lesions. He is healthy and is in the good condition.

Case 56. Mr. Lin, male, 68year-old, Wuhan, Professor, Medical record number:7701534

Diagnosis: the recurrence of the bladder cancer operation.

Disease courses and treatment conditions: After the removal of the bladder cancer was done in April 1994 in the hospital, Pathology showed: transitional cell carcinoma. After the operation the bladder was poured with chemotherapy. Because of the decrease of the white blood cells the chemotherapy stopped. In 1996 he came back to check up and found the cancer recurrence so that the second operation was done by the removal of eight tumors. After the surgery the patient's bladder was poured with XXX+XXXX twice every month for three months. After three months, repeat these medicine for another three months. Twice per month until 1997. In May 1998 the cystoscopy in the XXX hospital showed the xxx in the bladder. In December the ultrasound showed the bladder infection. In April 1999 because of the bloody urine, the cystoscopy showed that there were a four cm2 of the tumor and CT biopsy showed that bladder cancer. In May 1999 the arterial chemotherapy was poured. In June the second time of the poured the XXXX+XXXX+XXX was done. After that the white blood cells decreased into 2x109/l. In September the third time of the poured medicine with xxx+xxxx+xxx, the white blood cells decreased into 1.2x109/L, then inject the XXX to increase the white blood cells. His medical history: stroke in 1992, Hypertension(160/90mmHg), Diabete. In 1984 he had hepatitis and in 1998 had cirrhosis. Family history: two brothers had hepatitis B and then liver cancer, another brother had rectal cancer.

In July 1999 because of the white blood cells decrease after the chemotherapy, he started to take xxxx to protect the bone marrow and take XZ-C1+XZ-C4+XZ-C6. After taking them more than six months, the whole blood count come back again. His energy level is increased and his appetite is getting better and continue taking the medicine. In July 2000 the cystoscopy showed that the bladder was filled well and a 1.3cmx0.6cm xxxxx in the xxxx ranges, considering as the recurrence of the tumors and continued to take the medicine until June 2001, because of the prostate enlargement which caused the frequency and urgency of the urine. CT showed that this lesion was getting bigger than before(in February in 1999), then had arterialy poured once. He continued to take XZ-C1+XZ-C4+XZ-C6 untill July 2002 CT showed that the lesion in CT shrinkled. After taking the medicine, his general medical condition is better and his appetites is good without the bloody urine. He kept coming back to followup and take his medicine for more than six years. His lesion in his bladder is stable without metastasis and enlargement.

Comments: This case is transitional cell carcinoma. After the removal of the cancer, the long- time chemotherapy didn't stop the recurrence. Because of many years of the poured bladder and many times of the cystoscopy with the enlargement of the prostate and the narrowness of the urother, the cystescopy is difficult to be done. After taking XZ-C such as XZ-C1+XZ-C4+XZ-C6, the neoplasm in the bladder didn't develop and didn't metastes. Since he had this disease, it has been 11 years. His general medical condition is well and his appetite is getting better. When he walked more, sometimes the bloody urine occurred.

Case 57. Mr. He, male, 76year-old, Henan, officer, Medical record number:9201839

Diagnosis: left renal clear cell cancer.

Disease courses and treatment condition: in 1996 there is a kidney cyst, in 2000 on PE there is a 7.5cmx6.5cm cysts in the left renal. CT and MRI showed that left kidney tumor. On August 31 2000 the removal of the left kidney was done in Tongjing hospital. Pathology showed that middle degree of kidney clear cells carcinoma. After the surgery he started to take the xxxx without chemotherapy and radiactvie therapy. On September 28 2000 she started to take XZ-C1+XZ-C4+XZ-C6 to protect thymus ad bone marrow. After taking the medicine one month, he is vigour and his appetite is still low and contine taking the medicine for three months, his general condition is good and his energy level is high and his sleeping is good. After taking the medicine for one year, Ultrasound of the abdomen, Chest X-ray, and others regular tests are normal and he continues to take XZ-C1+XZ-C4+XZ-C6 to prevent the metastasis and recurrence. After five years of taking these medicine, his healthy condition is stable. On April 10 2005 when he follow-up with us, he is healthy and his face is glowing of the health and his voice is xxxx, and he is energetic and had the hear decrease due to his age.. His medical condition is100 by CCCCCC.

Comments: this case is left kidney clear cells. He was 76 year-old when he had his surgery. Because of his age, he didn't have the chemotherapy and radioactive therapy and only take the XZ-C immune therapy as the supplement therapy to protect his thymus and bone marrow to improve the immune functions and protect the recurrence and metastasits. He has been taking the medicine for more than five years and when he came back to followup he was 80 years old. His general medical condition is good and his appetite is good and his face is glowing of the health and his energy level is high and his voice is xxx as the normal healthy person.

Case 58 Mr. Yu, Male, 69year-old, Heilunjing, officer, Medical record number::6001181.

Diangosis: the bladder transitional cell cancer

Diseases courses and treatment condition: The bloody urine on Februay 27 in 1998. On March 2 the cystoscopy and ultrasound showed that there was the round lump in the front wall, which is 1.6cmx1.4cm and growed toward to the cavity of the bladder and is the neoplasum of the front wall of the bladder. On March 10 in 1998 the surgery removed the tumor tissues in the bladder and Pathology showed that the bladder transitional cell tumors. He was told that this tumor is the recurrence of the tumors. After the surgery, he had once chemotherapy(on May 26 1998). His reaction to chemotherapy is severe such as the vomiting, nausea, and the whole body is uncomfortable. The left testicule enlarges so that he stop chemotherapy. On June 18 1998 he started to take the XZ-C. He follow up with us very month and his condition is good and his urine is normal and he doesn't have any other symptoms. He follow up with us for more than six years and he is healthy.

Comments: in this case on March 10 1998 the surgery removed three tumors in the bladder and Pathology showed that bladder transitional cell carcinoma. After the operation once chemotherapy was done which the patient had severe reaction to this chemotherapy. On June 18 1998 he started to take the medicine XZ-C1+XZ-C4+XZ-C6. He continued to take this medicine for more than seven years and his healthy condition is good without other therapy and without the recurrence and metasatasis.

Comments:

Case 59. Mr. Zhong, male, 66 year-old, Wuxiu, officer, Medical record number:11602315

Diagnosis: right kidney clear cell tumors with the bone marrow metastasis and superclavaical lymph node metastasis.

Disease courses and treatment condition: Because of the pain in the right should, the diagnosis was "the inflamtion of the sourround shoulder", which there was a lump as big as XXX behind the right clavical and stern bone, the biopsy showed adenocarcinoma. After CT of abdomen and chest Ultrasound, there was no lesion found. On March 2002 he started to take the XZ-C such as taking XZ-C1+XZ-C4 and plastic XZ-C3. After the plastic gels, the lump was getting soft and shrinkle into small. On March 24

2002 Ultrasound showed a lump of 3.1cmx4.3cm in the right kidney. CT showed: L2, L4 had bone damage and still took the XZ-C and GEM+XXX chemotherapy once. On May 16 2002 the right renal was removed which there was a lump of the size of table tennis. Pathology showed clear cells. Because he was on the immune function medicine, his medical condition was stable and his appetite is good. Although he had the metastasis of his whole body, he still walked as the normal persons. In 2002,2003 and 2004 he came back every month to refill his medicine and his medical condition is stable. Until July 2004 he suddenly lost the ability of speech and headache. CT showed that the bleeding of the brain. After three weeks of the hospitalization, his medical condition was stable and CT showed that the brain bleeding was absorbed and he continues to take XZ-C1+XZ-C2+XZ-C6+LMS+XXX+XXX+xxxx etc. His medical condition is good and he is vigour and his appetite is good.

Comments: this case is the right metastasis lump of the clavic bone with L2 and L4 bone metastasis, the biopsy showed the metastasis adenocarcinoma. After the whole examination the right kidney tumor was found. On May 16 2002 he was diagnosed as right kidney clear cell cancer and the kidney was removed. On March 16 2002 he started to use the XZ-C by taking and plastic. After three years his medical condition is stable and his appetite is good and he is vigour.

Case 60. Mr. Shi, female, 61year-old, Hunan, Medical record number::790003989

Diagnosis: left kidney clear cell tumors

Disease courses and treatment condition: on Octocbr 27 2006 on PE the Ultrasound showed the left kidney lump. On November 8 2006 the left kidney was removed and Pathology showed that clear cell tumors with 0/2 lymph node. After the operation, the treatment of INF and IL-2 for three months without the radiactiv and chemotherapy. On May 10 2007 she started to take ZX-Csuch as XZ-C1+C4+C6+LMS+MDZ etc. She came back to refill up her medication every month for more than four years now. Her medical condition is ok and she is healthy now.

Comments: this case is left kidney clear cells tumor. After the operation, she took XZ-C only and persistently for more than four years. Her medical condition is good and after many tests she is healthy.

Sugguestion: XZ-C immune function medication can improve the immune function and to prevent the recurrence and metatastasis.

Case 61. Ms. Shi, female, 61 year-old, Hubei, Medical record number::790003989

Diagnosis: the kidney cell tumor

Disease courses and treatment condition: in October 2006 PE showe the right kidney lump and no other syptom. On October 2006 the right kidney lump was removed(partial) and Pathology showed the renal cell tumor. After theoperation, the chemotherapy was used. In September 2007 she started to take XZ-C such as XZ-C1+XZ-C4+XZ-C6+LMS+Vit and then every three month she came back to fill her medicine for more than four years now. She is healthy.

Comments: this case is the removal of the partial right kidney and Pathology showed that kidney cell tumors. Since September 2007 she started to take XZ-C1+XZ-C4+XZ-C6+LMS for more than four years. Her medical condition is stable.

10. Typical cases of assistant treatment after operation in Thyroid cancer and peritoneum carcinoma

Case 62 Ms Pen, female, 39 year-old, Shichuang Luchang, officer, Medical record number::7801545

Diagnosis: Thyroid cancer

Disease course and treatment: On April 27 1999 after the removal of the right neck lump, diagnosed as lymphocyte thyroid cancer. On May 6 1999 he had the radical total removal of the thyroid, then he had hourse voice and didn't have chemotherapy. On July 24 he started to take XZ-C: XZ-C1+XZ-C4, LMS, VS and follow-up with us every month and continue to use more than half years. Until Jan 2000 his voice gets better and after continue to take XZ-C another three months his voice come back to the normal. His general conditions get better and his emotion is stable and appetite is good and his energy level came back and he can go back his work. He persistently takes XZ-C1+XZ-C4 to improve his immune function and followed with us more six years and in May 2005 when he came back to us, his general condition is very good.

1999, 5	1999, 7	2000	2001	2002	2003	2004	2005
Thyroid operation	XZ-C						Follow-up

Comments: this patient has capillary thyroid cancer. After operation his voice was housral and didn't have radiology and chemoactive therapy. He only took the XZ-C to improve his immune function and to prevent recurrence and metastasis.

Case 63 Mr.Cheng, male, 64 year-old Hubei Xin Zhou, officer, Medical record number::7301454

Diagnosis: the tumor of the mesentaic membranexxxx.

Disease courses and treatment condition: On January 6 1999 the patient suddenly had the uncomfortable in chest and pain and vomit. The emergency diagnosis was "actual GI infection", the surgeons thought of that he had the pancreatitis. On March 3 EGD showed the obstractle of the duodenum. On March 6 1999 during the survey of the abdomen, the tumor which was behind the abdominal membrance including big vessals which during the operation a 6cmx9cm lump in the roots of the small intestine membreance xxxx of hard, stable, fixed and unsmooth on the surface, connected to aorta and the xxxx arterial and pressed the duodenum which it was difficult to remove so that the connection of the duodenus and colon was done because the tumor can not be removed and the patients was told to be treated by the combination of the western and Chinese therapy. On April 1999 she started to take XZ-C1Z+C4. From May 15 1999 to February 2002 she continued to take the medicine and refill her medicine. She is stable and her medical condition is good.

Comments: On March 6 1999 the tumor from the abdomen membrane was foundby the survey of the operation. Because it is connected to the small intestine membrance including the

Case 64. Mrs. Pu, female, 67year-old, Shiyiazhoung, worker, Medical record number::7601511.

Diagnosis: The recurrence after the surgery of the abdominal cavity serous tumors

Disease courses and treatment conditions: because of the belly was getting bigger and ascites, in May 1999 he was hosptilized in Tongjing and ascite(++) and his belly was like to frog and the tumor can be touched. On April 9 the surgery found that there were very many different sizes of the tumor, which were gel-like lump full of the abdominal cavity. One by one were removed, the total weight are 2.5g. During the operations, the chemotherapy tube was put with XXX 500mg. After the operation of four days xxx500MG once/per day and continued to use five days and xxx 100mg once/per day and continuing three days. On June 16 1999 he started to take XZ-C1+XZ-C4 andd after two months she is vigour and her appetite is good and her weight increases. PE: there were no lymph nodes in the superclavial, the abdomen is soft and flat, the ascite(-) and continue to take the XZ-C and refilled her medicine every month until November 26 2000, PE: there was a lump of the fit=size, hard, many nodual on the surface and deep and the clear edges which showed the tumor recurrence. The patient refused to the operation again and to chemotherapy, however he continued to take the XZ-C medicine: XZ-C1+XZ-C4+LMS+MDZ and the anticancer gel on the skin patched. Until Febrauay 24 2002 PE: there was on abnormal and her abdomen was soft and there was a lump which was hard, deep and clear edge and the size is smaller than before and her medical condition is stable. Until December 15 2004 her medical condition is good and her appetite is good and her abdomen is little enlarge and her ascite(++) and there is a fit-size lump with unsmooth surface and many nodule and deep and fix without the metastasis further. After her operation until now she has been following up with us more than six years and her medical condition is stable and the tumor is not metasatasis further.

Comments: This case is the serous tumor in the abdominal cavity. After the removal, the tumor recurrence. After the chemotherapy one week, the reaction is great so that in June 1999 she started to take XZ-C1+XZ-C3+XZ-C4 and she continued to take this medicine for more than six years and her medical condition is stable without the far metastasis and the tumors didn't grow big. She lives well with the tumors.

11. Typical cases of assistant treatment of non-Hodgkin lymphoma

Case 65 Ms. Liu, female, 34 year-old, Xinzhou, Medical record number::7701538

Diagnosis: Non-Hodgkin lymphoma in stomach and liver metastasis

Dieasce course and treatment: in Feb 1999 the patient has little difficulty swallowing and didn't pay attention to. In April he have significantly difficulty swallowing and have difficulty to swallow the water and other fluid foods. In May the endoscopy showed that stomach body and stomach pyloric cancer. And had total stomach removal in June 1999. Pathology showed: Stomach non-hodgkin lymphoma and liver metastasis and lymph node metastasis in the spleen and the stomach lesser and greater curvature. Because her condition is week, she didn't have any chemotherapy after her surgery. On August 18 1999 she started to take XZ-X1+XX-C4. After 2 months, her general condition get better and emotion is stable and her appetites get better. After taking this medicine for more than 3 years, there is not abnormal during her Ultrasond. In November 2002 he feel find and appetites get better so that he takes the medicine peroidly. On Jan 18 2004 When he came back to follow up, her general condition is good and appetites are great. On her PE, her abdomen is soft and there is no lump. Sometimes she felt weak on her right hand, however her left arm can work very well and do all of the chores. In April 2005 during her following-up, her general condition is well and everything is find, however she takes the medicince periodly to support her longt-term therapy.

Case 66 Ms Mei, female, 42 year-old, Wuhan, worker, Medical record number::400003599

Diagnosis: Non-hodgkin lymphoma

Disease course and treatment: in November 2005 the patient has pain in both of shoulder, fatigue and there is a thumb-size lump in low jaw. Then there are some egg-size lymph in both of inguinal areas. The lumps were not painful and the patient didn't have fever, however she felt fatigue. Pathology showed that non-hodgkin lymphoma, B cell large cells types which the immunohistochemistry showed: CD30(+), ALD(++), EMA(+), CD20(+), CD79(+), CD3(+), CD43(+), CD15(-). On Auguest 16 2006 the patient didn't have radiative and chemotherapy. On August 22 2006 She came to our office and started to XZ-C4+XZ-C2+LMS+MDZ=XX after PE which showed that the patient's general condition is fine and had a cutting scar in low jaw and there were xxx-size lymph nodes in the back of the neck and there were many lump in both of inguinal area. After 3 months she felt good and appetites increased and continued for three months to take XZ-C2+XZ-C4+XXS+DIANSHEN, the patient's energy level improved and continued to take XZ-C2+xz-c4+xx+dianshen+ganchao for three months, her medical condition turn better. She continues to take the medicine regularly and fills her medicine every month for more than 5 years, which she only takes. On September 26 2010 when she came back to follow up, she is fine and working and acting as the normal individual and her emotion is stable and her appetites are fine and is happy and playing card with her friends.

Comments: The patient had egg-sized lumps in both of inguinal area. Biopsy showed that non-hodgkin lymphoma with B large types. She didn't take chemotherapy and radioactive therapy. On August 22 2006 she started to takeXZ-C2+XZ-C4+LMS+Dianshen+qindai for more than five years which she fills up her medicine every month. Her medical condition is fine.

Suggestion: Non-hodgkins diseases can be treated by takeXZ-C2+XZ-C4+LMS. The patient continues to take her medicine only for more than 5 years and her medical condition is fine.

Case 67 Mr. Gao, female, 38 year-old, worker, Medical record number::550003745

Diagnosis: Non-hodgkin lymphoma, marginal zone lymphoma, recurrence after spleen removal and chemotherapy

Disease course and treatment: in June 2000 the 2cmx3cm lymph nodes on the right neck was biopsied and pathology showed that follicule lymphoma. The chemotherapy was given from June 29 2000 to July 10 2000, from September 2000 to March 2002, from June 2002 to May 2004 because of lung metastasis. In 2005 the spleen enlarged and was removed. Pathology showed: xx lymphoma, small cells types. CT showed that the lymph node in left lung and in both armpits and in diaphragm. After chemotherapy for three weeks, the lymph node disappeared. In November 2005 the lymph node in the back of right ears enlarged and chemotherapy was given for two weeks. In April 2006 the lymph nodes were enlarged in the back of right ear and the left neck. Biopsy showed: marginal Zone lymphoma. Ct showed that LN enlarged in the sizes and increased in the numbers in the entrance of the lungs and central veins.

After the spleen removal and many times chemotherapy this disease came back again. On Jan 7 2007the patient started to take XZ-C4+XZ-C2+LMS+MDZ+XX+XXX+Vit. After the patient took this medicine, her general medical condition is getting better and stable, her appetite is good and now she has been only using these medicine for more than four years regularly.

Common: This case is non-hodgkin lymphoma which was treated by chemotherapy. Since Jan 7 2007 She only took these medicine for more than four years. Her medical condition is stable and appetite is improved. She filled up her medicine regularly once per three month.

12. Typical cases of treatment of acute leukemia through chemotherapy +XZ-C

Case 68 Mr. Zhao, female, 34 year-old, Wuhan, officer, Medical record number:: 9801953

Diagnosis: Acute leukemia

Disease course and treatment: On Novermber 29 the patient was diagnosed as acute leukemia in Beijing hospital and was treated by chemotherapy for seven months. In August 2000 he was treated by bone morrow transplantation, however the results were not good after that because WBC, RBC and platelets are low. Such as wbc0.5x109/l, platelets were 5x100/l, HB46g/l. He depended on the blood transfusion, which were performed once per 8-9 days for 250ml. During his inpatient in Beijing, He had 10 times blood transfusion and 14 times platelets (once per 10 days).In Feb 2001 he came to Wuhan and on Feb 2, 2001 he started to use XZ-C1+XZ-C2+XZ-C8 to protect his thymus and his bone morrow. In April 2001 his WBC and RBC and Pletelets increase and stop to get transfusion. He takes XZ-C1+XZ-C2+XZ-C4 for more than one year and seven months and feel fine and he looked good and healthy and appetites increases and walking and runnig as the normal individual. In September 4 2003 he traveled to America and took his medicine XZ-C1+XZ-C2+XZ-C4 with him and he takes his medicine persistently.

In 2004 he immigrate into Canada and took his medicine XZ-C1+XZ-C2+XZ-C8 regularly and increase blood soups which will be filled once per 3 months. In April 2005 He called me and told us that he was healthy and his medical condition was controlled very well and appetite and sleep very well and started to work on business and energy level is perfectly well.

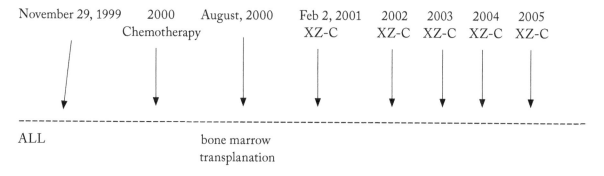

Comments: This patient has ALL and after seven months chemotherapy in August 2000, he had bono marrow transplantation. However the treatment results were not good because his blood counts were still low which he depended on the blood transfusion. On Feb 2 2001 he started to take XZ-C1+XZ-C2+XZ-C4. And increase blood soups etc. and after four months his blood counting went back the normal. After one year and seven months his blood counting keeps normal and he is healthy and has taken these medicine for more than 4 years and work in the business field and energy level is normal.

Suggustion: All can be treated satisfiedly by chemotherapy and XZ-C to protect the bone marrow and improve the immune system function. Now he has been followed up more than seven years and his healthy condition is very well.

Case 69 Ms. Hu, female, 64 year-old, Xisui, account, Medical record number::
850004087

Diagnosis: Hypothyroidism +multiple bone marrow tumor with toung amyloid change

Disease courses and treatment: In December 2005 the patient's low jaw was sollowed and snored heavily and on Physical exam: her tongue was big and after radiative treatment the enlargement tongue got better, howevery after stop treatment, the large tongue came back again. In December 2007 the soft tissue biopsy in the low jow was done and found that amyloid change of the low jaw amyloid change. Bone marrow biopsy showed that multiple bone marrow tumor. After six weeks chemotherapy, she came to our office. PE: her general condition is find and emotion is stable. Her tongue was enlargement and couldn't speak clearly and her low jaw was firm and bougle. She was in chemotherapy and start to take XZ-C on Octocber 10 2007. This patient had multiple bone marrow tumor and was treated by chemotherapy and had tongue amyloid change and her microcirculation need to improve and her blood need to be active and her swell needs to be treated. After taking XZ-C4,1,6+LMS+MDZ+Radix for three months, her medical condition is stable and after six months her medical condition is significantly improved and her appetites is good and general condition is fine. She fills up her medicine every two months for more than four years.

Part V More research papers and the meeting Poster Collection

Table of Contents

1. The experiment research of searching etiology of cancer factor and pathogenesis and pathological physiology to seek for the effective control methods

In 1985 the author visited 3000 of his patients who had general surgical procedures for their different types of cancers. He found that most of the patients had cancer recurrence and metastasis during two or three years after their operation. Some of them recurred and died several months after the operation. Therefore, the author found that even if the operation is successful, the long-term therapy isn't satisfied or is failure. The patients had a big surgery and only were alive for one or two years or three years. Apparently this is not the patient's goals and not our aim. Generally, we only pay attention to five year surviving rate, but five year death rate. For example, the five year survival rate of stomach cancer is 20%; in another side, the five year death rate of stomach cancer is 80% which made the patients' family surprised. After following up many patients we found that the key factors for long-term therapy are recurrence and metastasis. Meanwhile, we found that important questions: to look for the method and ways of preventing cancer from recurrence and metastasis is the key to improve the survival rate after surgery.

Currently there are very high metastasis rate which is related to many factors such as cancer's stage, grade, and differentiation, and the host immunology function. Now there are high recurrence rate in outpatient setting. Fo instance, during one week the author treated forty cancer patients including fifteen recurred patients after the operations so that in order to prevent the recurrence and metastasis after the surgery, we must start to do something since the operation time. Because the cancer removal operation can easily leave some remaining cancer cells, the tissue cells will seed and metastased easily.. Once there are remaining, the cancer cells wil recur and metastasis, which cause terrible results. Therefore, Oncology surgery must follow the basic oncology rules. To remove the tumor during the surgery is the same important and strict thing as the sterilized rules during the general surgery, even more strict. There are two goals of performing no-tumor rules: 1. Preventing spread; 2. Preventing planation. The key to the surgical long-term results is recurrence and metastasis. During 20 century the oncology surgery has made extremely success. The task during 21 century is to prevent recurrence and metastasis to improve the long-term surgical results.

If there is no out break on basic research, the clinical efficiency will not be improved. If there questions are resolved, the oncology surgery will have significantly success. There fore, in 1985 the author built his own experimental research laboratory to conduct the cancer research. First, to make the experiment tumor model, then to start the basic research from the clinical practice.

To look for the tumor pathogenic factors, pathogenesis and metastasis mechanism to search the preventive an treating methods through many steps of cancer cells metastasis. After seven years tudy, the research projects are all the clinical questions which got explanation from the basic research. After seven years animal research, the author finished the following research work by steps and steps.

1. The experimental research of making cancer animal models

   Why can human being get cancer? Under what condition can cancer happen? Why can some get cancer, others can not get cancer under the same condition can the same environment? Are there intrinis or extrinis factors or both of them? Therefore, we should make the animal cancer models to study?

   a. To make the cancer animal models in order to do tumor experimental research

   The author was the chairman in Department of surgery in the affility hospital of Hubei traditional medical University so that he could do clinical work and do animal experimental together such as the tumor samples from the patient in Operation room to place to the animal bodies after 30 minutes xxxx, however there were no tumor growth after 100 times experiment(more than 400 animals). After removing the thymus, then transplant the tumor again, the animal models were built up(210 animals models). Some of tumor animal models were set up by injection of steroid to reduce small animal immune function, then transplant the tumor.

   After removing thymus five days, the tumor were transplant to the body, then during 5 or 6 days the lump which size is yellow been-size will grow, during 12-21 days the lump size will become thumb-size. The tumor can be alive three or four weeks, however it cannot be passed from generation to generation.

   1. It was found that after removing thymus, the tumor animal model can be set up. The steroid injection can assist to make the animal tumor models set up.

2. The result showed that tumor growth and development are related to the host's immune response and has significant relation to host immune organs and immune tissue functions

3. The result showed that thymus and immune system have certain/sure relations to the cancer growth. After removing host's thymus, the cancer animal models can be set up.

   If the thymus didn't be removed, the animal model cannot be built. Alsoinjection steroid can decrease the host immune response, which is helpful to set up the animal model. If the immune system doesn't reduce, the animal models will not set up.

   The research result showed that the correlation between the immune response and cancer cell growth is negative. When the immune response difficiency or decrease, the tumor can grow, which will not be get rid of by hosts' immune response.

b. Which is the first happen: immune decrease caused the cancer or the cancer cause the immune response decrease?

There are 320 Quanming mice which are separated into A, B, C, D group. Each group has 80 mice. The methods of removing thymus and injection of tumor cells are the same as before.

In group A, first remove thymus, then five days later injection of 106 cancer cells; in group B, first inject the steroid, then seven day later injecting cancer cells; in group C, first inject the cancer cells, then 10 days later removing thymus; in group D, first injecting cancer cells, then 10days later inject steroid. The result showed: the tumor growed in group A, B; There are only 18 mice which grew the green pea-size tumor in the 14day. This experiment implied that first the host's immune function decreased, or immune organ thymus has difficiency, then tumor can grow. If the host has good immune function, the tumors will not grow so that we get the conclusion: first immune function decrease, then cancer can develop and grow. If the immune system doesn't decrease, we can not built the cancer model successful. From this research, to improve and to maintain good immune function and to keep the good immune organ function are the most important methods to prevent from cancer growth.

c. The research animal model of tumor metastasis:

In 1985 the author built his tumor metastasis animal models, which he injected human cancer cells into the mice whose thymus is removed. Later he built up tumor metastasis model through lymph system. In 60 mice0.2 ml / 106 /ml H22 cells fuild was injected into animals' claw skin. After seven or eight days, an xxxxsize tumor grew up and the whole foot and ankle started to swell. After 16 days there are 8 mice which the right inguinal lymph nodes started to enlarge so that the lymphatic drainage metastasis animal models were built. Later the author built blood metastasis animal models which 0.4ml 106/ml of H22 cell were injected into the vein, then caused multiple tumors growth in lungs. After that, the liver metastasis animal models were built. 80 Quanming mice are divided into two groups A, B. In A group, there 40 mice. First inject steroid, seven days later 10% 75mg/kg xxxx

Was injected into abdominal cavity, then open it through cutting in with 0.5cm opening, expose spleen. 10ul H22 liver cells were injected into it and pressure 3-5min to prevent cells from flow out so that cells can flow into lymphatic system and blood system. After 11 days

These animal were sacrificed to get the liver and to count the tumor nodes in liver. The result show that in A, B groups, the tumors grew, however, the tumor number in A group are much more than those in B group. In A group there are 3-5 nodule which sizes are around 1mm. In Bgroup there are 1-3 nodules.

The result showed us that metastasis is significantly related to immune syterm. When the immune system decrease s or when the medicine inhibits the immune system, the tumors will grow up.

2. The experimental research of searching the relation between tumors and immune organ to seek the methods of immune organ control

Removing thymus, decreasing immune or immune deficiency can build the liver meatatasis animal models so that thymus and tumors growth have certain relation. Thymus is the central immune organ and spleen is the biggest peripheral immune system. What is the relation between spleen and tumors? In order to find the relation between immune system function and the tumor growth and development, the experimental research were done:

a. The experimental research of the effects of spleen on tumor growth:

Spleen is peripheral immune organ which is very important during the anticancer. In order to seek the effect of spleen on the tumor growth and development, the following experiments were done.

270 quanming white mice were divided into spleen group and no spleen group. In no spleen group, the first cancer cells injection and them removing spleen; the first removing spleen and them cancer cells injection and then injecting the cells again. All of the results showed that: spleen inhibit the tumor growth in the early stages by 25%. In the late stage, spleen shrinkles and lost it inhabitation. After implanation of the spleen, the spleen anticancer function was recovered by 54%.

We found that spleen has two stages: in the early stage, it inhibit the tumor growth. In the late stages, it lost the inhibitaion, after implanation of the spleen, the inhibition function will be recovered.

b. The experimental research of seeking the effects of tumors on thymus and spleen:

As we discussed before, the centrol immune organ thymus and peripheral organ spleen can influence the cancer cells growth. However, do tumors affect the host thymus and spleen? The following research are done:40 Quanming white mice were divided into four groups, then measured the lymphocyte transferation rate before injecting the cancer cells and on the third, seventh and fourteen days after injection of the cancer cells, then sacrified the mice to observe the weight of thymus and spleen and to make the histological slides.

The result showed: in the early stages of the tumor growth, the spleen filled blood and enlargement, and the cells proliferation increases; in the late stages the spleen started to shrinkle and the cell proliferation was inhibited. The thymus started to shrinkle immediately after injection of the cancer cells and the cell proliferation was inhibited and the volume was significantly decreases and the weigh significantly decreased which showed the organ immune functions were inhibited.

This experimental results showed that the tumors will inhibit the thymus function significantly and also canuse the thymus shrinkle.

c. The experimental research of searching the anticancer function of the tranditional Chinese medicine of enhancing the spleen function soup

As the above the spleen has certain effect on tumor growth and spleen implanation can increase the the inhibition rate of the spleen on the tumor growth. The spleen in the trandition Chinese medicine is different from thespleen in western medicine. They are different in the theory, pathogenesis and clinical. However both of them are the same names "spleen", even if they have different functions, whether can we use the enhancing the spleen methods and combined with the above model medicine experimental research results to build the tranditional enhancing spleen function medicine and to do animal experiments to observe whether these medicine can inhibit the tumor growth or not. 40 Quanming white mice are divided into experimental groug(n=30) and control groug(n=10) both of which were injected 0.1x107 cancer cells. In the experimental group the enhancing spleen soup were given for 14 days to observe the tumor growth, mice live quality and the mice survival time.

The result showed that these enhancing medicine can delay the occurrent time of the tumor lump after the injection of the tumor cells and inhibit the tumor growth and increase the survival time and have certain anticancer function.

3. The experimental research of searching the methods of inhibition of thymus shrinkle during the tumor growth and reconstruction of thehost immune function

When the author made the tumor animal models, he found that the animal models were set up only after removing the thymus and after repeating the same experiments three times, the results are the same, which showed that thymus and the tumor growth have the relation. The above experiment of the relation between the immune organ and tumor growth showed that the tumor growth can inhibit thymus and caused the thymus shrinkle so that tumors not only inhibit the function of thymus but also cause thymus shrinkles.

Because of these, we have to search the ways to stop the thymus shrinkle and to recover the thymus function to rebuild the immune system function. Therefore, we must designe some ways to implant immune organs to rebuild the immune function such as implanation of the embryo liver, spleen, thymus. 200 Quanming white mice which were made into xxx tumor models were divided into six experimental groups and two contral groups which were implanted embryo spleen, thymus, liver to record the tumor growth, disappear, survival time, the immune function and the tissue pathology change and compared each experimental group number. The results showed that in three experimental groups the rate which the tumors were completely disappeared is 40% in the early stages and the rate which the tumors were completely disappeared in the later stage is 46.67%. After the tumors completely disappeared, the animals can survive for a long time. The partial disappeared rate is 26.67% in the early group and is 13.33% in the long-term group. In the partial group the average survival time is above one month which the immune function increase and immune organ enlarge. The immune organ histology slides showed that the organ cells proliferation increased. This result showed that the reconstitution of immunce system organ completely and partially can help the host to fight the tumor and to improve the treatment effects.

4. Searching the medicine of inhibiting the new vascular formation from nanetural drug

In 1986 when the author cultured the cancer cells, he found that cancer cells can proliferate, however cann't form the tumor mass, occasionally found that if one to two chicken soup drops was added in the tubes, the tumor cells form the cells masses. If one or two drops of xxxbasic was added, this mass will be dissolved. Currently, it is known that ther are several steps which the cancer cells metastase: 1. Cancer cells escape from the primary sites into blood through the vesscle then flow into microvascular, then into the organs, then stay in the organ as tumor mass without the vascular system which can not grow big. Later the new vascular system will form soon and the tumor will grow big. If any step can be stopped, the tumor metastasis will be stopped. Because the author considered that forming microvascular system is the key of metastasis and tumor growth and tumor nodes formation so that the experimental research of searching the medicine which can inhibit the formation of tumor vascular system from the natural herbs are designed as the following:

1. The observation of forming mice vascular after injection of tumors into abdominal muscle s

20 Quanming white mice were injected EAC cells fluid to form the tumor microvascular models, then use Olymphus microscopy to observe the microvascular formation and count the microvascular flow rate and flow

amounts. In the first day of implanation, we found that there is no vascular formation. On the second day, the host's microvascular system will grow out the thin and curve new vascule into the tumor masses. On three or four days, the density of the new microvascules ourtside the tumor will increase.

2. The effects of different TG dose on mice immune function:

40 Quanming white mice were divided into TG1, TG2, TG3 and TG4 for different doses groups. After 12 days feed, the mice were sarastified on the 13th day to weigh thymus, spleen, body weight. The result showed that the different doses of TG has different effects on immune organ. A small dose 20mg/kg can increase the thymus weight and a big dose 80mg/kg can cause the thymus shrinkle.

3. The experimental research of TG inhibition of the growth of tumor microvascules in abdominal muscles

40 Quanming white mice which was injected with EAC in abdomen muscle was put on the observation table. The observation table put on the microscope in the temperation machine to observe the microvascular system growth such as the shapes, numbers in the tumor masse or around the tumor masses and took the pictures and measures the dentisy of the microvascular which come into and go out from the tumor masses and the average dimaster of the tumor vascule of the artery and vien and blood flow rates.

The results showed that TG(20mg/kg) significantly inhibit the growth of tumor new vessels in the early stages.

This experimental result showed that TG can significantly inhibit the new microvascular growth inside the tumor and around the tumors and decreases the density of the microvascule which entrance and extrance the tumors.

Currently many scientist from our country and other counties pay attention to inhibiting the formation of tumor new microvascules to control the tumor growth and metastasis masses formation. In May 1998 American Folkman reported that two of his medication such as Angiostation and Endostatin can inhibit the formation of the tumor new microvascules. In the tumor animal models, they can decrease the tumors significantily, which these medicine will inhibit the growth of vascules and shrinkle microvascule and the supply for the tumor will cut off so as to kill the cancer cells. He was planning to use these medicine in the human being in 1999.

The author finished TG experimental research in July 1997 because TG is trandition medication for more than hundreds years in Chinese medicine and is used in the clinical for a long time, however in the past TG is never used in inhibiting the growth of the microvascules. Since September 1998 the author started to use it as anticancer medication to use in the clinical patients. Until December 1999 more than 80 cases which had stage II, III cancers used it, which showed the good results of controlling the reccurence and metastasis. Now TG is in clinical trail stage.

2. Experimental Observation of Effects on Thymus and Spleen from Tumor

It is usually considered that the immune functions of organisms affect the occurrence, development and prognosis, however at the same time tumors can inhibit the immune state of organisms. These two are mutually causal and intricate and complicated. When doing the animal experiments on the influences of spleen on the tumorous growth, the author have observed that the immune organs thymus, spleen of the cancer-bearing mice have changed a lot. It seems that this process presents a certain law. In order to study further on the relationship and laws between tumors and spleens or thymus, the following experiments are designed to observe dynamically the changes of conversion rates of thymus, spleen and lymphocyte of cancer-bearing mice in different phases and probe into the relationship between them.

【Material and Methods】

1. Experimental animal and grouping

Use 40 Kunming mice and divide into four groups at random with the age of 40~50days and the weight of 15~18g, ignoring the sexes.

Group I: Control group of healthy mice which are not inoculated with cancer cells. After executing them, take away their thymus, spleens and circumferential blood to do the experiment.

Group II: Inoculate the mice with $0.1*10^7$ ehrlich ascites carcinoma through abdominal cavity, execute them after 3 days and observe.

Group III: Inoculate the mice with cancer cells (as the above) execute them after 7 days and observe.

Group IV: Inoculate the mice with cancer cells, execute them after 14 days and observe.

Use the results of anatomizing 100 cancer-bearing mice after natural death as the alterant results of thymus and spleen in terminal period. In this period the average diameter of thymus of cancer-bearing mice is 1.2±0.3mm, average weight is 20±5 mg with a bit hard texture. While spleens are extremely easy to atrophy, whose average weight is 60±12mm, texture is hard, and its color is gray, with the germinal center reducing and fibrosing.

2. Experimental methods

Execute the mice of each group by digging out their eyes and blooding them at the preconcerted time. Reserve the whole blood of each mouse (using heparin for anti-coagulation) to do the experiment of lymphocyte conversion and then anatomize them immediately; observe the range of soakage, volume of ascites and the situation of all viscera; emphasize on observing the anatomical shape of thymus, spleens and lymph nodes and take out the thymus and spleen integrally, then measure their volume with a vernier caliper; weigh them respectively using analytical balance and send them to the department of defection.

3. Measuring the conversion rate of peripheral blood lymphocytes of mice in each group

Dig out their eyes and blood with heparin for anti-coagulation.

4. Making tumor model

As same as the experimental part as before Chapter.

【Experimental Result】

1. Thymic weights of mice in each group after inoculated with cancer cells in different phases (see table 1)

Do analysis of variance with the statistical data in table 1, see table 2. Using a curve to present the results of table 1 and table 2, draw the curve of change in the thymic weights (chart 1); the thymic weights of the 25th day and 30th day in the chart are quoted from the results of the experimental part in previous chapter.

Table 1 Comparison of thymic weights of mice in each group (mg)

Group	Group I healthy	Group II on the 3rd after inoculated	Group III on the 7th after inoculated		Group IV on the 14th after inoculated
组别	I 组正常组	II 组接种后第 3 天	III 组接种后第 7 天		IV 组接种后第 14 天
	72.8	78.2	90.0		40.0
	50.0	83.4	66.0		32.2
	56.4	89	85.4		39.8
	96.4	68	106.5		23.5
X_u	77.4	74.8	51.7		38.0
	100.7	95.4	77.8		36.0
	87.5	115.0	73.0		46.0
	76.8	56.4	60.0		20.0
	112.7	43.0	49.4		55
	51.0				20
ΣX	781.07	703.2	736.3	350.5	ΣX 2 571.7
N_i	10	9	10	10	N 39
$\bar{X}_i$	78.17	78.13	73.63	35.05	$\bar{X}$ 65.94
ΣX^2	6 6261.79	58 566.66	57 033.75	18 467.25	ΣX^2 191 324.75

Table 2 Analysis of variance of table 1

Resources of variation	SS	V	MS	F	P
Between groups	12967.10	3	4322.36	12.85	<0.01
Within groups	11777.12	35	336.48		
Total	24744.22	38			

It can be noticed that thymuses of the cancer-bearing mice present the regular change from table 1, table 2 and chart 1. Within 7 days after inoculation, thymuses have no obvious change observed by eyes; however their weights begin to lose weight. After 7 days, they present acute progressive atrophy; in the later period, the diameter of the thymuses reduce from the normal level 5~8 mm to about 1mm and the weights decrease from 76.1mg to 20mg with the texture becoming hard and the functions declining even lost, which indicates that the cellular immune functions are operated and inhibited increasingly with the development of tumors, and the immune functions are declined to a lower level with tumors growing more and more rapidly.

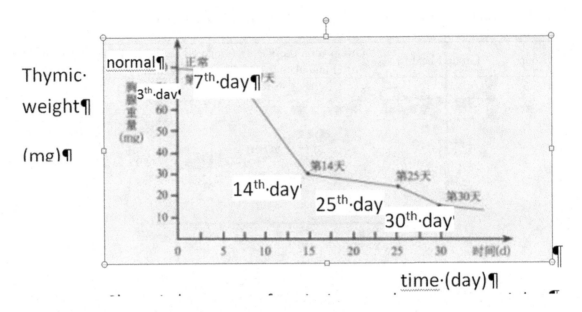

Chart 1 the curve of variation on the thymic weights

2. Splenic weights of mice in each group after inoculated with cancer cells in different phases (see table 3 and 4)

Table 3 splenic weights of cancer-bearing mice in each group in different phases

Group	Group I healthy	Group II on the 3rd after inoculated	Group III on the 7th after inoculated	Group VI on the 14th after inoculated

Table 4 Analysis of variance of table 3

组别	I 组正常组	II 组接种后第 3 天	III 组第 7 天	IV 组第 14 天		
	98. 4	103. 0	152. 8	120. 7		
	86. 0	110. 3	175. 8	96. 9		
	139. 0	153. 2	154. 5	103. 0		
	126. 0	96. 7	154. 0	102. 0		
	194. 4	206. 0	290. 4	91. 9		
X_i	130	137. 0	156. 0	122. 3		
	107. 4	174. 0	184. 0	88. 6		
	82. 8	143. 0	232. 0	109. 0		
	86. 0	160	86. 3	102. 4		
	82. 0			119. 0		
ΣX	1 258. 4	1 209. 0	1 720. 9	1 021	ΣX	5 210. 2
N_i	10	9	9	10	N	38
$\overline{X}_i$	125. 84	134. 43	172. 09	102. 1	$\overline{X}$	133. 59
ΣX^2	169 020. 88	175 088. 97	322 834. 65	106. 41	ΣX^2	773. 385

Resources of variation	SS	V	MS	F	P
Between groups	25345.12	3	8448	5.68	<0.01
Within groups	51983	35	1485.24		
Total	77328.12	38			

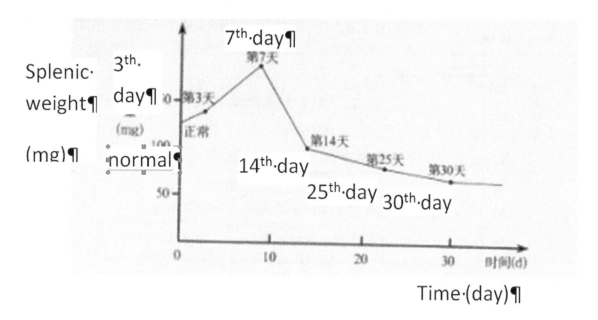

Chart 2 the curve of variation on the splenic weights

Inspect the 100 corpses in the experimental group in previous chapter and get the average splenic weight is 60±12 mg. Use a curve to describe the change in splenic weights (chart 2).

From the statistical data in table 3, 4 and chart 2, it can be found that spleens of cancer- bearing mice in the early stage the volume is enlarging gradually and the weight is increasing, while in the later stage, the spleens present progressive atrophy. The above indicates that in the early period, cellular proliferation is active and the effects of immune response are reinforced as well as the inhibition on tumors due to the tumor simulation so as to react on inhibiting the growth of tumors; while in the latter period, as the number has enlarged plentifully, a great of inhibitory factors are produced to inhibit cells and immunity to stop the proliferation of splenic immune cells and consume effector cells, which results in atrophy and fabric tissue hyperplasia, the inhibition on tumors is weakened even promote the growth of tumors.

3. Comparison of experimental results of peripheral blood lymphocytes of the cancer-bearing mice conversion at different time (see table 5 and 6)

Table 5 Comparison of the conversion rate of peripheral blood lymphocytes in each group at different time (%)

Group I healthy	Group II on the 3rd after inoculated		Group III on the 7th after inoculated		Group VI on the 14th after inoculated
I 组正常组	II 组接种后第 3 天		III 组第 7 天		IV 组第 14 天
45	53		43		31
40	62		32		28
51	48		26		19
42	43		45		21
60	52		30		22
39	51		32		23
	50				
ΣX 277	359	208	144	ΣX	988
N_i 6	7	6	6	N	25
$\overline{X}_i$ 46. 17	51. 29	24		$\overline{X}$	39. 52
$\Sigma_i X$ 13 111	18 611	7 498	3 560	ΣX^2	42 780

Table 6 Analysis of variance of table 5

Resources of variation	SS	V	MS	F	P
Between groups	2820.64	3	940.21	21.614	<0.01
Within groups	913.59	21	43.51		
Total	3734.23	24			

Using a curve to present the results of table 5 and table 6, draw the curve of lymphocyte conversion rate of the cancer-bearing mice at different time (chart 3).

Chart 3 curve of lymphocyte conversion rate

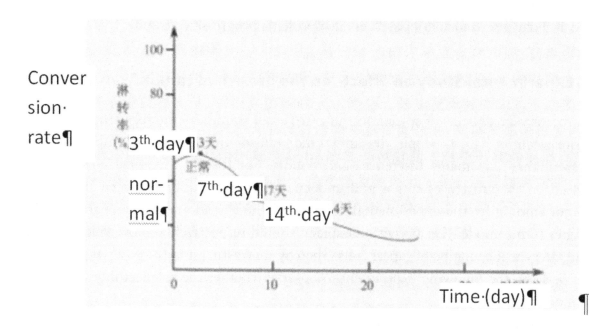

From table 5, 6 and chart 3, it can be seen that the change in lymphocyte conversion rate of the cancer-bearing mice presents certain regularity: after inoculation the conversion rate increase slightly and then presents an acute progressive decrease. Until 14th day (later period), it declines to normal level about 50% and continue declining after that, which indicates that in the whole course of diseases, tumors produce inhibitory effect on the cellular immunity; what's more, with the course of diseased this effect becomes more intensive and the immune functions are damaged.

From chart 1, 2 and 3 it can be known that the changes in thymic volume and weight are extremely similar to the curve of lymphocyte conversion rate presented as synchronism. By contrast, the changes in splenic volume and weight are different from them with increase in the early period and the decrease, which indicates that during the middle and later period, both the organismal humoral immunity and cellular immunity are damaged and inhibited.

4. Changes of thymic and splenic pathology

(1) Thymus presents progressive atrophy during the whole course of disease; on the 3rd day after inoculated with cancer cells, thymus shrinks slightly and the color is gray; on the 7th day, thymic volume shrinks obviously and the cellular proliferation is stopped with reduced mature cells; during the later period of tumors, thymus shrinks extremely and its volume is as big as a sesame with the diameter of 1 mm and hard texture.

(2) Spleen is congested and tumefied; the volume is augmenting with being black red and crisp. The number of germinal centers increase and mature decrease; while from the 14th day after inoculation, spleen also presents progressive atrophy.

3. Experimental Study on Effects on the growth of tumor from spleen

In recent years, effects of spleen on the anti-tumor immunity are receiving more and more attentions from people. Its anti-tumor effects are extremely complicated. At present there are many differences and doubts. For further investigating effects of spleen on the growth of tumor and understanding the relation between spleen and tumor immunity, the experimental surgical method is adopted to prepare Ehrlich ascites tumor model. Group without spleen should respectively remove spleen before and after the inoculation of cancer cells. Then by contrasting it to the group with spleen, we perform the following experiment to observe whether the splenectomy will affect tumor immune state.

[Material and Method]

1. Experimental Animal Grouping Kunming mice, no gender classification, mice age 50~60d, weight 15~20g, and quantity of 300. According to the group with or without spleen, different sequence of splenectomy and inoculation of cancer cells, they are divided into 5 groups. Then on the basis of various amounts of inoculated cells (1×10^4 ml or 1×10^7 ml) and different inoculated regions (abdominal cavity or subcutaneous), each group is further separated into subgroups A and B. The specific grouping is shown in the following table 1.

Table 1 Summary table of experimental animal grouping

Group Inoculation Method	cancer cells concentration 1×10^4/ml		cancer cells concentration 1×10^7/ml	
	percutaneous	transabdominal	percutaneous	transabdominal
Group I simulating spleen removal	I A$_1$ (15)	I A$_2$ (15)	I B$_1$ (15)	I B$_2$ (15)
Group II (spleen removal before inoculation)	II A$_1$ (15)	II A$_2$ (15)	II B$_1$ (15)	II B$_2$(15)
Group III (inoculation before spleen removal)	III A (30)		III B (30)	
Group IV (spleen removal before inoculation+ splenic cells)	IV A$_1$ (15)	II A$_2$ (15)	IV B$_1$ (15)	IV B$_2$ (15)
Group V (administration of Chinese medicine)	V A (15)		V B (15)	

The Fourth Section Experimental Study

Group I: Control group with spleen. Firstly simulating spleen removal, after 7d transabdominal or percutaneous inoculation of Ehrlich ascites cancer cells 0.1ml, the number of cancer cells is 1×10^4 or 1×10^7 (table 2).

Table 2 Control group of simulating spleen removal (Group I)

Group I	Inoculated Cancer Cell Number	Inoculated Regions	Mice Number
I A$_1$	0.1×10^4	right armpit subcutaneousness	15
I A$_2$	0.1×10^4	abdominal cavity	15
I B$_1$	0.1×10^7	right armpit subcutaneousness	15
I B$_2$	0.1×10^7	abdominal cavity	15

Group II: Group of spleen removal before inoculation. Firstly spleen removal, after 7d percutaneous or transabdominal inoculation of Ehrlich ascites cancer cells 0.1ml, the number of cancer cells is 1×10^4 or 1×10^7 (table 3).

Table 3 Group of spleen removal before inoculation

Group II	Inoculated Cancer Cell Number	Inoculated Regions	Mice Number
II A$_1$	0.1×10^4	right armpit subcutaneousness	15
II A$_2$	0.1×10^4	abdominal cavity	15
II B$_1$	0.1×10^7	right armpit subcutaneousness	15
II B$_2$	0.1×10^7	abdominal cavity	15

Group III: Group without spleen, i.e. group of inoculation before spleen removal. Firstly inoculation of cancer cells, after 7d spleen removal. Both are right armpit subcutaneous inoculations. The number of cancer cells is 1×10^4ml or 1×10^7ml (table 4).

Table 4 Group of inoculation before spleen removal

Group III	Inoculated Cancer Cell Number	Inoculated Regions	Mice Number
III A	0.1×10^4	right armpit subcutaneousness	15
III B	0.1×10^7	right armpit subcutaneousness	15

Group IV: Group of spleen removal before inoculation, and further transabdominal transplantation of splenic cells or clear liquid of splenic tissue. Firstly remove spleen, after 7d inoculate cancer cells. In another 1d, transabdominal injection of living spleen cell suspension or supernatant liquid of splenic tissue (table 5).

Table 5 Group of spleen removal before transplantation of splenic cells or clear liquid of splenic tissue

Group IV	Inoculated Cancer Cell Number	Inoculated Regions	Processing Factor	Mice Number
IV A$_1$	0.1×10^4	trans-sub right armpit	injection of supernatant liquid of splenic tissue	15
IV A$_2$	0.1×10^4	transabdominal	injection of supernatant liquid of splenic tissue	15
IV B$_1$	0.1×10^7	right armpit subcutaneousness	transplantation of splenic cells of newborn mice	15
IV B$_2$	0.1×10^7	abdominal cavity	transplantation of splenic cells of adult mice	15

Group V: Group of taking Traditional Chinese Medicine (TCM) complex prescription with efficacy of strengthening the spleen and replenishing qi (table 6).

Table 6 Group of taking Traditional Chinese Medicine (TCM) complex prescription with efficacy of strengthening the spleen and replenishing qi

Group V	Inoculated Cancer Cell Number	Inoculated Regions	Processing Factor	Mice Number
V A	$10^7 \times 0.1$	right armpit subcutaneousness	firstly take TCM for 10d, after inoculation continue to take medication for 3 weeks	15
V B	$10^7 \times 0.1$	right armpit subcutaneousness	after inoculation take medication for 3 weeks	15

2. Instruments and Materials

(1) An animal sterile operating room and a set of sterile surgical instruments.

(2) Hank liquid, improved Hank liquid, calf serum, PRH, triple-distilled water, 0.9% sodium chloride solution for injection, ketamine, soluble phenobarbital, heparin sodium, trypan blue stain, Giemsa stain, Wright's stain, hydrochloric acid baking soda, L-glutamic acid, sensitization and non- sensitization zymosan.

(3) Centrifugal machine with 400 rounds per minute, glass homogenizer, medicine vibrator, filtering metal gauze (size 1000), funnel, thermostat, baker, low temperature water tank, microscope, relative sterile workbench.

(4) Animal feed are refined pellet feed. The drinking water is tap water. Rearing cage is plastic mouse cage.

3. Tumor Inoculation and Model Preparation Ehrlich ascites tumor cell strain is introduced from Wuhan Biological Research Institute Cell Room. Ascites containing cancer cells are extracted from ascitic-type tumor animal abdominal cavity of mice Ehrlich ascites tumor. Firstly use improved Hank liquid to clean and centrifugate ascites for 3 times with 800 rounds per minute of centrifugal speed and five minutes. Remove supernatant liquid, and respectively combine deposited cancer cells with Hank liquid to make up the cancer cell suspensions, containing 1×10^4 ml or 1×10^7 ml inoculated cells. The trypan blue dead cells exclusion test proves that the living cell rate is above 95%. Then inoculate cancer cells to experimental mice through right armpit subcutaneousness and abdominal cavity. Each mouse is inoculated with cancer cell suspension of 0.1ml, i.e. amounts of containing cancer cells are 1×10^4 ml or 1×10^7 ml.

4. Splenectomy Combine ketamine with soluble phenobarbital to execute intraperitoneal anesthesia. Dosages are 0.4mg/10g and 0.2mg/10g. After anesthesia, fix the mouse on surgery board. Shear the belly fur. Use iodine (2.5%) and ethanol (75%) to disinfect the belly. Bespread the sterile cloth on it. An incision is made into each layer of abdominal wall tissue through left lower abdomen. Then enter into abdominal cavity. Expose and dissociate the spleen. Use silk thread of size 0 to ligate the splenic stalk. Excise the spleen. Ensure the strict sterile operation, gentle action and thorough hemostases. During the operation, notice whether there is a splenulus. In case there is, excise it together. For simulating spleen removal of control group, only open the abdominal cavity; pull but do not excise the spleen. Antibiotics are not used in and after the operation. Infection of incisional wound is 1.0%. After operation, continue to feed the mouse with refined pellet feed.

5. Preparations of Splenic Cell Suspension and Supernatant Liquid of Splenic Tissue

(1) Preparation of splenic cell suspension: Execute newborn Kunming mice of 24~48h or adult mice. An incision is made into abdominal wall to take out the spleen. Cut off peripheral envelope and adipose tissue of spleen. Use Hank liquid to irrigate them in sterile glass culture dish for 3 times. Then put spleen into the glass homogenizer. Add in Hank liquid for 5ml. Grind up the splenic tissue. Filter it with stainless silk net of size 100. Centrifugate the filtering medium (1000 rounds per minute, 10 min). Remove supernatant liquid. Use Hank liquid to dilute deposited cells and make up the splenic cell suspensions of 5×10^7/ml. Suspensions are dyed by trypan blue stain and proved that the living cell rate

is above 97%. Then transplant splenic cell suspensions into abdominal cavity of experimental mouse. Each mouse can only accept splenic cell suspensions of 2ml which belong to one receptor.

(2) Preparation of splenic cell homogenate: After excising the spleen, use quick freezing (-20 centi degree) and rapid rewarming to induce the cracking of dead splenic cells proved by trypan blue stain and microscopic examination. Then centrifugate the filtering medium (1000 rounds per minute, 10 min). Reserve supernatant liquid and remove deposits. Inject supernatant liquid through abdomen into the experimental mouse.

6. Observation Item

(1) Observe success ratio of cancer cell inoculation, occurrence time of subcutaneous tumor nodi and speed of tumor enlargement.

(2) Every day use vernier caliper to measure diameter and size of subcutaneous tumor nodi; measure mouse' weight; observe metastasis condition and moving degree.

(3) Observe the quality of life, fur color, vitality, state of nutrition, breath, mental state of tumor-bearing mice and survival time of bearing tumor.

(4) Observe abdominal shape and prohection of ascetic-type tumor-bearing mice. Also according to prohection state, divide ascites content into 5 grades.

Grade 0: the abdomen is not of fullness, without ascites, note as (-).

Grade 1: slight prohection of abdomen, with a little ascites, note as (+).

Grade 2: prohection of abdomen, with medium content of ascites, note as (++).

Grade 3: obvious prohection of abdomen, with more ascites, note as (+++).

Grade 4: shape of frog abdomen, with plentiful ascites, note as (++++).

During necropsy, measure the content of ascites, microscopic examination of cancer cell shape, count living cell rate and content.

(5) Determine immunologic functional condition of red blood cells of tumor-bearing mice: test for measuring C_3b receptor garland with semi quantitative method.

(6) Necropsy and pathological section: dissect each dead experimental mouse. Observe tumor's size and weight, infiltrating and metastatic condition, morphological structure and involvement condition of visceral organs; measure the content of ascites; extract tumor tissue, liver, spleen, thymus gland, lung and other visceral organs to carry out the examination of pathological section.

[Experimental Result]

1. Resulting comparison and analysis on different groups with right armpit subcutaneous inoculation of small dose of 0.1×10^4 ml Ehrlich ascites tumor cells.

(1) Comparison on occurrence time of tumor nodi with different processing method (T test), see table 22-7.

Table 7 Comparison on occurrence time (d) of tumor nodi with different processing method (T test)

Group	Group I A_1 (Control group with spleen)	Group II A_1 (Group of spleen removal before inoculation)	Group IIIA (Group of inoculation before spleen removal)	Group IVA$_1$ (Spleen removal before inoculation+supernatant liquid of splenic tissue)
Occurrence time (d)	8	7*	9	9*

Note: ① *. Compared with Group I A_1, $P<0.05$ has remarkable significance; ② In Group I A_1 (control group with spleen), one experimental mouse (accounts for 7.6%) suffers no tumor nodi after inoculation of cancer cells. It survives for a long term (i.e. survival time is above 90d). No tumor is found during dissection. Treat it as inoculation failure. Not for statistical treatment; also in Group IVA (group with transabdominal injection of supernatant liquid of splenic tissue), 3 experimental mice (accounts for 25%) fail to be inoculated.

According to table 7, the earliest occurrence time of tumor nodi in above groups belongs to group of spleen removal before inoculation (Group II A_1). Control group and group with injection of supernatant liquid of splenic tissue have the later occurrence time.

(2) For different processing methods, maximum diameter comparison of each group's tumor nodi on the seventh, fourteenth and twentieth day, see table 8.

Table 8 Size comparison of each group's tumor nodi on the seventh, fourteenth and twentieth day after subcutaneous inoculation of 0.1×10^4 ml cancer cells (maximum diameter mm)

Group	Group I A₁ (Control group with spleen)	Group II A₁ (Group of spleen removal before inoculation)	Group III A (Group of inoculation before spleen removal)	Group IVA₁ (Spleen removal before inoculation+supernatant liquid of splenic tissue)	P
seventh	0	3.3±0.48	0	0	<0.01
fourteenth	11.43±5.99	14.4±6.2	11.8±7.45	8±4.33	<0.01
twentieth	18.92±9.98	21.12±8.28	19.7±5.98	13.89±7.63	<0.01

Note: Values P in the table are gained through analysis of diameter variance (F test).

From above results in the table, the tumor which belongs to group of spleen removal before inoculation (Group II A₁) appears first and grows fast. Before the fourteenth day, its tumor volume reaches biggest. On the twentieth day after inoculation, tumors' sizes of control group (Group I A₁), group II A₁ (group of spleen removal before inoculation), group of inoculation before spleen removal (Group III A) reach unanimity. While tumors which belong to group of injecting supernatant liquid of splenic tissue (Group IV A₁) have the smallest volume. That explains that during early growing stage of tumor (before the seventh day), spleen has tumor inhibitory action. But during medium and advanced stages (experimental group sets: medium stage is from eighth day to fourteenth day since the inoculation; since the fourteenth day, it is tumor advanced stage), the inhibitory action of spleen weakens or disappears. Furthermore, it can be observed that after cancer cells inoculation of spleen removal group, since the fourteenth day, tumor nodi often bear liquefaction, necrosis and ablation, which result in the shrinkage of tumor volume. Even some incisions have healed. Why does such phenomenon appear? That needs to have a further observation.

(3) Comparison of mean survival time (MST) for groups of subcutaneous inoculation with 0.1×10^4 ml cancer cells, see table 9.

Table 9 Comparison of each group's mean survival time (MST)

Group	Group I A₁ (Control group with spleen)	Group II A₁ (Group of spleen removal before inoculation)	Group III A (Group of inoculation before spleen removal)	Group IVA₁ (Spleen removal before inoculation+supernatant liquid of splenic tissue)	P
MST (d)	41.61±12.24	38.73±19.63	44.8±15.95	50±27.21	<0.05

Note: Values P in the table are gained through F test.

From table 9, mean survival times of groups I A₁, II A₁, III A are close to each other. T test shows there is no difference among these three groups, $P > 0.05$. While for injection of supernatant liquid of splenic tissue, mean survival time of this group is obviously longer than those of other groups, $P < 0.05$. The significant difference exists.

2. Resulting analysis of each group's transabdominal inoculation with 0.1×10^4 ml cancer cells After inoculation of cancer cells, experimental mice can survive above 90d without any ascite or tumor nodus. Also a dissection of corpse shows no tumor. The above results are treated as inoculation failures. It explains the fact that vaccinal cancer cells are rejected by the organism and no tumor forms.

(1) Comparison of inoculation failure rate for each group's transabdominal inoculation of 0.1×10^4 ml cancer cells without ascites, see table 10.

Table 10 Comparison of each group's inoculation failure rate (T test)

Group	Group I A₂ (Control group with spleen)	Group II A₂ (Group of spleen removal before inoculation)	Group II A₂ (Spleen removal before inoculation+supernatant liquid of splenic tissue)
failure rate	26%	0**	54%*

Note: **. indicates the comparison with control group, T test $P<0.01$, with high degree of significant difference; *. indicates $P<0.05$, with significant difference.

Results of table 10 show that all experimental mice in the group of spleen removal before inoculation form ascites, and failure rate is zero. The inoculation failure rates of control group with spleen and injection group of supernatant liquid of splenic tissue are 26% and 54% respectively. It process that tumor is easy to grow in the mouse without spleen after inoculation of tumor. That is, the removal of spleen promotes the growth of tumor. On the contrary, injection of supernatant liquid of splenic cells will suppress the growth of tumor.

(2) Comparison of survival time for each group's transabdominal inoculation of 0.1×10^4 ml cancer cells, see table 11.

Table 11 Comparison of each group's survival time (F test)

Group	Group I A₂ (Control group with spleen)	Group II A₂ (Group of spleen removal before inoculation)	Group IVA₂ (Spleen removal before inoculation+supernatant liquid of splenic tissue)	P
survival time (d)	51.46±29.35	35.6±18.93	57.6±14.85	<0.05

From table 11, the mean survival time of group with spleen removal before inoculation is 35.6±18.93 days. While mean survival times of control group with spleen and injection group of supernatant liquid of splenic tissue are 51.46±29.35 days and 57.6±14.85 days respectively, and P<0.05. Significant differences exist among these three groups. In three groups, group of spleen removal before inoculation has the shortest survival time. Group with spleen owns long survival time; while group without spleen owns short survival time. That shows the removal of spleen promotes the growth of tumor and shortens survival times of tumor-bearing mice. On the contrary, injection of supernatant liquid of splenic cells will suppress the growth of tumor and prolong survival times of tumor-bearing mice.

3. Results of each group's subcutaneous inoculation with 0.1×10^7 ml cancer cells

(1) Comparison on occurrence time of each group's subcutaneous tumor nodi, see table 12.

Table 12 Comparison on occurrence time of each group's subcutaneous tumor nodi

Group	Group I B$_1$ (Control group with spleen)	Group II B$_1$ (Group of spleen removal before inoculation)	Group III B (Group of inoculation before spleen removal)	Group IV B$_1$ (Spleen removal before inoculation+transplantation of fetal mouse's splenic cells)	P
Occurrence time (d)	5.5	5	7.5	9	<0.05

Mice of group IIIB are removed spleens on the seventh day after inoculations. So after seven days group IIIB and control group with spleen (Group I B$_1$) are in the same condition. The table shows that for the group with spleen removal first, occurrence times of subcutaneous tumor nodi are slightly earlier than these of other groups. While for group IVB$_1$ (transplantation of fetal mouse's splenic cells), occurrence times of tumor nodi are obviously later than these of other groups. It proves that the removal of spleen promotes the growth of tumor. While transplantation of splenic cells intensively suppresses the growth of tumor.

(2) Comparison of maximum diameter average on each group's subcutaneous tumor nodi on the seventh, fourteenth and twentieth day after inoculation, see table13.

Table 13 Comparison of maximum diameter on each group's tumor nodi on the seventh, fourteenth and twentieth day (mm)

Group	Group I B$_1$ (Control group with spleen)	Group II B$_1$ (Group of spleen removal before inoculation)	Group III B (Group of inoculation before spleen removal)	Group IV B$_1$ (Spleen removal before inoculation + transplantation of fetal mouse's splenic cells)	P
seventh	5.07±1.847	10.88±5.278	2.83±1.948	3.0±1.56	<0.01
fourteenth	19.85±4.598	21.12±5.3	20.3±6.07	11±5.69	<0.01
twentieth	30.9±7.87	24±7.86	25.25±4.77	16±4.95	<0.01

Note: Values P in the table are gained through F test.

(3) Comparison of each group's mean survival time (MST), see table14.

Table 14 Comparison of each group's mean survival time (subcutaneous inoculation of $0.1×10^7$ ml cancer cells)

Group	Group I B$_1$ (Control group with spleen)	Group II B$_1$ (Group of spleen removal before inoculation)	Group III B	Group IV B$_1$ (Spleen removal before inoculation + transplantation of fetal mouse's splenic cells)	P
MST (d)	33.1±13.15	49.56±24.39	38.7±14.45	50.75±19.30	<0.01

From table 13 and 14, on the seventh day after inoculation, for the three groups-control group with spleen (Group IB$_1$), group of spleen removal before inoculation (Group IIB$_1$) and group of inoculation before spleen removal (Group IIIB), their maximum diameter averages of tumor nodi are $\overline{X}$(IB$_1$) = (5.07±1.847) mm, $\overline{X}$ (IIB$_1$) = (10.88±5.278) mm, $\overline{X}$(IIIB) = (2.83±1.948) mm respectively. $P<0.01$. Significant differences exist among these three groups. Tumors which belong to the group of spleen removal before inoculation (IIB$_1$) have the maximum volumes. Now on the seventh day, in fact groups IB$_1$ and IIIB have the spleen, which is in proliferative active phase. While group IIB$_1$ has no spleen. The tumor volume of group with spleen is smaller, and the tumor volume of group without spleen is larger. It indicates that the spleen can suppress tumor during early stage or the removal of spleen can promote the growth of tumor. While on the fourteenth day after inoculation, their average maximum diameters of tumor nodi are $\overline{X}$(IB$_1$) = (19.85±4.598) mm, $\overline{X}$(IIB$_1$) = (21.12±5.3) mm, $\overline{X}$(IIIB) = (20.3±6.07) mm respectively. $P>0.05$. Significant differences disappear among these three groups. On the twentieth day after inoculation, the tumor volume of control group with spleen is larger than that of other groups. The maximum diameter $\overline{X}$= (30.9±7.87) mm. At this time, the spleen of tumor-bearing mouse has extremely shrank, and lost the tumor inhibitory action. From the experiment, since the fourteenth day after inoculation, most mice tumors of group with spleen removal begin to bear liquefaction and necrosis. Some lumps ulcerate and ablate, whose volumes shrink. The reason that tumors in this period suffer from liquefaction, necrosis and ulceration is not clear at present. That needs to have a further observation.

Therefore, during the early stage of tumor, spleen can suppress the growth of tumor. For the group with spleen, the tumor growth rate is slower. Tumor volume is smaller. While on the advanced stage of tumor, the inhibitory action of spleen weakens or disappears. The tumor size of all groups reaches unanimity.

Furthermore, it can be seen from the stable that tumors of the group (IVB_1), which removes spleen before inoculation and transplants splenic cells of fetal mice, have obviously slower growth rate than that of other groups. The tumor volume is smaller. Its survival time is longer that that of other groups. These conditions prove that splenic cells of homogeneous variant fetus have obvious tumor-inhibitory action.

4. Results of each group's transabdominal inoculation with 0.1×10^7 ml cancer cells

(1) Comparison on occurrence time of ascites for each group, see table 15.

Table 15 Comparison on occurrence time of ascites for each group of transabdominal inoculation with 0.1×10^7 ml cancer cells

Group	Group I B_2 (Control group with spleen)	Group II B_2 (Group of spleen removal before inoculation)	Group IV B_2 (Spleen removal before inoculation+transplantation of splenic cells)
Occurrence time (median, d)	5	3*	4*

Note: **. indicates the comparison with control group, T test $P<0.05$, with significant difference.

(2) Occupying percentages of ascites content greater than (++) for groups on the fifth, seventh and fourteenth day after transabdominal inoculation of 0.1×10^7 ml cancer cells, see table 22-16.

Table 16 Comparison on ascites content of transabdominal inoculation with 0.1×10^7 ml cancer cells

Days after inoculation (d)	Group I B_2 (Control group with spleen)	Group II B_2 (Group of spleen removal before inoculation)	Group IV B_2 (Spleen removal before inoculation+transplantation of splenic cells)
2	0%	75% **	10% *
7	28%	100% **	70% *
14	100%	100%	100% *

Note: **. indicates the comparison with IB_2 (control group), T test $P<0.01$; *. indicates $P<0.05$; no *. indicates $P>0.05$.

(3) Comparison of survival time (d) for each group's transabdominal inoculation of 0.1×10^7 ml cancer cells, see table17.

Table 17 Comparison of each group's survival time

Group	Group I B$_2$ (Control group with spleen)	Group II B$_2$ (Group of spleen removal before inoculation)	Group IV B$_2$ (Spleen removal before inoculation+transplantation of splenic cells)
survival time (d)	20.15±4.59	15.56±10.94*	16.67±8.34

Note: *. indicates the comparison with IB$_2$, $P<0.05$, with significant difference; no *. indicates the comparison with IB$_2$, $P>0.05$, without significant difference.

Integrating tables15, 16 and 17, results show that for the group with spleen removal first (IIB$_2$), tumor growth rate is faster. Amounts of ascites are more. Survival time is shorter. Also visceral organs are easier to metastasize. Those explain that removal of spleen can promote the growth of tumor. Transabdominal transplantation of splenic cells of homogeneous variant adult mice can partially suppress the growth of tumor. But its inhibitory action is weaker than that of control group with spleen and group with transplantation of fetal mouse's splenic cells.

5. Results of necropsy and pathological examination Each mouse accepts the postmortem necropsy. Visually observe tumor shape, involved visceral organs and diffusion condition. And extract tissues for pathological section examination. The result shows that Ehrlich ascites tumor cell strain owns features of stable proliferation, strong invasiveness and so on. Subcutaneous inoculation is easy to induce the form of solid tumor. Necropsy proves that after inoculation tumors or ascites are easy to form in some regions, easily infiltrating to surrounding tissues. The metastases of cancer cells rarely happen to mice with subcutaneous inoculation. While for mice with transabdominal inoculation, cancer cells easily metastasize to liver, kidney and lymph node in advanced stage. Only two of two hundred and seventy experimental mice suffer from splenic metastases, proving the weak affinity of spleen to cancer cells. This group of experiments has also found phenomena that for the group of spleen removal before transabdominal inoculation, multiple carcinomatous metastases appear in visceral organs of abdominal cavity. Metastatic ratio is up to 50%. These metastases invade liver, kidney, pancreas and mesenteric lymph nodes, always implicating more than two visceral organs. While for control group with spleen and group with transplantation of homogeneous variant splenic cells, carcinomatous metastases rarely occur. Metastatic ratios are 20% and 25%, which are obviously lower than those of the group without spleen. It shows that spleen can suppress the growth of tumor. While the group without

spleens lose the inhibitory action, consequently leading to easy diffusion and metastasis of tumor.

Furthermore, dynamic observation of this group of experimental mice shows that thymus and spleen of tumor-bearing mice present a series of changes with the process of illness, which own certain regularity. About seven days after inoculation, the thymus presents acute and progressive atrophy. Its volume shrinks; the diameter of each normal lobule shortens from 5~8cm to about 1mm; the weight reduces from (70±10) mg to (20±5) mg. While soon after the inoculation of cancer cells, spleen becomes congested and tumid. The volume enlarges; weight increases; texture becomes fragile. Microscopic examination shows the increase of germinal centers and active cell proliferation. On the fourteenth day after inoculation, the spleen also quickly presents progressive atrophy. Its volume shrinks; the weight reduces from (140±15) mg to (50±10) mg. Germinal centers obviously decrease; cell proliferation is suffocated. The spleen also suffers from hyperplasia of fibrous tissues, fibrosis with gray color and rigid texture.

6. Testing results of erythrocytic immune function This group of experiments choose 100 mice to carry out the erythrocytic C_3b receptor garland test. The result shows that after the removal of spleen, bonding ratio of C_3b receptor garland of tumor-bearing mice is on a progressive declining tendency. That explains that after the removal of spleen, immunological adhesive competence of red blood cells drops to some extent.

[Discussion]

1. As seen from experimental results, spleen can suppress the growth of tumor. After the removal of spleen, compared with the control group, the growth rate is faster; the occurrence time and volume of subcutaneous tumor nodi is earlier and larger in the same period. For group with transabdominal inoculation of cancer cells and group with the removal of spleen, occurrence time of ascites is earlier; ascites content is greater; cells content is also higher. Survival time is shorter than that of control group. Necropsy finds that cancer metastatic rate of the group with the removal of spleen is 30% above that of control group (metastases to liver, kidney, pancreas and mesenteric lymph nodes). From table 22-13, group IIB_1 (spleen removal before inoculation) and group IIIB (inoculation before spleen removal) accept splenectomy in different time. On the seventh day after inoculation, maximum diameter averages of their subcutaneous tumor nodi are $\overline{X}(IIB_1) = (10.8\pm5.28)$ mm and $\overline{X}(IIIB) = (2.83\pm1.948)$ mm respectively. The former is obviously longer than the latter one. But on the fourteenth day after inoculation, the tumor of group IIIB quickly proliferates after the removal of spleen. The difference between them almost disappears. $\overline{X}(IIB_1) = (21.2\pm5.3)$ mm, $\overline{X}(IIIB)$

= (20.3±6.07), $P>0.05$, without significant difference. It prompts that the removal of spleen promotes the growth of tumor, i.e. spleen can suppress the growth of tumor.

In recent two decades, people find that spleen not only performs a great role in anti-infection, but also has the all-important influence on anti-tumor immunity. The active mechanism may be by producing Natural Killer cell, macrophage (MΦ), Lympholine-Activated Killer cell, TH/Ti cell, B cell, Ts cell, etc. to realize the cellular immunity; and by secreting lymphokines of Tufisn factor, TNF factor, IL-2, interferon, addiment, antibody, etc. to kill tumor cells. Ge Yigong once used rat Lw56 pulmonary sarcoma model to the effect of removing spleen on tumor growth. Mr Ge holds that success ratio of tumor inoculation after the removal of spleen is higher than that of group with spleen. The metastatic ratio increases. Results are similar to this group of experimental results.

This group of experimental results also prompts that after the removal of spleen, bonding ratio of C_3b receptor garland of organism peripheral blood is 40% below that of healthy group with spleen. It explains that erythrocytic immune function of organism reduces after the removal of spleen.

2. Spleen's inhibiting action on tumor growth mainly occurs in the early stage of tumor course. While in the advanced stage of tumor, spleen's inhibiting action on tumor growth weakens and disappears. As seen from tables 22-8 and 22-13, in the early stage of tumor (within 7d), the tumor of group without spleen has a faster tumor growth rate than that of control group with spleen. The volume of subcutaneous tumor nodi is large and ascites content is great. While in the advanced stage (after 14d) of tumor, tumor nodi of control group with spleen and group with the removal of spleen basically have the same volume. No significant comparability. No obvious difference between survival times. Necropsy and pathological examination of three hundred experimental mice find that spleen of tumor-bearing mice present a series of regular changes with the process of illness. In the early stage of tumor (within 7d after inoculation), due to the cytostimulation, the spleen becomes congested and tumid. The volume enlarges; cell proliferation accelerates; germinal centers increases. While in the advanced stage (since 14d after inoculation) of tumor, the spleen presents progressive atrophy. Its volume shrinks; germinal centers fall sharply. The spleen also suffers from hyperplasia of fibrous tissues. The fibrosis of spleen occurs; therefore, its anticancer immunization weakens or disappears. Even it can pass through the suppressor T cell. Macrophage and immune inhibiting factor can suppress the anticancer immunization of organism and promote the growth of tumor. That explains that spleen's effect on tumor immune state is bidirectional, has obvious time phase and is relevant to stadium. In early stage,

the spleen owns the anti-tumor action. In advanced stage, the spleen owns immune inhibiting action. But the basic reason that leads to the immune inhibiting state of organism is the tumor itself. Spleen just plays a certain part in the forming process of this state.

1. Transabdominal injection of supernatant liquid of healthy splenic cells and transplantation of homogeneous variant splenic cells can suppress tumor growth. For group of injection with supernatant liquid of splenic cells or transplantation of splenic cells (Group IV), comparative results with other groups show that the tumor growth rate is slower; the occurrence time of tumor nodi is later; the volume is smaller; ascites content is less. After the inoculation of small dose of 0.1×10^4 ml cancer cells, success ratio of inoculation for tumor-bearing mice is obviously lower than that of other groups. Moreover, after a little ascites or subcutaneous lesser tubercle firstly appearing in several mice, the tumor can disappear naturally. The survival time is above 90d (as long-term survivors). Especially splenic cells of homogeneous variant fetal mouse (group IVB_1) have obvious tumor-inhibitory action. The tumor inhibition rate is 54%. The survival time is 17d longer than that of control group. Pathological examinations of this group of tumor-bearing mice find that after transplantation of homogeneous variant fetal splenic cells, splenic islands grow on the abdominal cavity and (or) mesentery of seven mice (account for 50%). Pathological examination proves it as living splenic tissues. Fetal splenic cells have features of weak antigenicity, deficient quantity and strong cell proliferation, etc. After the transplantation of splenic cells of homogeneous variant mice, there is no sharp rejection. And moreover, it is not subject to blood group ABO. Do not need the cross test of different blood groups. Here in China some people use traumatic splenic cells to prepare LAK cells for treating advanced malignant tumors, which achieves better curative effects on inhibiting tumor growth and prolonging mouse's lifespan.

At present, adoptive immunotherapy of tumors with transplantation of fetal splenic cells has not yet been reported in the literature. This group of experiments needs to have a further observation.

4. Negative correlation between anti-tumor immunological action of the organism and the quantity of cancer cells This group of experiments finds that anti-tumor immunological action of the organism is obviously affected by the quantity of inoculated cancer cells. The less the quantity of cancer cells, the stronger and more significant the anti-tumor effect; on the contrary, the weaker the anti-tumor effect. As for 0.1×10^7 ml inoculated cancer cells, immunological action of the organism is obviously suppressed. The tumor growth rates of group without spleen and group with spleen have bigger

difference in the early stage. While after medium stage (after 7d), the difference will quickly disappear. There is also no significant difference in survival time. But for $0.1×10^4$ ml inoculated cancer cells, anti-tumor action of the organism is relatively significant. The inoculated failure rate of group with spleen is obviously higher than that of group without spleen. The growth rate of tumor is slow; the volume of tumor nodi is small; and the survival time is long. Furthermore, after the transplantation of homogeneous variant splenic cells for small dose of inoculated cancer cells group, anti-tumor immunological action goes up remarkably. The growth rate of tumor decreases obviously. Some tumor nodi even can naturally disappear after its formation. Also the survival time is long. These results show the negative correlation between anti-tumor action of the organism and the quantity of inoculated cancer cells. While there is a positive correlation between cancer's immunological inhibiting action on the organism and the quantity of inoculated cancer cells. The spleen participates in tumor immunoregulation, which has double influences on immune state of tumor-bearing mice. In early stage, the spleen shows a certain anti-cancer action. As the development of tumor, the number of tumor cells is increasing. The spleen is shrinking gradually. Then the anti-cancer action is converted into immunological inhibiting action. But the basic reason of immune inhibiting state is the tumor itself. The progress of cancer, an increase in the number of cancer cells and the reinforcement of inhibiting action lead to the atrophia of spleen, thymus gland and other immune organs.

5. Experimental result prompts of this group

(1) The spleen has certain anti-tumor effects. In tumor's early stage, spleen can suppress the growth of tumor. While in advanced stage of the course of disease, the anti-tumor action of spleen weakens or disappears. The spleen even can promote the growth of spleen.

(2) Adoptive immunotherapy of tumors with transplantation of homogeneous variant splenic cells of fetal mice can reinforce anti-tumor immunological action of the organism, and suppress the growth of tumor.

(3) There is a negative correlation between anti-tumor action of the organism and the quantity of inoculated cancer cells. The more the quantity of cancer cells, the more easily the immunological action of the organism is suppressed or damaged. The faster the growth rate of tumor, the worse the prognosis.

4. EXPERIMENTAL STUDY ON TREATMENT OF MALIGNANT TUMOR BY ADOPTIVE IMMUNOLOGIC RECONSTITUTION THROUGH COMBINED TRANSPLANTATION OF FETAL CELLS

I. Experiment on Adoptive Immunologic Reconstitution of Fetal Liver, Spleen and Thymus Cells through Combined Transplantation

In this paper, the author introduces the experiment on the systematic adoptive immunologic reconstitution with the mice bearing Ehrlich ascites cancer (EAC) subcutaneous solid tumor through combined transplantation using the same kind of fetal liver, spleen and thymus cells. In this experiment, set up groups of monomial transplantations of fetal liver, spleen and thymus respectively; the groups of bigeminal transplantation of fetal liver and spleen cells, fetal liver and thymus cells as well as fetal spleen and thymus cells, and then observe the time of the growth, regression and survival, index of cellular immunity as well as all items of pathological examination in each group respectively; compare the curative effects of each groups. The research results show that the curative effect of trigeminal group is better than that of the bigeminal group which is better than the individual groups in turn. For the experimental group of trigeminal cell transplantation, the complete regression rates of the tumor in near and forward future are 40% (n=15) and 46.67% (n=15) respectively, and the partial regression rates (the percentage of the tumor regression is more than 50%) are 26.67% and 13.33% respectively. Those whose tumors regress completely can survive for a long time and the lifetimes of those whose tumors regress partially are prolonged for more than a month on average, and their immune index improves obviously and the immune organs are of hypertrophy. The sections of immune organ tissue reveal the active cell proliferation. Moreover, the pathological sections of tumor tissue show that a large amount of lymphocytes soak around the tumor tissue and in stroma, and then form parcel; flaky concretion, liquefaction necrosis, karyorrhexis and other pathologic phenomena emerge in the central tumor tissue. For the experimental groups of bigeminal cell transplantation, except a few cases of partial regression, there is no complete one. All the improvement of the immune indexes, the prolonged lifetime, and the soakage of lymphocytes in tumor tissue are less obvious than those of the experimental trigeminal group. As to monomial groups of cell transplantation, the results of regression, lifetime and immune indexes as well as the pathological examination results are less apparent than the former two groups, but better than the control group of the tumor-bearing mice. It can be implied that compared with partial reconstitution, systematic adoptive immunologic reconstitution can develop the anti-carcinomatous immunologic function and improve the curative effects though overall systematic synergism.

Thanks to the theory of biological response modifier (BRM), treatment of tumor has been experiencing a profound reform. The fourth generation of the modality of tumor therapy, biological treatment of tumor has become the focus in the field of tumor therapy after surgeons, chemotherapy and radiotherapy. According to a large number of clinical and experimental researches, it can be found that the organismal immune state exhibits progressive inhibition with the evolution of the stadium. Therefore, how to restore and reconstitute the anti-carcinomatous immunologic function is the core of the research of tumor biological treatment. The adoptive immunotherapy developed by Rosenberg who is the representative has got outstanding achievement in this field. Except transferring the active factors amplified in vitro and various kinds of artificial immunologic factors, fetal immune organs and cell transplantation are promising researches. Although the technique of biotherapy is expensive, it possesses several advantages like economy, convenient technique and easy popularization in that the sources of embryo are broad in China, which is worthy of thorough research and exploration. In recent years, many scholars at home have developed the research on transplantation of fetal liver, spleen and thymus from the level of cells to tissue and then to the level of organs for curing advanced malignant tumors and they have achieved some curative effects. The thorough researches can explain the source, proliferation, differentiation and the function of lymphocytes as well as the function and effects of reconstituting immune organs and peripheral immune organs clearly. Currently, in many cases of adoptive immunologic treatment with transplanting fetal immune organs, only single fetal organs is utilized, cell transplantation of fetal liver, spleen and thymus cells as well as tissue transplantation, etc. there is no similar literature or reports on the question that it is possible to carry out adoptive reconstitution systematically and integrally. The combined transplantation of fetal liver, spleen and thymus cells, in which the transplantation of fetal liver cells has analogous function of marrow transplantation and is combined with the transplantation of fetal thymus and spleen cells, can make the adoptive reconstitution approach to the systematical and integral level. But it is worthy of researches and exploration that whether it can bring synergism into play and improve curative effects.

1. 【Material and Methods】

Animals and tumor model

Experimental animals: 200 cross bred Kunming mice in closed flock, 5 to 6 weeks old, 18±2.1g in weight, no gender limitation.

Facilities for model of planting tumors: prepare mice of ascitic type after the anabiosis of the root of Ehrlich ascites tumor; when the ascites are formed, draw out the ascites of the cancer cells and centrifuge washing with Hank for three times(800r/min), five minutes for one time; remove the supernatant liquid, then dilute the liquid with the precipitated cancer cells to the concentration of 10^7/ml; use eosin exclusion teat to verify that the percentage of living cells is above 95%; inoculate the experimental mice under the skin of the right hollow viscera, 1ml for each mouse; after a week, all the mice have tumor nodes with the diameter of 9.5±1.5mm in the point of inoculation to make the subcutaneous solid tumor model bearing Ehrlich Ascites tumor.

Grouping

Group the experimental animals with random into control group bearing tumors (Group B, n=9), observation group for combined transplantation of fetal liver, spleen and thymus cells in forward future (Group CI, n=15), observation group in near future (Group CII, n=15, carry on combined transplantation to this group once a week for successive 5 weeks and then execute the mice), treatment group with transplantation of fetal liver cells (Group F), treatment group with transplantation of fetal spleen cells (Group G), treatment group with transplantation of fetal thymus cells (Group H), treatment group with combined transplantation of fetal liver and spleen cells (Group I), treatment group with combined transplantation of fetal liver and thymus cells (Group K), $n_F=n_G=n_H=n_I=n_J=n_K=$ 12. When the model is prepared, carry out correspondent cell transplantation once a week for each group respectively for five times in a row. As to the control group, use Hank as comparison.

Preparing of the suspension of fetal liver, spleen and thymus

Use the female mice that copulate naturally by stages and have been pregnant for 15 to 18 days; paunch them aseptically to take out the fetal mouse, liver, spleen and thymus; rinse them through the Hank individually under 4℃, then individually mix them with aseptic homogenate to the full; dilute the mixture with Hank under 4℃ and filter them to collect the suspension with adequate cells; Sample the suspension and do bacterial culture and pyrogen experiment; if the experimental results are negative, divide them and package as standby.

The approach and method for cell transplantation

Transplantation of fetal liver cells: use the prepared suspension of fetal liver cells for caudal vein injection, 0.2ml for each mouse at a time.

Transplantation of fetal spleen cells: use the prepared suspension of fetal spleen cells for intraperitoneal injection, 0.2ml for each mouse at a time.

Transplantation of fetal thymus cells: use the prepared suspension of fetal thymus cells for intramuscular injection in the back leg, 0.2ml for each mouse at a time.

The treatments for the experimental mice mentioned above begin after a week from cancer cell inoculation, once a week for successive five weeks. As to the control group, use the same amount of Hank as comparison.

Observation item

General items: after cancer cell inoculation, observe the time when tumor emerges; measure the size of the tumor nude with a vernier caliper every two days (the average vertical diameter, mm), the quality of life, the situation of the tumors and the lifetime (d).

Dynamic observation on T cells in peripheral blood: in this experiment, use Alpha Naphthyl Acetate Esterase (ANAE) staining method to take count of the T cells in peripheral blood. Prepare six pairs of nitrogen magenta solution and 2% ANAE solution respectively, store them in the shade under 4℃; before using the prepared solution, add 89ml, 1/15mol/L, pH=7.6 phosphate buffer into the 6ml nitrogen magenta solution gradually and mix up fully, then add 2.5ml, 2% ANAE solution gradually, then mix up to the full. The final sample is amber with pH being 6.4 as solution for incubation. Put this into the water bath of 37℃ for warm-up. Cut the tip of the mouse's tail, and get the section. After the section has dried by natural wind, soak it into the solution for incubation for 1 to 3 hours, then wash it clear by tap water and air it. Use 1% methyl green to dye for 1 to 3 minutes, wash with tap water. After airing, observe the section under microscope. There are black red granules, namely ANAE positive cells in different size and quantity (the amount generally is 2 to 5). Count 200 lymphocytes and then calculate the percentage of T lymphocytes. Observe the percentage dynamically after a week from having built the model and from treatment respectively and measure it every two weeks.

Dynamic observation on the conversion rate of lymphocytes: Measure the conversion rate with the morphologic method of microdose whole blood culture in vitro. Prepare RPMI 1640 complete medium (1640 is the product of Japanese Juchheim, containing 10.4g dry powder in each bag), which consists of 1ml, 20%, 30.0g/L L- glutamine of killed calf blood serum, 3ml 60.0g/L aseptic $NaHCO_3$, 10000U penicillin and 10000μg streptomycin. Sanitize the tail strictly and cut the tip for 0.2mm; collect blood aseptically for 0.1ml with heparinization microdose sampler; add 1.8ml complete medium and then o,1ml PHA; cultivate the sample in the water-jacket incubator under constant temperature of 37℃ for 72 hours and stir it once a day. After the cultivation, draw most of the supernatant liquid out and add 4ml 8.5g/L NH_4Cl to mix up; place the mixture in the water-bath of 37℃ for 10 minutes, then centrifugalize it in 2500r/min, discard the supernatant liquid; Add 5ml fixation fluid (9 units of methanol and an unit of glacialaceticacid; place the sample under ambient temperature for 10 minutes and centrifugalize it in 1500r/min for 5 minutes, discard the supernatant liquid and reserve the precipitate. Add Hank to the precipitate to the volume of 0.2ml, mix the precipitate and Hank and drop on a clean glass to stretch uniformly. After natural airing, dye it with Giemsa for 5 minutes, then wash with tap water. After drying, observe 200 lymphocytes under the microscope and calculate the percentage of the conversion rate of the metrocyte. As same as T cells, observe the percentage dynamically after a week from having built the model and from treatment respectively and measure it every two weeks.

Measuring the green weights of immune organs: do comprehensive autopsy in detail for each dead or the executed mouse, cut the thymus and spleen and observe their sizes, then weight them with a torsion balance; calculate the ratio of the green weight of the immune organs to the body weight for each mouse.

Pathological examination: do systematic pathological autopsy to each dead and the executed mouse, observe the tumor soakage and tumor metastasis; reserve tumor tissue, thymus, spleen, lung, liver, kidney, etc. for tissue pathological section ant attach importance to observe the lymphocyte soakage in tumor tissue and the pathologic changes in the immune organs.

2. 【Experimental Results】

1. Comparison of the average lifetime of the mouse in each group (geometrical average) and the persistence in different ages of tumors

According to Table 1, the lifetimes of all treatment groups are prolonged obviously compared with the control group with P being less than 0.05. Especially, the effect of the treatment group of trigeminal cell transplantation is most obvious, with P being less than 0.01. Other treatment groups have significant difference compared with the trigeminal treatment group with P being less than 0.5. In Group CI, the tumors in 7 cases regress completely, which gain a long- term survival and no tumor relapse. The rate of tumor regression in 2 cases is more than 50%, in which the two mice survive for 2 months and die of tumor relapse. Regarding the persistence in different ages of tumor, in the third week after bearing tumor, all treatment groups have significant differences compared with the control group. With the extent of the stadium and observation period, compared with the control group, Group CI shows notable differential all along, but other treatment groups lose the difference from the control group gradually and show the significant difference from that of Group CI.

Table 1 comparison of the average lifetime of the mouse in each group and the persistence in different ages of tumors

Group	N	Lifetime(d) $\overline{X}$+S	The persistence in different ages of tumor							
			1week	2week	3week	4week	5week	6week	2weeks	3months
GroupB	9	13.3±1.2	100	55.6	11.1	11.1	0	0	0	0
GroupF	12	22.5±1.6△*	100	83.3	58.3*	50	33.3	33.3	0△	0△
GroupG	12	21.4±1.9△*	100	75	75*	50	33.3	16.7△	0△	0△
GroupH	12	26.2±1.4△*	100	100	100*	58.3*	41.7	33.3	0△	0△
GroupI	12	27.4±1.7△*	100	91.7	91.7*	50	33.3	33.3	8.3△	0△
GroupJ	12	28.3±1.8△*	100	83.3	83.3*	66.7*	41.7	41.7	16.7	0△
GroupK	12	23.5±1.5△*	100	100	100*	58.3*	33.3	25	16.7	0△
Group CI	15	47.2±2.0**	100	93.3	93.3*	73.3*	66.7*	60*	46.7*	46.7*

Note: ①in Table 1, Group B is the control one bearing cancer; Group F is the treatment group with fetal liver cells; Group G is the treatment group with fetal spleen cells; Group H is the treatment group with fetal thymus cells; Group I is the group of combined treatment of fetal liver and spleen cells; Group J is the group of combined treatment of fetal liver and thymus cells; Group K is the group of combined treatment of fetal spleen and thymus cells; Group CI is the group of combined treatment of fetal liver, spleen and thymus cells; ②*means that comparing the each treatment groups with the control group, P <0.05; **means P <0.01; △ means comparing the treatment groups with Group CI, P <0.01.

2. The curative effect and the analysis on the effect

Table 2 the analysis on the curative effect

Group	N	Curative rate	The rate of apparent effect	Effective rate	Rate of inefficiency	Total effective rate
GroupB	9	$0^{\triangle\triangle}$	0	0	100	0
GroupF	12	$0^{\triangle\triangle}$	0	34.4(4)	66.4(8)	33.4(4) $^{\triangle\triangle}$
GroupG	12	$0^{\triangle\triangle}$	0	25(3)	75(9)	25(3) $^{\triangle\triangle}$
GroupH	12	$0^{\triangle\triangle}$	8.3(1)	33.4(4)	58.3(7)	41.7(5) $_{\triangle}^{*}$
GroupI	12	$0^{\triangle\triangle}$	8.3(1)	33.4(4)	58.3(7)	41.7(5) $\triangle$*
GroupJ	12	$0^{\triangle\triangle}$	26.67(2)	41.7(5)	41.7(5)	58.3(7)*
GroupK	12	$0^{\triangle\triangle}$	26.67(2)	33.4(4)	50(6)	50(6)*
GroupCI	15	46.7**	13.3(2)	20(3)	20(3)	80(12)**

Note: *means P <0.05 compared with the control group, ** means P <0.01 compared with the control group; △ means P <0.05 compared with Group CI, △△ means P <0.01 compared with Group CI

The standards of curative effects:

① Cure: The tumors regress completely, the suffers regain long-term survival without relapse;

② Apparent effects: The tumors regress partially (the regression rate is more than 50%), and the survival time is more than 2 months;

③ Being effective: The lifetime is prolonged for more than one time without obvious tumor regression.

④ Inefficiency: The tumors grow progressively leading to death in short term (3 to 4 weeks).

According to Table 2, the curative effect of Group CI reaches 46.67%, and is obviously different from other groups with P <0.01. There is no obvious difference among each group as to the rates of apparent effect and being effective respectively. The comparison of the total effective rate shows that except the treatment groups of unitary fetal liver or spleen cells, the total effective rate of all other treatment groups have visible distinction from the control group, with their curative effects being in the rank that the trigeminal is better than the bigeminal which is above the monomial. Moreover, in the groups of monomial cell transplantation, the curative effect of TH cells treatment group is the best, and in the groups of bigeminal cell transplantation, the curative effect of the group containing TH cells is better than that of the groups without TH cells, which indicates that thymus cells play an important role in the course of treatment, but sole liver or spleen cell transplantation have little effects. However, if two of liver, spleen or thymus cells are combined, the curative effect can be improved. And the combination of the three can improve the curative effect significantly.

1. Observing and comparing the growth rate of tumors, the regression and prognosis

In this experiment, the mimic clinical method is used to file case history for all the experimental mice in each groups to record their growth rate of tumors, regression and the prognosis. Measure the average vertical diameter every two days. For the cases of death, all the terminal measured values are regarded as effective sample parameter in the following measures within the same group. After a week from the establishment of the model, tumors grow rapidly with the average vertical diameter being 9.5±1.5mm. After a week from beginning the treatment, tumors continue to grow. Until the second week, the results of each group become differential that the mice bearing tumors have progressive exhaustion with the tumors growing rapidly in the control group; within four weeks, all mice are dead. In the group of sole cell transplantation, the life quality of the experimental mice are improved apparently with their tumors growing slowly, but all the mice bearing cancer die within two months. In the groups of bigeminal cell transplantation, the growths of the tumors are inhibited obviously. Five cases have partial regression but all the mice die with three months. In the group of trigeminal cell transplantation, there are nine cases with apparent tumor putrescence, fall off and ulcer, then scab. In other seven cases, the tumors regress completely, and then canker, scab. In two cases, the regression rate of tumors is more than 50%. As to other cases, except the mice in two cases die in the second and the third week respectively, tumors in the residual cases are in dead state until the death from exhaustion. The sufferers whose tumors regress completely regain long-term survival without relapse for more than six months, and they have normal capacities to become pregnant and give birth. From the above observation, it can be found that the sole or bigeminal cell transplantation is able to inhibit the growth of tumors, improve the life quality and prolong the lifetime; the trigeminal cell transplantation can not only inhibit the growth of tumors, but also result in apparent complete or partial regression and prolong the lifetime.

2. Dynamic observation on the number of T lymphocytes in peripheral blood and the conversion rate of lymphocytes

From table 3 and 4, after a week from the establishment of the model, the cellular immune indexes of the experimental groups decline obviously with the average decrease being more than 50% compared with that of the control group (the number of T cells in the normal group X is 62.5±1.7 and that of lymphocyte transformed X is 66.8±4.8), indicating that the development of tumors does inhibit immune function. After a week from beginning treatment, all immune indexes are improved (P<0.05) and there are no apparent differential among all treatment groups from the comparison between the treatment groups and the control group as well as the comparison of the indexes before and after the treatment. Seen from the growth of tumors, the immune indexes are improves, but the inhibition of tumors is not apparent. The continuous dynamic observation shows in the groups of sole and bigeminal cell transplantation, the inhibition of tumors and the improvement of immune indexes last for a certain period (3 to 4 weeks), after that period the immune indexes tent to decline, so that the state of the mice bearing cancer deteriorates, which is consistent with the reports on the clinical monitor of immunologic functionand the prognosis. In the group of trigeminal cell transplantation, the immune indexes have persistent improvement, especially the tumors regress obviously. For those who regain long-term survival, the above indexes measured two months later are still close to the indexes of normal mouse. By contrast, for those suffering deterioration, the indexes measured before their deaths have declined below the level before treatment. The above indicates that the cellular immune indexes do reflect the curative effects and can be regarded as a good prove for prognosis; at the same time it can indirectly prove that immunocyte transplantation is able to achieve the aim of immunologic reconstitution for cancer-bearing organisms.

Table 3 dynamic observation on the number of T lymphocytes in peripheral blood (ANAE)

Group	N	The number of T lymphocytes ($\overline{X}\pm S$)							
		n	1 week	n	2 weeks	n	4 weeks	n	6 weeks
GroupB	9	9	3.42±4.8	5	29.1±2.9	1	32	0	
GroupF	12	12	31.4±3.6	10	54.6±5.12△*	6	48.7±2.2△	4	36.7±4.9
GroupG	12	12	35.5±3.9	9	52.5±4.7△*	6	46.6±3.3*	2	33.4±5.1
GroupH	12	12	32.6±4.1	12	56.6±4.1△*	7	50.9±2.1△	4	40.7±3.8△
GroupI	12	12	36.2±2.7	11	53.4±3.5△*	6	55.3±3.6△	4	39.3±4.2△
GroupJ	12	12	30.8±4.3	10	55.8±3.8△*	8	56.4±1.9△	5	42.6±2.7△
GroupK	12	12	33.7±3.4	12	57.3±4.4△*	7	55.8±2.8△	3	41.3±4.5△
GroupCI	15	15	31.8±3.1	14	59.6±2.6△*	11	62.5±1.7△	9	67.8±3.4△

Note: * means P<0.05 compared with the control group; △ means P<0.05 in the comparison before and after the treatment

Table 4 the dynamic observation of the conversion rate of the lymphocytes in peripheral blood

Group	N	The conversion rate of lymphocytes ($\overline{X} \pm S$)							
		n	1 week	n	2 weeks	n	4 weeks	n	6 weeks
GroupB	9	9	3.25±5.4	5	25.51±3.6	1	28	0	
GroupF	12	12	31.6±3.7	10	51.2±2.7△*	6	54.2±6.1△	4	36.1±5.4
GroupG	12	12	29.8±4.3	9	48.4±4.6△*	6	52.8±1.8*	2	33.5±2.5
GroupH	12	12	34.1±4.1	12	56.5±2.1△*	7	52.4±3.7△	4	40.7±1.9△
GroupI	12	12	28.5±5.1	11	53.4±3.5△*	6	50.5±2.9△	4	37.3±3.2△
GroupJ	12	12	29.4±2.9	10	58.1±3.5△*	8	60.6±3.4△	5	46.5±4.5△
GroupK	12	12	30.7±1.8	12	54.9±5.2△*	7	57.5±4.3△	3	45.8±3.9△
GroupCI	15	15	31.5±3.2	14	55.8±2.8△*	11	63.9±3.2△	9	66.8±4.8△

Note: * means P<0.05 compared with the control group; △ means P<0.05 in the comparison before and after the treatment

5. Anatomic observation of immune organ and comparative analysis of immune organ's green weight

The observation results are seen in table 5 and table 6. In this experiment, in order to see the changes in immune organs of cancer-bearing organisms and the relevance to the curative effects, another near-future observation group of trigeminal cell transplantation is set up (Group CII, n=15, the tumors in six cases regress completely and the regression rates in four cases are more than 50%). After building the model, give the treatment to the mice in Group CII for five times and then execute them. At the same time, set a normal group for comparison, using Hank to simulate the model and execute the mice in the sixth week. Anatomize the mice and observe the changes in their immune organs; measure the green weight of the immune organs and calculate the ratio of immune organs to the body weight; compare the values in Group CII with those of the other groups. From the results, it can be found that in all the cases that in all experimental groups, the tumors develop progressively and lead to death, the thymus shrink apparently and the degree of atrophy is relevant positively to the tumor development. The atrophied thymus is dull-colored and of crisp texture. As to spleen, its change is not as obvious as that of the thymus. In most cases, the spleens are congested and swelling. Only in a few cases the spleens are atrophied. However, in Group CII in all the cases that the tumors regress completely and partially, the thymus and spleens are hypertrophied, so as the indexes of thymus and spleen increase. Through statistical disposition, these indexes are not only differential apparently from the death cases in each group (or the cases without tumor regression), but also different from the normal control group.

Table 5 the comparison of the green weight of the immune organs between the death cases and the normal control group.

Group	N	Thymus(mg)/body weight(g) $\overline{X}\pm S$	spleen(mg)/body weight(g) $\overline{X}\pm S$
Normal	10	2.97±0.38	3.80±0.23
Group B	9	1.02±0.32**	4.01±1.32
Group F	8	1.21±0.41**	4.213±0.87
Group G	10	1.18±0.46**	4.45±1.63
Group H	8	1.28±0.25**	4.47±1.24
Group I	8	1.34±0.43**	4.67±0.48
Group J	7	1.47±0.28**	4.56±0.62
Group J	9	1.43±0.35**	4.89±1.47
Group CII	5	1.96±0.37**	5.12±1.56

Note: * means P<0.05 compared with the control group; ** means P<0.01 compared with the normal control group

Table 6 the comparison of the green weight between the cases of complete or partial tumor regression and the cases without apparent regression in Group CII

Immune organ(mg/g)	Normal group (N=10, $\overline{X}\pm S$)	Group with tumor regression (N=10, $\overline{X}\pm S$)	Group without tumor regression (N=10, $\overline{X}\pm S$)
thymus	2.79±0.38	4.65±2.21**△△	1.96±0.37
spleen	3.80±0.23	10.15±2.29**△△	5.12±1.56

Note: ** means P<0.01 compared with the normal control group; △△means P<0.01 in the comparison between the group with tumor regression and the group without tumor regression.

1. The comparison of pathological examination

In this experiment, anatomize the mice in each group and observe the pathologic section. Observe the tumor soakage and metastasis as well as the changes in immune organs like thymus, spleen, etc. Reserve the viscera like tumor tissue, lung, kidney, thymus and spleen as tissue pathological section for observation. The results show that with the course developing, the range of local tumor soakage expends and the tumor becomes hypertrophied without apparent remote organ metastasis. The thymus shrinks obviously, which has positive relevance to the evolution of the tumor. As to the spleen, it is congested and swelling. In the near-future observation group of trigeminal cell transplantation, the thymus, spleen and liver in the cases of complete or apparent partial regression do not become hypertrophied obviously, which exhibits significant differences from the normal group. When the mice in the cases of complete regression are anatomized, no residual cancer cells can be found in the part of tumor inoculation with both naked eyes and microscope. At the 3rd or 4th week when the tumor putrescence is the most apparent, reserve the tumor tissue as pathological section for observation. It can be found that there are large amount of lymphocytes soakage around the tumor tissue and in the stroma which wrap the tumor tissue resulting a wide range of tumor cells are liquefied and solidified to be dead. The sections of immune organs show that the thickness of the thymus cortical area and the denseness of lymphocytes as well as the increase in epithelial reticular cell, phagocytotic phenomenon and thymus corpuscles. In the spleen, the white pulp area enlarges and the lymph nodes increases, also the lymphocytes become dense. In the control group, the sections of tumor tissue show that the tumor cells soak into the deep-layered muscular tissue and there are cancer embolus formed by tumor cell transplantation in the blood vessels but no lymphocytes soakage. As to the thymus, the cortex atrophy and the cells are sparse, the blood vessels are congested. In the spleen, the amount of lymphocytes decreases significantly and the cells are sparse. In other treatment groups, the tumor sections show that the boundary of the tumor are clear with a little lymphocyte soakage and the changes in thymus and spleen is between the group of trigeminal cell transplantation and the control group. Moreover, the arrangement of the cells is dense with light atrophy.

【Discussion】

1. Therapeutic evaluation

It can be found from the results of the above experiment that the adoptive immunological therapy through transplantation of immunocyte with the origin of embryo can inhibit the growth of tumor and improve the life quality in different extend and force the tumor to regress completely or partially, and then improve the immune indexes apparently and prolong the lifetime, which indicates that immunocyte transplantation with the origin of embryo can reconstitute the anti- carcinomatous immunologic functionfor cancer-bearing organisms. The combined reconstitution of central immunity and the peripheral immunity at the same time is the best and better than the partial reconstitution of bigeminal and monomial cell transplantation.

2. Possible mechanism

The possible mechanisms to take effect are mainly the following: ①After the cancer-bearing organisms accept the same kind of xenogenous embryo cell transplantation, the immune system of the organism gets non-specific simulation to produce immune hyperplasia so as to improve the immunologic function to resist tumors. ②Cell transplantation belongs to organ transplantation, which can keep active for a certain period of time in the acceptor. By immunocyte transplantation with the origin of embryo, fetal liver cells can provide stem lymphocytes, which is combined with thymus and spleen cell transplantation so as to achieve the combined reconstitution of central immunity and peripheral immunity and enable the organism to gain adoptive immunity. A large number of researches home and abroad on the proliferation, differentiation and function of fetal immune organs and histiocytes show that when fetal immune organs are in their 16 weeks, they put up obvious proliferation to the original simulation of division, which becomes more intensive in the 24th week. In the 8th week of pregnancy, lymph tissue begins to emerge in the fetal thymus and lymph nodes as well as the cells with secretion in the 20th week. All these researches indicate that fetal immunocytes are able to bring immunoreaction into play. ③Some researches show that both the supernatant liquid from fetal thymus tissue cultivated outside the body and thymus extractive have the ability to promote the formation rate of the acceptor's E- wreath and the transformation of lymphocytes obviously. Therefore, fetal immunocyte transplantation can strengthen the cellular immunity of the cancer-bearing organism for cancer-bearing organism. ④ low immunogen of the fetal organs and the homology between the transplanted fetal organs and the acceptor's immune organs are in favor of forming immunologic tolerance to the transplanted for the acceptor, which can not only avoid rejection or have light rejection, but also simulate each other to achieve synergetic effects so as to reconstitute immunity. Moreover, as the curative effects of the trigeminal cell transplantation group are much better than those of the other groups, it is be believed that the effects result from the relatively complete reconstitution of central immunity and peripheral immunity at the same time which lead to the synergetic effects. In a word, the mechanism is much more complex than the above mentioned. It will be useful to step further to make the mechanism clear if the level of the immune factors that are closely relevant to anti-tumor immunity like IL-2, TNF, INF, etc. and the activity of the immunocytes that relate directly to anti-tumor immunity like NK, LAK, TIL, etc. in peripheral blood can be detected and the transplanted cells can be marked to make clear their distribution and survival inside the acceptor.

1. Problems about the barrier of transplantation

Although fetal organs have low immunogen, it is still impossible to avoid rejection, just in different degree. Therefore, the problem about the barrier of transplantation exists and directly relate to the success of transplantation and that whether the transplant can continue to act inside the acceptor. In this experiment, the animals used belong to the hybrid species in closed flock, which ensures largely that the mice in each experimental group have relatively close genetic background. It is probably the important reason for the success of transplantation with tissue matching except the low immunogen of embryonic tissue. Apart from those, it is possible that the mismatch of histocompatibility leads to the cases with inconspicuous curative effects in Group CI and Group CII. Thus, the key of improving curative effects may lie in studying and solving the barrier of transplantation.

2. The choice of the approach and method of transplantation

The transplantations of fetal immune organs from the level of cells, to tissue, then to the level of entire organ belong to adoptive immunity. In terms of the current repots, for fetal liver and spleen, blood cell transplantation is the best; for thymus, spleen and tissue, omentum embedding is the best. Although the technique of cell transplantation is simple and easy to be successful, it can only last for a short time. Therefore, the best approach of transplantation needs further observation and research.

II. Progress of Study on Treatment of Tumor by Adoptive Immunity through Transplantation of Immunocyte with the Origin of Embryo

According to a large amount of clinical and experimental researches, the immunity of the tumor-bearing organisms tent to be in progressive inhibition with the course the disease. So how to reconstitute the anti-tumor immunity is the core of the research on immunological therapy. In 1980s, the fourth generation of tumor treatment mode, namely biological treatment of tumor, brought tumor therapeutics into a new era, when the adoptive immunotherapy was the most outstanding achievement. For those whose tumors were in the advanced stage, several kinds of the conventional therapies were of no effects. However, adoptive immunotherapy of LAK, TIL and gene-modified TIL, which is represented by Rosenberg gained prominent curative effects, attracting the attention all over the world. In this technique, it is needed to gain a great amount of artificial synthesized IL-2 with high purity by biotechnology and plentiful immune competent cells through cultivate and proliferation in vitro in a long term to reach the aim, so the cost was very expensive. Currently, this project is still in depth research. As only a few institutes at home have developed the research in this area, there is no doubt that the above mentioned therapy is an extremely prominent research direction in treatment of tumor, however it is some difficult to become popularized in China. Besides, treatment of tumor by adoptive immunity through transplantation of immune cells, tissue and organs with the origin of embryo is another prominent research in the treatment of tumor by adoptive immunity, which is featured by simple technique, low cost and popularity. In recent years, some researchers have used embryonic liver, spleen and thymus to do transplantation from the level of cellular tissue to organs with vessel pedicles, which has been applied in the treatment of advanced malignant tumor gaining some curative effects, and paid much attention gradually.

i. Research status of fetal liver cell transplantation (FLT)

In 1958, Uphoff was the first one to fetal liver cells into the mice who died from ray of fatal dose with the remarkable effects of regaining hematopiesis. From then on, that fetal cell transplantation can be applied in curing the diseases in hemopoietic system and in the therapy of regaining hematopiesis after chemotherapy and radiotherapy for those with malignant tumors is researched extensively. In the following researches it has been found that FLT can not only reconstitute hematopiesis, but also reconstitute immunity. Wu Zuze and other researchers have found that FLT is able to reconstitute T and B lmphyocytes. They have also found that founder cells in fetal liver and spleen nodes are possessed with the basic features of several kinds of hematopoietic stem cells or lymph myeloid stem cells through the comparative research on the proliferation and differentiation between fetal liver cells and myeloid hematopoietic stem cell. Fetal liver cells contain a small amount of macrophages and lymphocytes. After 5 months from being pregnant, the amount of T lymphocytes begins to increase gradually, which is thought to be the substantial foundation of applying FLT to cure hematopoietic disorders immunologic deficiency disease to reconstitute hematopiesis and immunity. These features of fetal liver cells, especially the ability to reconstitute immunity make FLT play an important role in improving immunity. In recent years, there have been more and more researches on applying FLT to treatment of tumor.

ii. Research status of treatment of tumor through fetal spleen cell transplantation

1. Research on the relationship between spleen and the growth of tumor

It has been thirty years since Old and others began to study the influence of spleen to the growth of tumor. During this period, many scholars have done a large number of experiments and clinical researches on the effect of spleen in anti-tumor immunity, but they can not get a consistent conclusion as they hold that spleen has both positive and negative effects on anti-tumor immunity. With more deep researches on splenic surgery and its function, most scholars tent to confirm the anti-tumor immune function. As spleen is the biggest immune organ in bodies, it is the place where Th and Ts cells become mature. The antibodies, Fibronetin, Tufftsinr-1NF and IL-2, etc. immune factors secreted by Th and Ts cells as well as killer cells like LAK and NK, etc. play an crucial role in anti-tumor immunity. Ge Yigong, etc. have found when researching the effect of ablating spleen to the growth of W256 rat's sarcoma that in the group of spleen ablation, the survival rate of the tumor inoculation and the diameter of tumor are higher apparently than those of the control group. Meanwhile, in the former group, the postoperative changes of T cell subgroup in peripheral blood are manifested by the reduction in T and Th cells and slight increase in Ts cells which is on the low level continuously after inoculation and have remarkable differential from the group without tumor and the tumor-bearing control group($P<0.001$). That is consistent with the research on the effects of spleen to the growth of tumor that was done before. They have also found that after ablating spleen, there was positive correlation between the decline in the ratio of Th/Ts in T cell subgroup and the diffuse and metastasis of tumor. Lersch has reported that lymphocytes inside the spleen of tumor-bearing mice decline progressively with the growth of tumor, which is consistent with the experimental results mentioned above. All these researches can indicate that spleen plays an important role in anti-tumor immunity.

2. Researches on treatment of tumor through fetal spleen cell transplantation

Based on the understanding of the action of spleen in anti-tumor immunity, many scholars have begun to develop the experimental and clinical researches on treatment of tumor through fetal spleen cell or tissue transplantation. Ma Xuxian, etc. report that fetal spleen cell transplantation has been used in nine cases of advanced malignant tumor. All sufferers in these cases feel better after the treatment. The author also has found that fetal spleen cell transplantation can inhibit the growth of tumor apparently when studying the effects of spleen to the growth of tumor. What's more, some scholar has studied the feature and approach of fetal spleen transplantation and found that transplantation through vein is the best, intramuscular injection and celiac injection follow. For tissue transplantation, omentum embedding is the best; both HVGR and GVHR are few. The mechanism of spleen cell transplantation is still in research.

iii. Research status of treatment of tumor through fetal thymus transplantation

Among immune organs, thymus has the closest relation to anti-tumor immunity and the researches on thymus are the most profound. Thymus plays a decisive role in cellular immunity and even the entire immunoregulation as thymus is the central immune organ where T cells develop and grow up.

1. Research on the relationship between thymus and the growth of tumor

The function of thymus has close connection with the occurrence of tumor that can lead to thymus atrophy, low level of thymosin or lack of analogous thymic factor. For those experimental animals, that the thymus are ablated or irradiated by dead dose ray can promote the tumor metastasis. Therefore, fetal thymus transplantation or thymic epithelial cell transplantation as well as injection of thymosin can put off thymus atrophy and reconstitute immune function. The above researches indicate that thymus plays an extremely important role in anti-tumor immunity.

2. The application of fetal thymus transplantation in treatment of tumor

Many scholars have done plentiful researches on treatment of tumor through fetal thymus transplantation. Zhou Shifu, etc. have performed the treatment of tumor through fetal thymus transplantation for 14 tumor cases. After 46 hours, the immune indexes have been improved and the conditions of the sufferers have been remitted and improved. Song Ruze, etc. have used the treatment of advanced malignant tumor through fetal thymus tissue omentum transplantation and gained the same curative effects. Liu Dungui, etc. have used cell transplantation, tissue transplantation and transplantation of thymus with vessel pedicle to treat advanced liver cancer resulting in that tumors in some cases shrunk significantly and the lifetime was prolonged for six months. All these can indicate that fetal thymus transplantation is an effective approach of immunotherapy of tumor.

Moreover, some scholars have studied on the features of the immune organs in different ages with the origin of embryo like the activity and the saving time, etc. They have found that the activity of fetal organs after five months' pregnancy is best. The researches on the approach of transplantation show that fetal liver and spleen cell transplantation through vein is the best, and omentum embedding is best for spleen and thymus tissue transplantation.

All these researches provide precious theoretic and experimental basis for treatment of tumor by adoptive immunity through immune organ transplantation with the origin of embryo and contribute to further studies.

5. TG'S INHIBITION ON ANGIOGENESIS OF TRANSPLANTATION TUMOR OF MICE

Since Folkman presented the concept that the growth of tumor depends on vascularization in 1971, the following researches further confirm that angiogenesis is a key factor for the growth of tumor. Thereafter researchers have brought forth the concept of anti-angiogenic therapy, that is, by preventing neovascularization and (or) spread of new-born rete vasculosum and (or) destroying new-born blood vessels to stop the production or establishment of small solid tumor, and finally to prevent the growth, evolution and metastasis of tumor. At present, foreign experts have done a lot of studies in this respect and made gratifying progress. Therefore anti-angiogenic therapy is expected to be an effective means to cure tumor. But domestic relative studies start fairly late; and very few reports are given to it except some counts about capillary density of tumor tissues.

Along with the deepening research of Common Threewingnut Root, its new pharmacological actions are constantly to be found, such as anti-tumor action and two-way regulating action on immune system. Especially the recently discovered Common Threewingnut Root, which inhibits in vitro the formation of lumen that induced by the migration, proliferation and differentiation of vascular endothelium cells, has a better inhibiting action on neovascularization. In order to further explore the inhibiting action of Common Threewingnut Root on new-born blood vessels of tumor in vivo, the writer adopts transplantation tumor model of mouse's abdominal muscles. Based on the observation of formation characteristics of tumor blood vessel and its relation with tumor, researchers' new findings in recent years and the writer's experimental results both prove that Common Threewingnut Root has the two-way regulating action with dose dependent on immune system. Choose adequate doses of TG with no effect on the body's immune function to carry out the experimental study of TG's inhibiting action on new-born blood vessels of transplantation tumor of mouse's abdominal muscles. The study is to know about TG's inhibiting capability on tumor angiogenesis, which can provide experimental references for further anti-tumor study in terms of blood vessels.

I. Experimental Study on Observation of Angiogenesis of Transplantation Tumor at Mouse's Abdominal Muscle

This experiment depends on the anatomical position and structural features of mouse's abdominal muscle, adopts EAC transplantation tumor model of abdominal muscle, fixes and displays blood vessels with transparent specimen, which are all for finding out the formation characteristics of tumor blood vessel and its relation with tumor.

[Material and Method]

1. Materials

(1) Animals: 20 Kunming mice, 18~22g, a 50:50 proportion of male and female.
(2) Cancer-bearing mouse: Kunming mouse with the intraperitoneal inoculation of EAC cells.
(3) Instrument and apparatus: mouse retaining plate, 1ml injector, test tube and heparin tube, glass slide, ophthalmic scissors, microsurgery scissors and surgical

clamps, small cutting needle, 1-0 silk thread, ophthalmic needle holder, glass petri dish, light microscope, Olympus Japanese microscopic observation and photographic system of type BH-2.

(4) Reagent: Wright stain, 0.2% physiological saline of trypan blue, Hank solution, depilatory, 1% pentobarbitale sodium solution, 10% formaldehyde solution, tertiary butyl alcohol solution of 70%, 80%, 90%, 95% and 100%, methyl salicylate.

2. Method

(1) Prepare EAC cell suspension (6.0×10^7/ml): Aseptically draw ascites of cancer-bearing mouse with the inoculation for 7~9d; put ascites in a sterile tube; draw another little ascites in a heparin tube for cell count; store tubes in ice blocks. Drop remaining ascites in the empty needle on a glass slide, cover with another slide and stain the specimen with Wright stain, finally use it for differential counting of cells, the proportion of cancer cells $\geqq$ 95% (if insufficient, choose another cancer-bearing mouse). Dilute ascites in the heparin tube with physiological saline to 10 times and 100 times; respectively take 0.95ml blending with 0.1ml trypan blue physiological saline of 0.2%; use the counting method of white blood cells to count the total number of tumor cells and dead tumor cells, calculate the survival rate, which should be $\geqq$ 95% (if insufficient, choose another cancer-bearing mouse). Finally dilute ascites in the tube with sterile pre-cooling Hank solution to 6.0×10^7/ml and use it for the inoculation.

(2) Inoculation in the area of peritoneum: Use depilatory in advance to clean a mouse's ventral seta two days ago; anaesthetize it injecting with 1% pentobarbitale sodium (0.3mg/10g weight) into the abdominal cavity; lie on its back and fix it on mouse retaining plate; sterilize the abdominal skin; cut open the skin about 1.2cm long from the middlemost place about 1cm below the processus xiphoideus; conduct the blunt separation to one side gently and carefully, then find an area on this side with few blood vessels in the abdominal muscle; inoculate 0.04ml EAC cell suspension with the concentration of 6.0×10^7/ml, then present a full small "swelling" without any collapse, which explains the correct inoculation location without penetrating the peritoneum. Finally stitch the skin and isolate this mouse for protection until it regains consciousness safely.

Note: During the process of inoculation, always store the test tube with cancer cell suspension in ice blocks so as to ensure the constant survival rate. And also require a fast and stable manipulation.

(3) Group and make transparent specimen: 20 inoculated mice, randomly divide into 10 groups with 2 mice of each group. Since the first day after the inoculation, pull off the cervical vertebra to execute one group each day for making transparent specimen. The specific making procedures are as follows.

Submerge and fix the execute mice in formaldehyde solution with the concentration of 10% for 24h. Take out the mice, cut open their skin, peel off the whole abdominal muscle membrane, rinse it with distilled water for 1 min, and submerge it orderly in the tertiary butyl alcohol with different concentration (70%, 80%, 90%, 95% and 100%) to dehydrate for 6~8h. Finally submerge it directly into the methyl salicylate until the tissue is completely transparent.

(4) Observe and shoot tumor vessels: Use Olympus microscope of type BH-2 to observe the transparent specimen in the small petri dish with methyl salicylate. Note the shape, quantity and distribution of new born capillary around tumor tissues and in the tumor. Then take microscopic photos and use Olympus microcirculation microscopic photographic system to observe the flow rate of new born capillaries.

[Experimental Result]

On the first day after the inoculation, there is no new born vessel in the inoculation area, around which the original host's capillaries slightly exude. On the second day, tumor cell mass swells. It is clear that original host's capillaries put forth slim but crooked new vessels, which invade into the tumor. There is no continued vessel segment. On the third and fourth day, the tumor tissue has a further growth. The density of new vessels outside the tumor increases; the caliber is irregular; vessels array in disorder. In the tumor, incontinuous and imperfect new vessels with maldistribution and various thicknesses are obviously in the direction of muscle fiber. Some vessels are comma-shaped or bud-shaped, and irregular bud-shaped vessels connect each vessel. On the fifth and sixth day, the tumor presents the progressive growth. Capillaries outside the tumor twist or distend or cluster to distribute with various thicknesses; vessels in the tumor start to interlace with each other or show irregular sinusoid dilatation. On the seventh and eighth day, the color in the tumor becomes red. Capillaries outside the tumor distend, twist and come in different shape and size; in the tumor only a few incontinuous and short vessels present an irregular distribution, most vessels have no any figure and fuse in the shape of flake or mass. On the ninth and tenth day, there is only a red mass-shaped zone in the tumor, which is fused by vessels. Brown area of hemorrhage and necrosis appears in the centre of the tumor. Vessels with extreme dilatation and distortional appearance can be made out in some areas.

Transplantation tumor model of mouse's abdominal muscles helps to have a more intuitional observation, from inflammation changes of stimulating the angiogenesis since the first day after inoculation to tumor vessels that gradually appear later. It reflects the formation characteristics of tumor's new-born capillaries and their relations with the tumor. That is, new-born capillaries generally register as the abnormal route, irregular arrangement, irregular diameter, the lack of continuity and integrity, and even comma-shaped or bud-shaped immature differentiation and growth. The relation between capillaries and tumor is the continued proliferation and enlargement of tumor cell cluster along with the formation and growth of new-born capillaries in the inoculation area. Simultaneously, the tumor mass characterized by progressive growth causes the blood vessels in the central part to bear the rise in blood pressure, dilatation, and necrosis, which appear as a red fused mass.

II. Experimental Study on Effects of TG with Different Dosages on Immunologic Function of Mice

In recent years, reports about Common Threewingnut Root having the two-way regulating action with dose dependent on immune system have continued to arise. TG is a refined product that separated and abstracted repeatedly from the crude drug— Common Threewingnut Root. In order to have a better understanding of the two-way regulating action, this experiment chooses three different doses of TG to act on the phagocytic function of mice celiac macrophages (MΦ) and immune organs. Their drug reactions can basically reflect TG's effect on the immune function of mice.

TG's effect on the phagocytic function of mice celiac macrophages (MΦ)

[Material and Method]

1. Materials

(1) Animals: 40 Kunming mice, 18~22g, a 50:50 proportion of male and female.

(2) Drugs and reagents: ① TG turbid liquor: Pulverize TG tablets; use 0.5% Carboxythmethyl Cellulose (CMC) to respectively prepare turbid liquors of three different concentrations, TG_1 10mg/10ml, TG_2 10mg/20ml and TG_3 40mg/10ml; ② 0.5% CMC solution; ③ 2% chicken red blood cell (CRBC) suspension: Sterile venous sampling of 2ml under the chicken wing; put the blood sample in a heparin tube; clean it for three times with physiological saline; after centrifugation, abandon the supernatant fluid and white blood cell layer at the interface; when the specific volume of blood cells keeps stable, use physiological saline to prepare 2% (V/V) red

cell suspension; ④ Sterile calf serum; ⑤ 1:1 acetone- methanol solution; ⑥ 4% (V/V) Giemsa-phosphate buffer.

(3) Instrument and apparatus: Gastric lavage needle, thermotank, and for the rest, please sees "Experimental Study on Observation of Angiogenesis of Transplantation Tumor at Mouse's Abdominal Muscle".

2. Method

(1) Grouping: 40 mice are randomly divided into 4 groups with 10 mice of each group, group TG_1, TG_2, TG_3 and control group.

(2) Gastric lavage: According to the proportion of 0.2ml/10g (weight), respectively inject TG suspension into the stomach with corresponding concentrations (group TG_1 20mg/kg, TG_2 40mg/kg and TG_3 80mg/kg) and 0.5% CMC solution for 12 days.

(3) Induction and functional examination of celiac Mφ: On the tenth day after gastric lavage, sterile injection of 0.5ml calf serum into each mouse's abdominal cavity. On the thirteenth day, inject 1ml CRBC suspension with the concentration of 2% into each mouse's abdominal cavity. 30min later pull off the cervical vertebra to execute the mouse. Cut open the abdominal wall skin from the middlemost place. Inject 2ml physiological saline into the abdominal cavity and turn the mouse's body. Aspirate 1ml celiac lotion, averagely drop it on two glass slides and put slides into an enamel box with wet paper cloth. 30 min after moving the box into 37°C thermotank for warm cultivation, rinse the two glass slides with celiac lotion in physiological saline, dry by airing, fix in 1:1 acetone- methanol solution, dye them with 4% Giemsa-phosphate buffer, rinse with distilled water and dry by airing. Finally conduct the count of Mφ (200 Mφ on each slide) under the oil immersion lens of microscope. See the following mathematical equation to calculate the phagocytose percentage.

$$\text{Phagocytose Percentage} = \frac{\text{Amounts of M}\phi \text{ that phagocytizes CRBC}}{200 \text{ M}\phi} \times 100\%$$

(4) Statistical treatment: The data is represented by average ± standard error $(\overline{X} \pm S)$, and analyzed by t test.

[Experimental Result]

Determination result about TG's effect on the phagocytic function of mice celiac Mφ can be seen in table 1.

Table1 TG's effect on the phagocytic function of mice celiac Mϕ ($\overline{X}\pm$S)

Group	Dosage(mg/kg)	Case load	Amounts of Mϕ that phagocytizes CRBC (%)
Control group	–	10	44.83±0.41
TG$_1$	20	10	47.20±0.35*
TG$_2$	40	10	45.72±0.25
TG$_3$	80	10	44.40±0.45*

Note: Compare to the control group, *$P<0.05$

As seen from the table 1, in low doses of 20mg/kg, TG can obviously activate the phagocytic function of Mϕ ($P<0.05$); in median doses of 40mg/kg, TG has no obvious effect on the phagocytic function of Mϕ ($P>0.05$); in high doses of 80mg/kg, TG will inhibit the phagocytic function of Mϕ ($P<0.05$). The above results indicate that TG can affect the phagocytic function of mice celiac Mϕ and have the obvious characteristic of dose dependent, that is along with the gradual increase of TG dosage, the phagocytic function of mice celiac Mϕ can respectively present three different effects of being activated, no obvious effect and inhibition.

TG's effect on immune organs of young mice

[Material and Method]

1. Materials

   (1) Animals: 40 three-aged Kunming mice, 10~12g, a 50:50 proportion of male and female.

   (2) Drugs and reagents: TG suspension and 0.5% CMC solution: Preparation is same as stated before.

   (3) Instrument and apparatus: Analytical balance and for the rest, please sees "Experimental Study on Observation of Angiogenesis of Transplantation Tumor at Mouse's Abdominal Muscle".

2. Method

   (1) Grouping and gastric lavage: see "Experimental Study on Observation of Angiogenesis of Transplantation Tumor at Mouse's Abdominal Muscle".

   (2) Weighing of thymus gland and spleen: On the thirteenth day after the experiment, pull off the cervical vertebra to execute the young mouse. Cut open

its skin, chest cavity and abdominal cavity. Excise the whole thymus gland and spleen. Use filter papers to suck dry the blood and finally weigh thymus gland and spleen on an analytical balance.

(3) Statistical treatment: The data is represented by average ± standard error ($\overline{X}$±S), and analyzed by t test.

[Experimental Result]

Weighing results of thymus gland and spleen can be seen in table2. As seen from the table 2, TG at different dosages has different effect on immune organs of young mice. In low doses of 20mg/kg, TG can stimulate the weight gain of young mouse's thymus gland ($P<0.05$); in median doses of 40mg/kg, though there is a trend in weight loss, no obvious difference exists when compared with control group ($P>0.05$); in high doses of 80mg/kg, thymus gland appears as obvious atrophia compared with control group ($P<0.01$). Only in high doses, TG can inhibit the growth of young mouse's spleen ($P<0.05$); while in median and low doses, there is no obvious effect ($P>0.05$).

Table2 TG's effect on immune organs of young mice ($\overline{X}$±S)

Group	Dosage(mg/kg)	Case load	Thymic weight (mg/10g weight)	Spleen weight (mg/10g weight)
Control group	-	10	26.38±1.22	70.43±0.76
TG$_1$	20	10	30.20±0.74*	72.65±0.83
TG$_2$	40	10	23.48±0.88	69.88±0.56
TG$_3$	80	10	21.12±0.76**	68.44±0.42*

Note: Compare to the control group, *$P<0.05$, ** $P<0.01$

Experiments about TG's effect on the phagocytic function of mice celiac Mφ and weight of young mice's immune organs can basically reflect TG's two-way regulating action with dose dependent on mice's immune function. That is, along with the gradual increase of TG dosage, there are three different immune effects of enhancement, no obvious effect and inhibition. It prompts that the application range of TG can be expanded by different effects of choosing different dosages of TG on immune system.

III. Experimental Study on Inhibition of TG of Different Dosages on Angiogenesis of Transplantation Tumor at Mouse's Abdominal Muscle

i. Observation on new-born capillaries of transplantation tumor at mouse's abdominal muscle

Researches in recent years have found that Common Threewingnut Root has the characteristic of inhibiting migration and proliferation of endothelial cell to suppress angiogenesis. In order to have a further exploration of its inhibiting action on tumor angiogenesis, this experiment bases on the previous experiment and chooses adequate doses of TG (40mg/kg) that have no effect on mice's immune function. Through observation in vivo by microcirculation microscope, experts can carry out an experimental study on angiogenesis of transplantation tumor at mouse's abdominal muscle.

[Material and Method]

1. Materials

(1) Animals: 40 Kunming mice, 18~22g, a 50:50 proportion of male and female.

(2) 6.0×10^7/ml EAC cell suspension; see [Experiment 1] for preparation.

(3) 20mg/10mg TG suspension and 0.5% CMC solution; see [Experiment 2] for preparation.

(4) HH-1 microcirculation detection system (microcirculation microscope, photomicrography system and display system, video light mark blood flow meter, etc.), other required reagents and instruments are same as those mentioned in the previous experiment.

2. Method

(1) Inoculation: see this chapter "Experimental Study on Observation of Angiogenesis of Transplantation Tumor at Mouse's Abdominal Muscle".

(2) Grouping: 40 inoculated tumor-bearing mice are randomly divided into medication administration group and control group with 20 mice of each group. Then each group is also randomly divided into four groups with 5mice of each group, which is the third day, sixth day, ninth day and twelfth day.

(3) Gastric lavage: Since the first day after inoculation, medication administration group and control group begin to undergo the gastric lavage of 20mg/ml TG suspension and 0.5% CMC solution according as the proportion of 0.2ml/10g (weight).

(4) Observation of new-born tumor capillaries: Respectively on the third day, sixth day, ninth day and twelfth day, observe new-born capillaries of tumor at mouse's abdominal muscle among the proper group of medication administration group and control group (groups of the third day, sixth day, ninth day and twelfth day). Specific method and procedure are as follows: ① Carry out the anesthesia with the injection of 1% sodium pentobarbital (0.3mg/10g weight) in abdominal cavity before operation, carefully cut open the skin below the processus xiphoideus to the lower abdomen, conduct blunt separation of skin to the middle axillary line of one side, and then cut open the abdominal muscle along the white line. This operation should be careful and gentle. If there is a little oozing of blood, use small gauze dipped in tepid physiological saline to stanch the bleeding. ② Make the mouse lie on side on the self-made observation platform, overturn the abdominal muscle that is detached from one side of the skin, and fix incision edge on the outer margin of the window of observation platform, which lets the half-side abdominal muscle cover the whole window and makes the tumor mass be located in the middle of the window. ③ Put the observation platform with mouse on the microscope carrier that is in a thermotank (Refer to the preparation of Tian Niu and make an improvement), and drop 37°C Ringer-Locke liquor in the overturned abdominal muscle to moisten it. ④ Start the cold light source and bring into focus for observation.

(5) Observation project: Use HH-1 microcirculation detection system to observe the shape and quantity of new-born capillaries in and around the tumor, and take microscopic photos. Measure the density of new-born capillaries which enter and leave the tumor, as well as the average diameter and flow rate of tumor arterioles and venules. Use a vernier caliper to measure the maximum diameter and transverse diameter of tumor, and calculate its maximum transverse section.

(6) Statistical treatment: The data is represented by average ± standard error ($\overline{X}\pm S$), and analyzed by t test.

[Experimental Result]

1. Changes in the shape and quantity of new-born capillaries in and around the tumor. See table 3.

2. The density of new-born capillaries which enter and leave the tumor (the number of new-born capillaries around tumor cell cluster/mm^2). See table 4.

The above results indicate that the density of new-born tumor capillaries of group TG is obviously lower than that of control group ($P<0.05$), which shows that TG has an inhibiting action on tumor vascularization. Especially on the third and sixth day, this manifestation is more apparent ($P<0.05$). The angiogenesis speed of control group is faster during the previous six days, but then it gradually slows down. While the angiogenesis speed of group TG during the previous six days is slower than that during the next six days and capillaries are obviously smaller that those of control group, indicating that TG significantly slows down angiogenesis speed during the previous six days and suppresses the angiogenesis. During the next six days, the angiogenesis speed of group TG gradually increases to that of control group on the tenth day to twelfth day. It shows that during the next six days TG's inhibiting action on tumor vascularization begins to remit. But as seen from table 25-4, on the twelfth day the density of new-born tumor capillaries of group TG is still obviously below that of control group, indicating that the comprehensive effect of drugs still appears as the inhibition of tumor vascularization up to now.

Table 3 TG's effect on the shape and quantity of new-born capillaries in and around the tumor

Observation Date	Control Group	Medication Administration Group of TG
The Third Day	Obvious, unbalanced and new-born capillaries in the tumor; unbalanced and crooked capillaries around the tumor; capillaries unevenly enter and leave the tumor. The whole tumor body is light red.	No crooked new-born capillaries enter and leave the tumor; capillaries around the tumor grow straight in the original direction; no obvious, unbalanced and new-born capillaries in the tumor. The whole tumor body is milky white.
The Sixth Day	Abundant capillaries with various thicknesses around the tumor branch from minute blood vessels of the host, twist into the tumor and form a nodular capillary network, which make the whole tumor body become light red.	Slender earthworm-shaped capillaries grow around the tumor; there are new-born capillaries without dilatation and distortion in the tumor. The whole tumor body is light red.

| The Ninth Day | Abundant twisty and spreading capillaries grow around the tumor; abundant unbalanced and new-born capillaries appear in the tumor and intertwine with each other to form the shape of fasciculation and twist. There are new-born vascular buds resembling a pointed cone or cyst. The whole tumor is flesh-colored. | A small quantity of new-born circuitous capillaries start to grow around the tumor; capillaries in tumor grow in number and begin the irregular dilatation. The whole tumor body is light red. |
| The Twelfth Day | Abundant capillaries around the tumor look like a string of beads, or intertwine with each other to cause an irregular arrangement, or penetrate the tumor and form into concentrated clumps; capillaries in the tumor extremely distend and fuse into the shape of mass or anal sinus, which form a vast light-tight area of hemorrhage and necrosis in the centre of the tumor. The whole tumor body is maroon. | New-born slender capillaries around the tumor grow in number without interlaced phenomenon. Capillaries in the tumor distend and fuse, but there is no the area of hemorrhage and necrosis. The whole tumor is flesh-colored. |

Table 4 TG's effect on the density (the amount of capillaries/mm²) of new-born tumor capillaries ($\overline{X}\pm S$)

Group	Case load	The Third Day	The Sixth Day	The Ninth Day	The Twelfth Day
Control Group	5	3.40±0.14	8.34±1.05	11.26±1.28	13.1±0.90
TG Group	5	1.84±0.12**	3.64±0.64**	6.58±1.20*	9.90±0.92

Note: Compare to the control group, *$P<0.05$, ** $P<0.01$

3. The average diameter and flow rate of tumor arterioles and venules

Results can be seen in the table 5, 6, 7 and 8.

Table 5 TG's effect on the diameter (μm) of tumor arterioles ($\overline{X}\pm S$)

Group	Case load	The Third Day	The Sixth Day	The Ninth Day	The Twelfth Day
Control Group	5	15.0±0.71	18.8±1.07	20.8±0.84	21.4±0.75
TG Group	5	14.2±0.97	19.0±1.14	18.0±0.71*	19.2±0.58*

Table 6 TG's effect on the diameter (μm) of tumor venules ($\overline{X}\pm S$)

Group	Case load	The Third Day	The Sixth Day	The Ninth Day	The Twelfth Day
Control Group	5	22.6±0.68	24.0±0.71	25.6±0.51	26.8±0.58
TG Group	5	22.4±0.93	23.2±0.86	23.4±0.75*	19.2±0.68*

Table 7 TG's effect on the flow rate (mm/s) of tumor arterioles ($\overline{X}\pm$S)

Group	Case load	The Third Day	The Sixth Day	The Ninth Day	The Twelfth Day
Control Group	5	0.42±0.014	0.45±0.022	0.39±0.011	0.36±0.015
TG Group	5	0.43±0.018	0.47±0.013	0.42±0.012	0.41±0.013*

Table 8 TG's effect on the flow rate (mm/s) of tumor venules ($\overline{X}\pm$S)

Group	Case load	The Third Day	The Sixth Day	The Ninth Day	The Twelfth Day
Control Group	5	0.35±0.016	0.32±0.014	0.28±0.014	0.23±0.016
TG Group	5	0.34±0.014	0.35±0.013	0.32±0.012	0.29±0.015*

Note: Compare to the control group, *$P<0.05$

As seen from the above tables, on the ninth and twelfth day, diameters of tumor arterioles and venules of TG group are obviously thinner than those of the control group ($P<0.05$); on the third and sixth day, there is no significant difference between the two groups ($P>0.05$). On the twelfth day, flow rates of tumor arterioles and venules of TG group are faster than those of the control group ($P<0.05$); on the third, sixth and ninth day, there is no significant difference between the two groups ($P>0.05$). It indicates that TG also has an influence on minute blood vessels (feeding the tumor) of the original host. Especially during an advanced stage, narrowing the diameter and quickening the flow rate can affect the amount of tumor blood supply.

4. The maximum cross section of tumor

Results can be seen in the table 9.

Table 9 TG's effect on the tumor size ($\overline{X}\pm$S, mm)

Group	Case load	The Third Day	The Sixth Day	The Ninth Day	The Twelfth Day
Control Group	5	9.46±0.65	21.78±1.90	34.11±1.62	65.99±2.21
TG Group	5	4.91±0.76**	14.01±1.27**	27.09±2.16*	62.64±2.45

Note: Compare to the control group, *$P<0.05$, ** $P<0.01$

The above results indicate that in the previous nine days TG inhibits the growth of tumor ($P<0.05$); especially in the previous six days, this effect is more obvious ($P<0.06$). On the twelfth day, there is no significant difference between the tumor size of TG group and that of control group ($P>0.05$). It prompts that TG can obviously inhibit the growth of tumor in an early stage. While in the middle-late stage, this effect decreases. Finally in the advance stage, there is no significant inhibiting action.

Determination of plasma endothelin (ET) in mice with transplantation tumor at abdominal muscle

ET is a kind of biologically active peptide synthesized by epidermic cells with extensive biological effects. Recently, increasing researches indicate that ET has an intimate relation with the growth and development of tumor, and also can participate in and promote the vascularization. In order to have a further understanding of tumor, ET and TG's effect on ET of tumor mice, experts carry out the following experiments.

[Material and Method]

1. Materials

(1) Animals: 60 Kunming mice, 18~22g, a 50:50 proportion of male and female.

(2) EAC cell suspension of 6.0×10^7/ml, 20mg/10ml TG suspension and 0.5% CMC solution: Preparation is same as stated before.

(3) Endothelin radioimmunoassay kit.

(4) The gamma (γ) radioimmunoassay counter of SN-682.

Other required reagents are same as those mentioned in the previous experiment.

2. Method

(1) Grouping and gastric lavage according to the table 10.

Table 10 Grouping and gastric lavage of experimental mice

Animals (mice)	Grouping	Gastric lavage (0.2ml/10g)
20 uninoculated mice	Normal group ① 10 mice	physiological saline×6d
	Normal group ② 10 mice	physiological saline×12d
40 inoculated mice	Control group ① 10 mice	0.5% CMC×6d
	Control group ② 10 mice	0.5% CMC×12d
	Administration group ① 10 mice	20mg/10ml TG×6d
	Administration group ② 10 mice	20mg/10ml TG×12d

*. The inoculation method refers to "Experimental Study on Observation of Angiogenesis of Transplantation Tumor at Mouse's Abdominal Muscle".

(2) ET determination: Six days after gastric lavage, collect specimens of blood from the eye socket of mice with 2ml of each mouse in normal group ①, administration group ① and control group ①. Put the blood sample in the tube

with 10% EDTA · Na 230μl and 40μl aprotinin. Lightly shake the mixture well. Centrifuge for 10min with 3000 revolutions per minute at 4°C. Separate plasma and store it at -20°C for determination. Twelve days after gastric lavage, for the mice of remaining groups to adopt the same method to collect specimens of blood, separate plasma. Use the specific radioimmunoassay and gamma (γ) radioimmunoassay counter of SN-682 to measure both the present and previous plasma. Operating procedures should be seriously carried out according to instructions of radioimmunoassay kit.

(3) Statistical treatment: The data is represented by average ± standard error ($\overline{X}\pm S$), and adopt analysis of variance — F test to carry out the comparison among groups.

[Experimental Result]

Determination results of plasma endothelin (ET) in mice can be seen in the table 25-11.

Table 25-11 TG's effect on the plasma endothelin (ET) in mice with transplantation tumor at abdominal muscle ($\overline{X}\pm S$, pg/ml)

Group	Case load	The Sixth Day	The Twelfth Day
Normal group	10	93.6±4.72	93.4±4.83
Control group	10	126.4±3.87**	132.8±4.02**
Administration group	10	106.4±4.49*ΔΔ	114.6±5.41*Δ

Note: Compare to the normal group, *$P<0.05$, ** $P<0.01$; while compare to the control group, Δ $P<0.05$, ΔΔ $P<0.01$

The above results indicate that ET of administration group and control group is obviously higher than that of normal group ($P<0.05$), which shows that the tumor can increase the plasma endothelin (ET) of mice. While ET of administration group is apparently lower than that of control group, and this phenomenon is significant during the previous six days ($P<0.01$), which shows that TG can reduce the increase of plasma endothelin (ET) caused by the tumor and effects in the early stage are stronger.

Results of observation on new-born capillaries of transplantation tumor at mouse's abdominal muscle with microcirculation detection system indicate that TG can inhibit the growth of new-born capillaries in and around the tumor, reduce the density of new-born capillaries which enter and leave the tumor and suppress the growth of tumor. Furthermore, those effects of TG are significant in the early stage, and TG can change the diameter and flow rate of tumor arterioles and venules in the advanced stage to narrow the diameter and quicken the flow rate. Determination results of plasma endothelin (ET) show that the tumor can increase the plasma endothelin (ET) of mice. But TG can reduce the increase of plasma endothelin (ET) caused by the tumor with stronger effects in the early stage.

[Discussion]

1. Analysis and evaluation on the observation method of new-born capillaries by building the transplantation tumor model of mouse's abdominal muscles

At present, the methodology of tumor capillaries research is still in the process of constant exploration and improvement. Generally choose the rabbit cornea, chorioallantoic membrane (CAM) and yolk sac of chick embryo, and hamster cheek pouch for in vivo techniques; and also insert manual apparatus into rabbit ear chamber and subcutaneous air pouch of rat's back, which are called "sandwich" observation room, as the location of transplantation tumor for viviperception. In recent years, corrosion casting and immunohistochemistry are also used to display and identify vascular composition. Each of the above methods has its merits and drawbacks. At present, experts are still exploring to find a kind of simple, economical model and method with high quantitative feature and repeatability for the angiogenesis research. Therefore, combining concrete conditions of this laboratory, the writer has studied and designed the transplantation tumor model of mouse's abdominal muscles, applying improved microcirculation observation techniques to observe new-born capillaries of tumor. This method is easy, convenient and intuitional, and finally becomes a new approach for the tumor capillaries research on the methodology.

(1) Model evaluation: The approach of transplanting tumor at mouse's abdominal muscles is adopted to study and observe the relation between tumor and capillaries, as well as the drug effect on tumor capillaries, which has the reliable theoretical and practical basis.

The abdominal muscle layer of mouse is thinner. A thin layer of aponeurosis lies between the exterior of abdominal muscle layer and skin. The interior of abdominal muscle layer links closely with the abdominal membrane. The Hunter's line divides the abdominal muscle layer along the centre position into right and left halves, which are provided blood circulation by inferior epigastric arteries and veins. The right and left halves diverge one more into tiny branches (arterioles and venules) and capillary branches, which form rich anastomoses around the abdominal muscle of each side. The center position has fewer vascular branches and ramus anastomoticus and becomes an area with rare vessels, where is convenient for the observation of new-born capillaries.

When EAC cell suspension is injected into the abdominal muscle layer, tumor cells will quickly begin the infiltrative growth and expand along the flat surface of abdominal muscle without any adhesion of skin and organs in the abdomen. When the tumor grows up to a certain extent, it will gradually break through the abdominal muscle layer, penetrate inward through the abdominal membrane, move into organs in the abdominal cavity through implantation metastasis and finally produce ascites.

Consequently, the better choice is to inoculate in the area with rare vessels and observe tumor capillaries during the period of the tumor not yet penetrating through the abdominal membrane, which can both make a clearer observation of the emergence and change of new-born capillaries and avoid many factors' combined effects on new-born capillaries, such as ascites and tumor diffusion caused by the tumor's penetration through the abdominal membrane.

Combined with this experiment content, in order to have a better reflection and observation of the transplanted tumor in abdominal muscle and the whole growing and developing process of new-born capillaries, the writer has carried out repeated trials and finally chosen EAC cell suspension with the concentration of 6.0×10^7/ml for inoculation. According to the growth status of tumor, the writer arranges 10 days' observation and 12 days' treatment. Divide four time spans of the third day, sixth day, ninth day and twelfth day to reflect the tumor's reaction to drugs in the early, intermediate and advanced stages.

The transplantation tumor model of mouse's abdominal muscles can intuitively and clearly reflect the formation and change of new-born tumor capillaries, and it also provides new idea and method for studying new-born tumor capillaries' selection of transplantable parts and preparation of animal model. There are a few points that should be remembered when preparing the model: ① Inoculation site should be chosen in the abdominal muscle with rare vessels, not penetrating the peritoneum. The mark is a full small "swelling" without any collapse on the inoculation site. ② The experimental operation should be gentle and careful. Try to keep away from the tiny venous tributary (generally only 1~2 vessels) that links skin and abdominal muscle, so that no local hemorrhage is caused. Then the inoculation effect and the growth of new-born tumor capillaries after inoculation will be unaffected. ③ Appropriately increase the number of experimental mice to reduce errors of different location of rare vessels of abdominal muscle caused by individual difference.

(2) Evaluation of observation method

① Observation of transparent specimen: The tissue of abdominal muscle membrane is thinner. After transparent treatment, other sites are all transparent except vessels are red. Naked eyes can clearly see vessels' routes. Microscope observation can show the shape, distribution and interrelation of capillaries. The transparent specimen is not only convenient and intuitive but also preserves the natural form of vessels and associative perception. When preparing the transparent specimen, do not inject with Chinese ink or other pigments, but directly display vessels through natural color of blood, which prevent particle size, dispersion degree and viscosity of perfusate from affecting the specimen quality and changing the shape of vessels due to improper injection pressure. The transparent specimen must completely reflect the condition in vivo so as to make displayed vessels be closer to the reality.

The transparent specimen of abdominal muscle- membrane can clearly display various vessels in the abdominal muscle, involving the route, shape and distribution of capillaries around and in the tumor as well as localized congestion, oozing of blood and bleeding, which make it more convenient for observing new-born capillaries inside and outside of the tumor. The transparent specimen can only show the change of capillary form after animals have died, but it cannot reflect their blood flow state. Therefore, combined with the dynamic state of vital blood flow and functional parameters to have observation, it will be more favorable to have a complete understanding of new-born tumor capillaries' features.

② In vivo observation with microcirculation microscope: The mouse's abdominal muscle membrane is thinner with the shape of film and is easy to transmit light, whose vascular form and fluid state can be clearly seen through the microcirculation microscope. Inoculated tumor cells begin the infiltrative spreading growth in the abdominal muscle. In the early stage, the abdominal muscle membrane still can transmit light and display the vascular form in tumor tissue due to unobvious increase in thickness. In the advanced stage, the tumor tissue grows and thickens; the pressure of central part increases; necrosis and hemorrhage arise, which appear as a light-tight solid mass; vessels in this part cannot be seen, but the form of vessels in other transparent parts of tumor can be seen at present. The microcirculation microscope is used to observe new-born capillaries inside and outside of transplantation tumor at abdominal muscle and those which enter and leave the tumor as well as tumor arterioles and venules, which can completely reflect the relation between tumor and vessels as well as drugs' effect on new-born tumor capillaries in the respect of vascular form and fluid state.

The above two observation methods can complement each other with joint application. Observation of transparent specimen can cover the shortage of not observing vessels in a light-tight part of tumor in vivo; while in vivo observation makes up for the observation of dynamic state of blood flow. The above methods can only make one-off observation and cannot have a continuing dynamic monitoring in a long term, so they also remain inadequate. In order to have a more accurate and deeper research, the methodology needs the further improvement and completeness.

2. Evaluation of experimental drugs Common Threewingnut Root generally refers to the plant belonging to Tripterygium of Celastraceae. There are three varieties in China, which are Common Threewingnut Root, Tripterygium Hypoglaucum and Common Threewingnut Root of North-East (Tripterygium regelii Sprague et Take). This kind of drug has an acrid-bitter flavor and medicinal properties of cold and hot. The drug passes through main channels of liver and spleen as well as twelve regular channels, which has efficacies of clearing away heat and toxic material, expelling wind and removing dampness, relaxing the muscles, stimulating the blood circulation and removing obstruction in channels, reducing swelling and alleviating pain, destroying parasites and relieving itching. This drug, which contains about 70 components, is recorded in *Sheng Nong's herbal classic* at the earliest. Since the 1970s, it has been used in treating rheumatoid arthritis, which results in certain curative effect. In recent twenty years, it has been widely used in treating chronic nephritis, hepatitis, purpura haemorrhagica and all kinds of skin diseases. At the same time, the research of pharmacological action also becomes deeper, widely covering adrenal gland, immunity, generation, micturition, central nerve and blood system. Experts all agree that this drug can enhance adrenal cortex function, relieve inflammation and alleviate pain, resist fertility and prevent tumor activity. Only as to its effect on immune system, experts each sticks to their own viewpoint. There were many controversies and inferences. In an early period, experts embarked on the research of its effect on immune system because of its unique effect on treating rheumatoid arthritis. The earliest result indicates that this drug can suppress immunity. As more and more researches are done deeperly, most researchers gradually tend to the viewpoint of "two-way regulation". They hold that Common Threewingnut Root has the two-way regulating action with dose dependent on immune system. For instance, Zheng jiarun, Yan Biyu, Luo Dan, Lei Yi and Fan Yongyi respectively report that Common Threewingnut Root has the two-way regulating action on mouse's thymic weight, human thymocyte hyperplasia, NK activity of mouse's spleen cells, T and B cell function of mouse's spleen and proliferation of T cells in vitro. Through the experiment of the effect of TG with different dosages on MΦ function of mice abdominal cavity and immune organs by the writer, it reflects that Common Threewingnut Root has the two-way regulating action on immune

system. The above results indicate that Common Threewingnut Root does not have the only effect of immunological suppression. Many experiments have proved that a small dosage of Common Threewingnut Root can enhance the immunization to some extent. While within a certain limits, there will be a reversible manifestation between enhancement and inhibition. It can also show nearly no appreciable effect on immunologic function. When further increasing the dosage, this drug will show the complete inhibiting action on immunization. The inhibiting action of Common Threewingnut Root is obviously related to its dosage.

Given the above conclusions, the writer chooses the dosage of TG, which has no appreciable effect on immunologic function, to carry out the experiment. It can avoid drugs' influence on immunologic function, which may complicate the research of TG's inhibiting action on tumor capillaries. At the same time, it can provide experimental considerations and exploring foundations for experiments and clinical researches of TG's anti-tumor action on the premise that Common Threewingnut Root will not damage the body's immunological function.

The drug of this experimental research is a kind of prepared product after repeated separation and abstraction. The amount of active principle is higher and the untoward effect is less. In order to have a further exploration of angiogenesis inhibition of active principle in this drug, various chemical compositions and monomers after the second separation and purification still need further study.

3. Features of tumor angiogenesis Under normal conditions, the angiogenesis only limits in embryonic development, repair in trauma and endometrial regeneration. Furthermore, the host can strictly control its growth with various mechanisms. But in the recent twenty years, experts haven't found any mechanism which can suppress tumor angiogenesis. It indicates that tumor angiogenesis has its own features.

Through the observation on new-born capillaries of transplantation tumor at mouse's abdominal muscle, it is easy to find that as the formation and growth of capillaries in the inoculation area, tumor cell cluster constantly proliferates and its volume continually expands. It starts with the exudation of original host's capillaries, and then slender and crooked new-born capillaries gradually come out with the characteristics of disorganized arrangement, uneven distribution and irregular diameter. Especially these capillaries, which enter into the tumor, have incontinuous routes, lack completeness and present the shape of comma or bud. The above signs indicate that those capillaries are not fully mature and cannot form complete and continuous basilar membrane. Furthermore, they are not blocked and packed by well-differentiated vascular walls with multilayered structure, which make vessels expand irregularly in the shape of nodositas or sinus. Along with the progressive growth of tumor, dust-color area of hemorrhage and necrosis appears in the centre of the tumor. Capillaries in adjacent sites are hard to be seen because of extreme dilatation, which may be due to the constantly rising pressure within tumor caused by the continuous proliferation of tumor cells. The pressure of central part in tumor is relatively highest, and the central part is far away from new-born capillaries that penetrate from the outside of tumor, so the central part is easy to suffer from necrosis because of ischemia, involving the necrosis and hemorrhage of vessels. But there still are different-shaped tumor capillaries with active proliferation at the margin of tumor, which can ensure the required nutrition for the further infiltrative growth. This phenomenon also indicates that the tumor grows indefinitely and cannot be adjusted and controlled.

At present, experts have been adopting various methods to study tumor vessels. The existing achievements have proved that the formation of tumor vessels is different from the angiogenesis in a normal physiological state. It has its own special uniqueness, such as infantile differentiation, incomplete vascular wall and out of the body's control, etc. While the whole process and regulatory mechanism of tumor angiogenesis remains obscure and are still in further exploration. This experiment just superficially reflects the relation between tumor and vessels, as well as some features of tumor vessels. The deeper study also needs the breakthrough of methodology, and the continued clarification of biological characteristics of tumor vessels in terms of the physiology and pathology of angiogenesis, biochemistry and molecular biology.

4. Exploration of TG's inhibiting action on new-born tumor capillaries Since Common Threewingnut Root is explored and applied, domestic and foreign medicine circles have been starting to pay great interest and attention to it and carrying out multi-disciplinary study and exploration one by one for broadening the application range. The recent researches show that Common Threewingnut Root can inhibit the migration and proliferation of vascular endothelial cells (EC). Zhu Jinbo and another two Japanese scholars utilize self-made F-2 and F-2C of EC strain to study the effect of Common Threewingnut Root on the process of angiogenesis. The result shows that Common Threewingnut Root can directly act on EC and inhibit its migration, proliferation, differentiation and the formation of lumen, which prompts that Common Threewingnut Root has a better inhibiting action on angiogenesis. The experimental study of TG's inhibiting action on new-born capillaries of transplantation tumor at mouse's abdominal muscle finds that TG can suppress tumor angiogenesis with

stronger effects in the early stage. Presumably TG's active mechanisms may include the following respects.

(1) Directly act on new-born tumor capillaries: The experimental results indicate that TG can obviously suppress the growth of capillaries in and around the tumor and reduce the density of new-born capillaries which enter and leave the tumor. Thus it can be inferred that TG may directly act on endothelial cells of tumor vessels, suppress the migration and proliferation of cells and reduce the formation, differentiation and growth rate of tumor vessels.

(2) Directly act on tumor cells: TG's direct damaging effect on tumor cells has been proved in an early period. It is generally acknowledged that TG comes into the effect of cell toxicant by directly interfering with DNA replication of tumor cells and suppressing RNA and protein synthesis. During the process of angiogenesis, the tumor cell itself can produce multiple angiogenesis factors, such as fibrocyte growth factor (FGF), angiogenine, transfer growth factor (TGF) and tumor necrosis factor (TNF-2), etc. Furthermore, the tumor cell can release some chemical mediators to induce the angiogenesis of host and tumor. The above substances that are released by tumor cells and can induce angiogenesis are collectively called "tumor angiogenesis factor (TAF)" by Folkman. TG can reduce the production of TAF by directly killing tumor cells, which indirectly inhibits the angiogenesis.

(3) Change of tumor blood flow: Determination result of the average diameter and flow rate of host's tumor arterioles and venules shows that TG can change the blood flow in the tumor and affect the growth and change of tumor and its new-born capillaries by acting on the blood supply of tumor.

(4) Reduction of plasma ET content: The recent researches indicate that ET has the effect of growth factor on promoting cell proliferation, which can stimulate the growth of endothelial cell and the proliferation of vascular smooth muscle cells. ET has an intimate relation with the tumor, which can promote the transcription and expression of proto-oncogene and the growth and differentiation of tumor, increase the blood flow of tumor tissue and stimulate the angiogenesis. The determination result of mouse's plasma ET indicates that ET of inoculated group is obviously higher than that of normal group. It proves that ET has an intimate relation with tumor and the tumor can increase mouse's plasma ET content. While ET of TG group is apparently lower that that of control group,

which indicates that TG can obviously lower mouse's plasma ET content and reduce the growth effect on promoting tumor and angiogenesis caused by ET.

Furthermore, TG has a feature in this experiment that its inhibiting action on tumor angiogenesis in the advanced stage is weaker than that in the early stage. In addition to TG's pharmacological characteristic of suppressing angiogenesis, its inhibiting power is also related to drugs' accumulative action. It is conjectured that TG accumulates in vivo and plays an extensive pharmacological effect with prolongation of medication time, and thus affects its inhibiting action on tumor angiogenesis.

This research result indicates that TG can suppress tumor growth by inhibiting tumor angiogenesis with no significant effect on the immune system, and moreover, TG's effect in the early stage is significant. This study provides references for the further multi-field and multi-angle TG researches, and also new ideas for the research of TG anti-tumor mechanisms. Without doubt, this conclusion still needs extensive repeated experiments to be verified. At the same time, drug purification and methodology improvement are necessary for the further deeper study.

Inhibiting the formation of new-born tumor capillaries to suppress the tumor growth is a new idea on oncology that emerges in recent years.

This topic is on the basis study of formation features of new-born capillaries of transplantation tumor at mouse's abdominal muscle as well as capillaries' relation with tumor and TG's two-way regulating action with dose dependent on the immune system of mouse, and thus by choosing the TG dosage (40mg/kg weight) of no obvious effect on mouse's immune function to carry out experiments of TG's effect on the shape and quantity of new-born capillaries of transplantation tumor at mouse's abdominal muscle, the density of new-born capillaries which enter and leave the tumor, the average diameter and flow rate of tumor arterioles and venules, tumor size and plasma ET. The above experiments find that TG can inhibit tumor angiogenesis through various mechanisms of direct action on new-born tumor capillaries as well as tumor cells, the change of tumor blood flow and the reduction of plasma ET content, and moreover, TG's effect in the early stage is significant. This research result shows that the anti-tumor study of TG from the angle of vessels has certain significance and needs the further study confirmation and deepening.

IV. The Significance of Inhibition of Angiogenesis in Treatment

Tumorigensis is a complicated process and is affected by many factors, involving the foundation of tumor vascular net. Many researches have proved that tumor growth must depend on angiogenesis. By inhibiting certain steps or the whole process of tumor angiogenesis to control tumor growth is of great importance to tumor therapy and prevention of tumor's distant metastasis.

i. The relation between tumor angiogenesis and the generation and growth of tumor

At present, the question about tumor generation mainly focuses on the study of oncogene; nevertheless, malignant change of tissues, tumor formation and tumor gene activity are just necessary conditions instead of the whole. Folkman Judah and other scholars in Children's Hospital of Harvard Medical School do a series of studies about the generation of pancreatic islet B cell tumor of mutant mice. The study result finds that tumor gene activity is related to the proliferation of B cells, and moreover, angiogenesis plays an important role during the generation of B cell tumor. The generation of tumor is caused by getting angiogenic ability of hyperplastic tissue. The research proves that one of evident characteristics of most precancerous lesions is the lack of obvious neovascularization. Compared with the tumor with abundant new-born vessels, the transition from precancerous condition and lesion to blood vessel phase may be the "switch" for tumor generation. It indicates that the induction of angiogenesis and the consequent neovascularization are both ahead of the tumor generation. Once the tumor is found, its further growth must depend on the continuous generation of vessels. This concept has been put forward by Folkman in 1971. He holds that tumor cells and vessels combine into a highly integrated ecological system. If there is no angiogenesis, the tumor will not swell. Many experimental research evidences in recent years further support the above views.

The growing period of solid tumor cells can be divided into invading prophase without vessels and invading growth phase of vascularization. During the invading prophase, the growth of tumor cells mainly depends on diffusion to gain nutrition. When the diameter of solid tumor exceeds 1~3cm and cell number is up to about 10^7, tumor's central part and its continued growth must be provided with oxygen and nutrient substance by vessels. ① Observe the black tumor cell cluster of mouse that is cultured in agar. When the cluster grows to 1mm³, the proliferation of its peripheral cells and the necrosis of central cells are equivalent. When the tumor body continues to swell, the proliferation and necrosis achieve a dynamic equilibrium. If the tumor grows in the organism, then this phase can also be called the blood vessel phase of tumor growth. Breaking this state needs the growth of new and functional capillaries so as to provide adequate oxygen and nutrient substance. ② Observe the growth rate of transplantable tumor in the subcutaneous transparent cavity of mouse. The tumor shows a slow linear growth before angiogenesis. While after angiogenesis, the tumor shows a rapid exponential rise. ③ Implant tumor tissue masses into the rabbit cornea. The tumor stands back from the host's vascular bed. The new-born capillaries around the cornea are found to gather toward the tumor. The growth rate averages 0.2mm/d. After new-born capillaries grow into the tumor, the tumor mass begins to grow rapidly and exceeds 1cm³. ④ The tumor grows in the isolated perfused organ of mouse. Because there is no vascular proliferation, the tumor limits in 1mm³. If this tumor is transplanted into the mouse, it will rapidly grow to 1~2cm³ after angiogenesis. ⑤ Suspend tumor cells in the aqueous humor of anterior chamber of rabbit eyes. Because there is no vessel, the tumor size is less than 1mm³. If this tumor is transplanted into iris vessels, it will grow rapidly with 1.6 times of its original volume in two weeks. ⑥ When the human retina blastoma is transplanted into the vitreous body or anterior chamber, the growth of this tumor will be limited due to the lack of vessels. ⑦ Use ³H- thymine to label tumor cells of fixed cancer. The label index of tumor cells reduces with the increase of distance between the nearest open capillaries and tumor cells. The mean value of label index of tumor cells is the function of label index of tumor vascular endothelial cells. ⑧ Transplanted tumor in CAM. During the avascular period (≥72h), the growth of tumor is restricted. A set of experiments show that the tumor diameter is no more than (0.93±0.29) mm. In 24 hours after the vascularization, the tumor starts growing rapidly. On the seventh day, the average diameter of tumor is (8.0±2.5) mm. ⑨ Oophoroma metastasizes to the abdominal membrane. Before the vascularization, this tumor grows slowly and its size seldom exceeds 1mm³. ⑩ If the tumor diameter is less than 1mm, there will be no vascularization in the metastatic cancer of rabbit cornea. All other metastatic cancers, whose diameter is greater than 1mm, have the formation of vessels.

All these above can indirectly or directly prove that tumor growth must depend on vascularization and the vascularization is a key factor for tumor development.

ii. The anti-tumor action of angiogenesis inhibitors

In the early 1970s, along with the presentation and research of the concept that tumor growth depends on vascularization, researchers also bring forth the relevant concept of anti-angiogenic therapy. That is to say, by preventing neovascularization and (or) the expansion of new-born vascular net and (or) destroying new-born vessels to stop the generation or establishment of small solid tumor and also arrest the growth, development and metastasis of tumor. Ways of adopting anti-angiogenic therapy: ① Suppress tumor to release tumor angiogenic factors (TAF); ② Neutralize the tumor angiogenic factors (TAF) that have already been released; ③ Inhibit the reaction of vascular endothelial cells (EC) on angiogenic factors; ④ Disturb the synthesis of basilar membrane; ⑤ Destroy the formed new-born tumor vessels, etc. In conclusion, ideal tumor angiogenesis inhibitors must be able to suppress one or more procedures or the whole process of tumor angiogenesis.

At present, people have done a lot of researches in this respect. Experimental results indicate that angiogenesis inhibitors (AI) can inhibit the growth of tumor. ① According to more domestic reports, the combination of heparin and hydrocortisone is acknowledged as an effective angiogenesis inhibitor. Experiments prove that their combined application can suppress the angiogenesis in CAM, promote tumor regression, prevent metastasis and inhibit the neovascularization of rabbit cornea that caused by tumor. That this kind of inhibitor is used to cure some mice tumors can bring about a striking effect. For instance, after the oral administration of heparin (200U/ml) and subcutaneous injection of hydrocortisone (250mg), 100% reticulum cell sarcoma, 100% Leuis lung cancer and 80% B16 melanoma can have a complete regression. What's more, 80% tumors will not suffer from the relapse after regression. ② Fumagillin is a kind of antibiotic which is naturally secreted by aspergillin. For the in vitro experiment, Fumagillin can inhibit the proliferation of endothelial cells. For the in vivo experiment, Fumagillin can inhibit the angiogenesis caused by tumor and also suppress the tumor growth of mice. For example, 30mg/kg of Fumagillin can inhibit the growth of Lewis lung cancer and B16 melanoma. ③ 1μg/ml TNP-470 (a kind of Fumagillin synthetic analogue) can inhibit the growth of cultural endothelial cells of human umbilical vein. 3~10mg/kg TNP-470 can suppress the growth of nude mice's transplanted tumor of human oophoroma. ④ Platelet factor 4 (PF_4) is a kind of 28kDa protein that is released by the dense body when blood platelets aggregate together. There is a great affinity between PF_4 and heparin. Taylor and other scholars have found that PF_4 can effectively inhibit the growth of CAM vessels. Recently Maione and others have discovered that recombination of human PF_4 ($rHuPF_4$) can suppress the reproduction and migration of human endothelial cells, and also produce an avascular area in chick embryo CAM. Sharpe has carried out the research about mice melanoma and human colon cancer, which proves that human PF_4 ($rHuPF_4$) has an inhibiting action on the growth of solid tumor. ⑤ α-Difluoromethylornithine (DFMO) is a kind of nonreversible ornithine decarboxylase inhibitor. It can inhibit the angiogenesis caused by melanoma in chick embryo CAM, and then inhibit the tumor growth in CAM. ⑥ The latest approved angiogenesis inhibitor - Angio stain is a kind of 38kDa protein, which can inhibit the generation of endothelial cells and angiogenesis in the Lewis mice tumor. When Folkman injects Angio stain into the mouse with transplanted tumor, this new type of inhibitor can keep this transplanted tumor in a state of dormancy, that is to say, the multiplication rate of tumor is equal to the death rate of cells. In addition, Angio stain can suppress the growth of human tumor.

At present, people have realized that the anti-tumor effects of many anti-tumor methods directly or indirectly act on the structure or function of tumor vessels, such as anti-tumor angiogenesis, the change of tumor blood flow and its regulation, etc. That by inhibiting the angiogenesis of malignant tumor to suppress the growth and metastasis of tumor is a new way to fight against cancer, and meanwhile adopting angiogenesis inhibitors to cure tumors will open up a new and promising therapeutic area clinically. For instance, cooperating operation, chemotherapy, radiotherapy and immunological therapy will certainly improve the overall tumor treatment level.

Tumor cells produce multiple tumor angiogenesis factors (TAF), such as basic fibroblast growth factor (bFGF), acid fibroblast growth factor (aFGF), endothelial cell growth factor (ECGF), vascular endothelial cell growth factor (VEGF), platelet derivation endothelial cell growth factor (PDECGF), epidermal cell growth factor (EGF), transforming growth factor (TGFα, TGFβ), tumor necrosis factor (TGF-α), granulocyte colony stimulating factor (G-CSF) and granulocyte macrophage colony stimulating factor (GM-CSF), etc. TAF has the promotional effects on tumor generation, development and metastasis. Exploring the generative mechanism of tumor capillaries and the inhibition of capillaries' formation and growth is one of the effective measures to prevent and cure tumors, and may also become a new promising anti-cancer therapy after the surgical treatment, radiotherapy, chemotherapy and biological therapy.

Two of my five posters which were posted in American Association Cancer Research(AACR) meeting:

Thymic Atrophy and Decreased Immunologic Function: Possible Factors behind Cancer Development

Jie Xu M.D.[1], Ze Xu M.D.[1], Shiping zhu M.D.[1], Shaoming Qio M.D.[1], Mona Mohamed M.D.,Ph.D[2], Bin Wu M.D.,Ph.D[1]

[1]Research Institute of Experimental Surgery of Hubei University of Traditional Chinese, Wuhan, Hubei, China, [2]the Johns Hopkins University, Baltimore, MD

Introduction

Immune system plays extremely roles in preventing our body from getting any disease such as virus, bacteria and cancers, etc. In the past many attentions were on genetic and other reasons. Dr. Xu Ze in China did many experiments which described the relations between immune functions and cancers, especially the central immune organs bone marrow and thymus. Dr. Xu Ze is the first one in the world who did these thymus animal experiments and found that thymus atrophy and decreased immunologic function are the possible factors involved in cancer growth and metastasis. His clinical immunotherapy strongly supports his basic experiments. T-cells are matured from thymus, which have naturally capable of killing cancer cells, especially naive T-cells who can become a specific CD8 killing T cells after they meet the specific antigen in the periphery immune organs and this ability can be supressed by the tumor. Dr. Xu did a series of experiments to search the relation between immune functions and cancers. In this poster we summarized one of our research results of the relations between thymus atrophy and decreased immunologic function and the cancer development.

Objectives

The objective of this work was to investigate the relations of the immune system and the development of cancers.

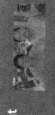

Cancer-bearing Animal Model

Materials and Motheds

Over a 7-year period, 680 Kunming mice, age 8-10 weeks divided into 4 groups: 1) 140 controls; 2) 105 Mice had tumor cell inoculation in the armpit; 3) 105 Mice had tumor cell inoculation in their armpits and received 10 ml steroid injection (for 30 days) to lower the immuno function, and 4) 330 Mice had tumor cell inoculation in the armpit after excision of their thymus. In group 3, 80 of them were sacrificed to observe the thymus a month later while the tumors grew up to the size of a thumb and removed these tumors. In group 4, the mice were anesthetized and their skin and muscles were incised along the second, third and fourth ribs to expose the thymus which was gently separated and was excised. Each mouse was put in a separate cage and the mice were taken care of very carefully. We used H₂₂ cells to make a unicell suspending liquid. After dyeing the cancer cells with lichenin and counting them (averaging 1x106/ml), we made the hypodermic inoculation of cancer cells with 0.2 ml normal saline which was injected to the mice at the left side of their antorfor armpit skin. We weighed the tumor under their armpit skin. and measured the diameter of the tumor every 3 days and measured the diameter of the tumor under their skin with the caliper. Cancer development was monitored and assessed by observing the injection site for tumor growth by monitoring the tumor sizes. We resorved the whole blood of each mouse to do lymphocyte conversion. The mice were then euthanized and the thymuses, spleen were then excised, weighed and their size and volumes were recorded

Results

1. Group 3 and 4 showed cancer-bearing signs 7 days after removing their thymus and after receiving steroid injections.

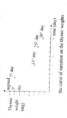

2. Group of cancer-bearing mice with thymus showed progresive atrophy of the thymus on gross and histology and developed advanced cancer sooner. If the tumors were removed, thymus stopped atrophy. However, the thymus of the control group did not show progressive atrophy. In the cancer later stage thymus weight decreased from 78.13+13.2 mg to 20-5mg, the diameter of the volume decrease from 5-6mm to 1mm. The cell proliferation clearly decreased.

3. The numbers of metastatic nodules in the liver in the group which received steroid injections were 35% more than the ones in the non-steroid injection mice group.

4. In thymus- reserved group receiving steroids, the spleen showed initial increase in its size on the 7th day, but then decreased in its size on the 14th day.

Discussion

Thymus is the central immune organ in which T cells mature and develop and have a critical role in immune regulation. The occurrence and metastasis of the tumor have close connection with the thymus functions and spleen functions such as the thymus progressively atrophy during the tumors growth (1, 2, 3). Hiroshi et al (4) found that the IPSCs cells generated fully active, cancer-specific T lymphocytes. It is well established that immune cells called T cells are naturally capable of destroying cancer cells and this ability can be suppressed by the tumor which possibly secrets the immune inhibiting factors which function on the thymus and made it shrink which consequently caused loss of its function (5,6). The spleen was initially enlarged suggesting its reaction and response to inhibit the growth of the tumor in its early stage, however, at a later stage, the spleen regressed 50%.

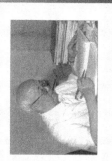

Conclusion

Thymus resection—immunologic deficiency—decreased immunological surveillanco-immunologic escape are the main possible factors of cancer development. First, the immune function decrease, then cancer can develop and grow. If the immune system doesn't decrease, the cancer model can not be set up successfully. The occurrence and metastasis of cancer has an obvious relation with the immune function of the immune organs such as thymus, spleen and other immune organs.

References

1. Xu Ze Jie Bin Wu. New Concept and New Way of Treatment of Cancer. AuthorHouse press in March, 2013.

2. Carrio R, Torroella-Kouri M, Iragavarapu-Charyulu V, Lopoz DM. Tumor-induced thymic atrophy: alteration in interferons and Jak/Stats signaling pathways. Int J Oncol. 2011;38(2),547-53.

3. Loromo-Bor On A, Zipori D, Hanau Ghara H. Increased regulatory versus effector T cell development is associated with thymus atrophy in mouse models of multiple myeloma. J Immunol. 2008;181(5)3714-24.

4. Hiroshi et al. Cancer-Killing Stem Cells Could Be Used To Treat Cancer. Accessed at
http://www.medicalnewstoday.com/articles/256609.php

5. A New day for immunotherapy In<-AACR Cancer Progress Report 2012: making research count for patients: a new day>> Published by AACR American association for cancer research. Clin Cancer Res 2012:18(suppl 1),61-63.

6. Kaiserlian D, Savino W, Hassid J, Dardonne M. Studies of the thymus in mice bearing the Lewis lung carcinoma: Possible mechanisms of tumor-induced thymic atrophy. Clin Immunol 1984:32(3),316-25.

Contact Informations

1. Dr. Xu Ze: xuze8@cnil@gmail.com
2. Dr. Bin Wu: wxyc@gmail.com

Observation of Experimental and Clinic Curative Effect on Z-C Medicine Treating Malignancy

Ze Xu M.D.[1], Jie Xu M.D.[2], Shiping Zhu M.D.[2], Shaoming Qio M.D.[2], Bin Wu M.D. Ph.D.[3]

[1]Department of Surgery of Affiliated Hospital of Hubei College of Traditional Chinese Medicine, Wuhan, China. [2]Research Institute of Experimental Surgery of Hubei University of Traditional Chinese, Wuhan, Hubei, China. [3]The Johns Hopkis Universit, Baltimore, MD.

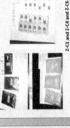

Introduction

In order to look for the traditional herb medicine with actually curative effect and without toxicities and adverse reactions, our surgical tumor research institute has screened, 200 kinds of Chinese herbal medicine with so-called anticancer reaction recorded on Chinese herbal medicine books for tumor-inhibition reaction on the solid carcinoma In the tumor-bearing animal models one by one in the past years. Through long-term in-vivo tumor-inhibiting animal experiments, we have screened 48 kinds of Chinese herbal medicines with relatively good tumor-inhibition rate that can prolong the survival time, protect the immune organ and obviously improve the immunologic function. According to the clinical conditions, the anticancer medicines screened are combined into 2 compounds including Z-C₁ and Z-C₄ with better anti-cancer reaction than each single medicine. In the original screening, we carried out the tumor-inhibiting animal experiment for each single medicine and now we further carry out the experimental study on these two groups of compounds for the tumor-inhibiting reactions in the solid tumor of the tumor-bearing rats.

Z-C₄ therapy group | Control Group
30 days after inoculation of hepatic carcinoma H₂₂

Z-C₄ therapy group | Control group
Thymus was hypertrophic | Thymus was atrophic
30 days after inoculation of hepatic carcinoma H₂₂

Objectives

To find Traditional Chinese Medicines(TCM) of treating carcinoma which are good curative effect and have no side effect.

Materials and Methods

A. Hepatic carcinoma H₂₂ cell strains from fresh tumors in rats were prepared into the single cell suspended liquid, after dyeing and counting of the cancer cells (1x 10⁶/ml), 0.2ml of cancer cells were inoculated subcutaneously into the front axilla of the right side of each rat ; 260 Kunming white rats, weight: 21±2g, 8-10 weeks of dividing rats for groups ① traditional herb medicine Z-C₄ group (90 rats). The rats were given to 0.8ml/rat, equivalent to 1.4mg of the dried medicinal herbs by gastriclavage once every day after 24h of transplantation of cancer cells ②Traditional herb medicine Z-C₄ group (90 rats), the dose and methods tho same as Z-C1. ③Chemotherapy group (50 rats), CTX 50mg/kg weight every other day from the next day after transplantation of cancer cells by gastriclavage. ④Control group (30 rats), 0.8ml normal saline /rat were given via gastriclavage every day from the next day after transplantation of the cancer cells, then measure the weight of the rats every 3d, measure the diameter of the tumors, measure the immunologic function and complete blood counts. Half of each group as Group A, regularly killing of the rats in batches, separation of tumor and weighing of the tumor and then calculation of tumor-inhabiting rate, pathological section and ultra-structural organization. The rest half of each group as Group B were given to medicine for a long time until natural death, then tumors were separated and weighed, the long-term tumor inhibition rate and life elongation rate of the tumor was calculated.

B. These medicine are applied into clinics since 1994. Z-C₁ is the compound 150ml to be taken once/day and Z-C₄ is powder, 10g to be taken once/day and observe the short-term curative effect and iconography indexes as well as the survival time of long-term curative effect, quality of life and immunologic indexes.

Results(1)

1. Animal experiment:

a. The repression rate of mice H22 in liver cancer to of group Z-C1 for 2, 4, 6 weeks is 40%, 45% and 58%, and repression rate of mice H22 in liver cancer to of group Z-C4 for 2, 4, 6 weeks is 55%,68% and 70%, while repression rate of group CTX for 2, 4 and 6 weeks is 45%, 45% and 49%.

b. The survival time: the average survival time of Z-C₁, Z-C₄ and CTX was longer than the one of the normal saline control group (P<0.01), compared with the control group, the life elongation rate of Z-C₁ group was 85%, the one of Z-C₄ group was 200% and the one of CTX group was 9.8%. The rats in Z-C₁ and CTX in Group B met with death in 75d.

c. Both Z-C₁ and Z-C₄ medicine improved the immunologic function, especially Z-C₄ obviously improved the immunologic function, increased the white blood cells and red blood cells, without any effect on the hepatic function and kidney function and without damage to the hepatic and kidney section. CTX decreased the white blood cells and reduced the immunologic function with the renal damage to the kidney section.

d. Pathology: the thymus in the control group was obviously atrophic and the cells were discrete and the blood vessal met with sludge while Z-C₄ therapy group displayed that the cortical area of the thymus built up, the lymphocyte was dense, the epithelium reticulocyte increased and the thymus corpuscles increased.

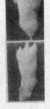

Control group | Z-C₄ control group
HE x 100 cortex atrophia | HE x 100 the cortex
Lymphocyte obviously | lymphocyte was highly dense
decreased | the thymus built up

Results(2)

2. Clinical Application:

1.Z-C medicine has good effect to prolong survival time and has no side response for a long time taking. The symptom was improved, the diseases state was stable, the quality of life was improved, the survival time was prolonged In 4277 medium and advanced cancer patients, and the patients live with tumors in balanced state for a long time.

Conclusion

Z-C1 and Z-C4 medicine have remarkable curative effects and no side effects for long-term administration and can improve survival time and life quality and immunity in the medium and advanced cancer patients, control the patients' pain and soften and shrink body surface metastasis tumors.

Z-C1 and Z-C4 and Z-C6

References

1. Han Rui, editor-in-chief, Study and Experimental Technology of Anti-cancer Medicines. Beijing: Joint Press of Beijing Medical University and Peking Union Medical College, 1997

2. He Xinhuai, Xi Xiaoxian, editor-in-chief, Immunology of Traditional Herb Medicine, Beijing: People's Military Medical Press, 2002, 341-348

3. Zhou Jinhuang, Immunopharmacology of Traditional Herb Medicine. Beijing: People's Military Medical Press, 1994: 134-157

4. Xu Ze, New Concept and New Mode of Carcinoma Therapy, Wuhan: Hubei Science and Technology Press, 2001,171-173

Contacts

1. Dr. Xu Ze email: xuze8cn@email.com
2. Dr. Bin Wu email: seascyl@hotmail.com

1. Our research team:

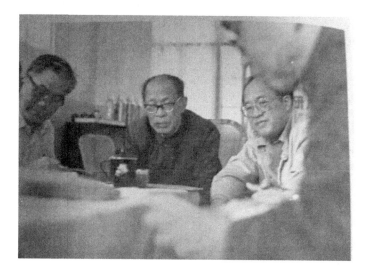

Academician Qiu Fazu(middle), Honorarry President of Tongji Medicine University, medical leading scientist of general surgery in China, directed the scientific research design in Experimental Surgery Lab

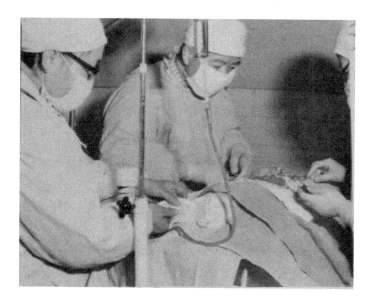

Experimental research on non-tumor technic in Radical operation

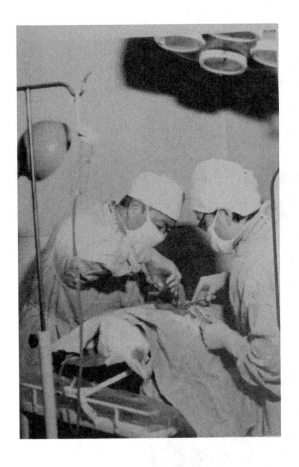

This experiment is to research the non-tumor technic in operation and make the experimental obsrvation and research in operation throught the cancer-bearing animal model. Observe the number of the exfoliative cancer cells, detect and number the cancer cells in the nevous blood of tumor in operation. Experimental observation of the dyeing of the gastric lymph nodes by tracing.

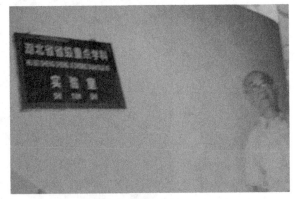

Our research lab

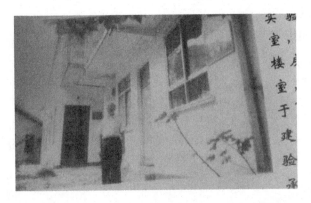

This is a research
and clinic lab

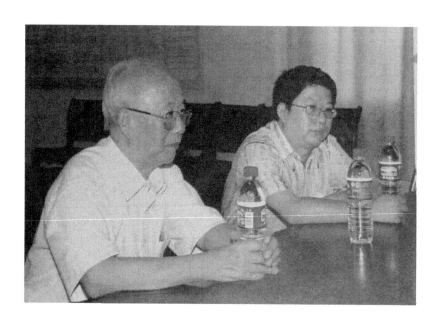

The meeting for our research

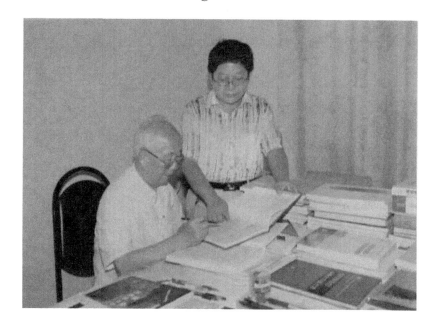

The research meeting

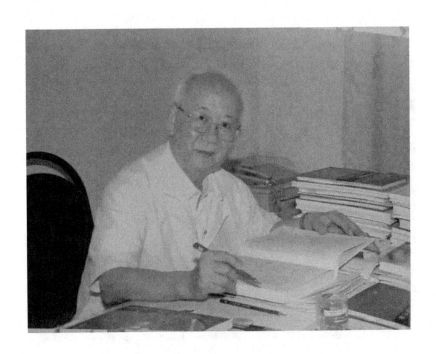

writing the books

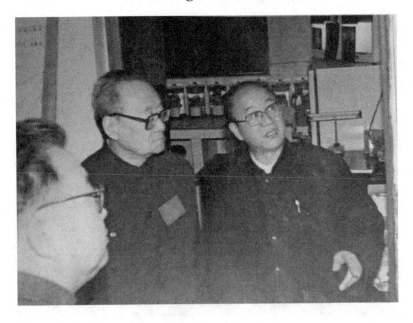

Academician Mao Shoubai(middle), Vice president of Chinese Academy of Preventive Medicine Science, Vice Group Leader of Parasitology of the united Nation inspected Experimental Surgery Lab

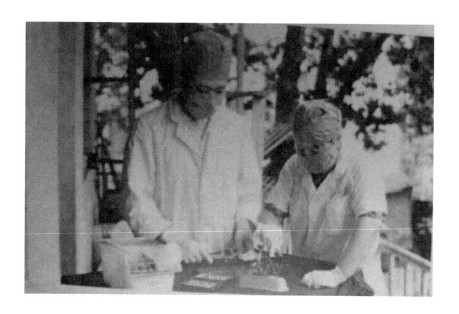

Experiment on anti-cancer metastasis and recurrence in experimental surgery research institute

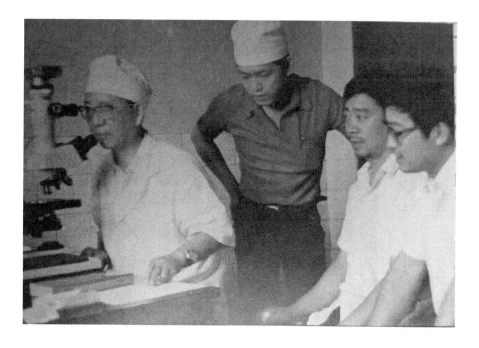

Prof Xu Ze(left), Postgraduates(Right 1, 2, 3)

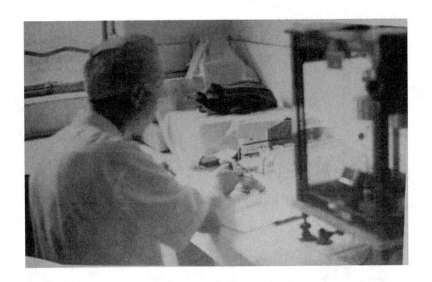

Experimen on anti-cancer metastasis and recurrence in experimental surgery research
Institute

Observe ultrastructural organization of the experimental model cancer cells with
electron microscope

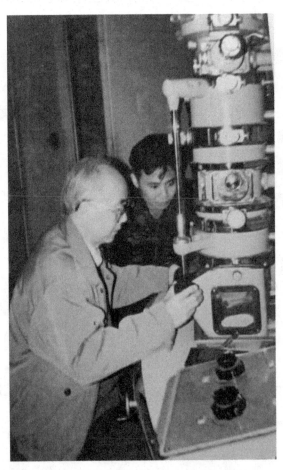

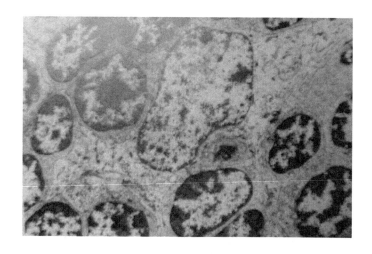

Ultrastructural organization of H22 liver cancer cells of cancer-bearing mouse

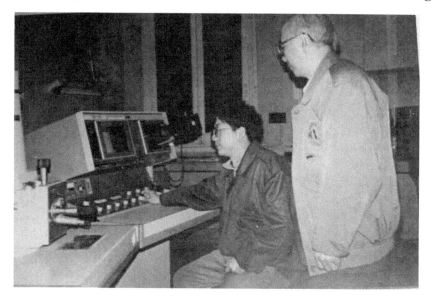

Observe ultrastructural organization of the experimental model cancer cells with electron microscope

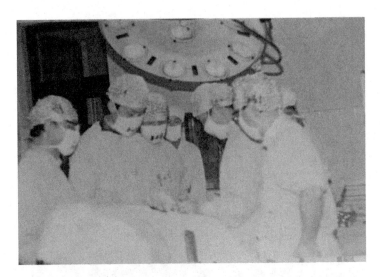

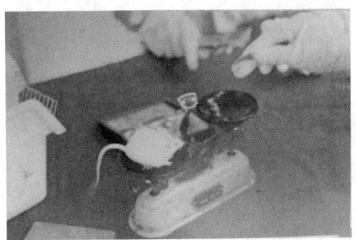

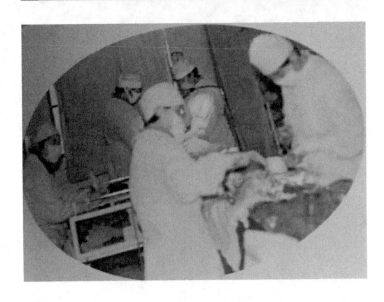

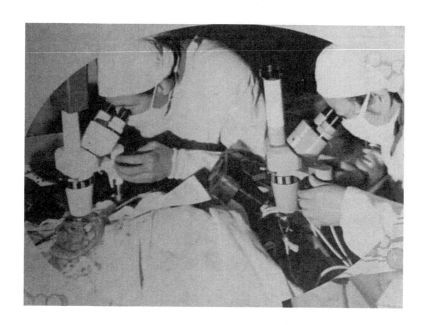

Experimen on Anti-cancer metastsis and recurrence in experimental surgery
research institute

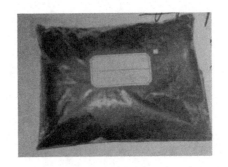

Z-C3

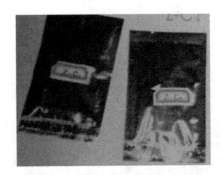

Z-C4

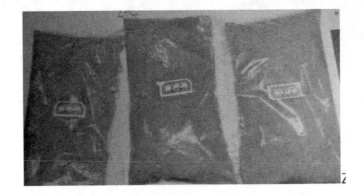

Z-C1

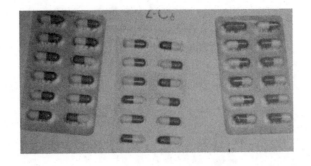

Z-C6

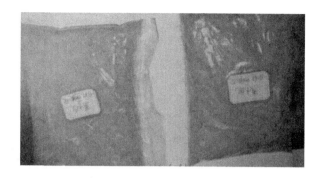

Medications of reducing edema

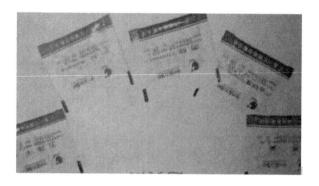

Medications of reducing jaudice

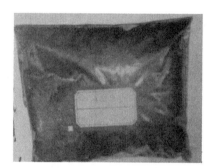

Z-C3

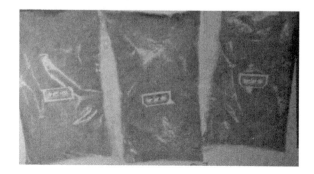

Z-C1

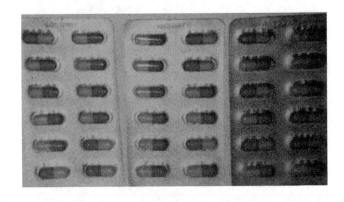

Z-C7

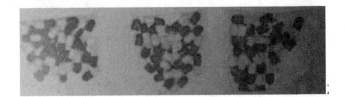

Z-C2

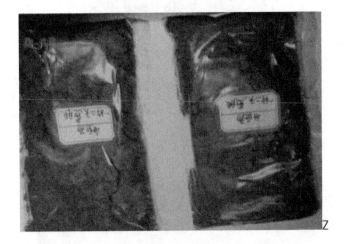

Z-C8

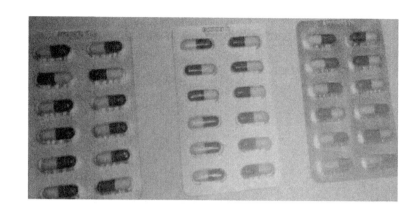

Z–C10

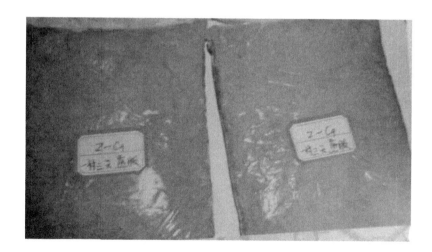

Z–C9

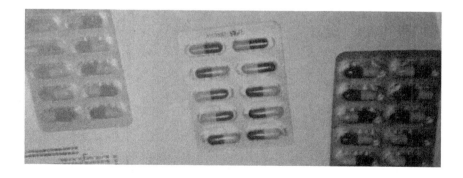

3. Experimental research on Protecting Thymus and Upgrading Immunity as well as protecting Bone Marrow and Hematopoiesis

Treatment Group and Group of Z-C1 Medicine

C1   Treatment group   Control group

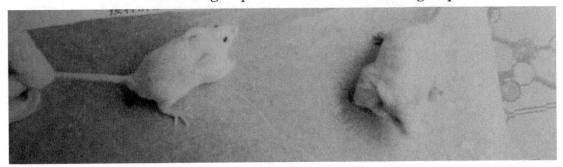

Tumor   Thymus   Spleen   Kidney   Liver

C4   Treatment   Control

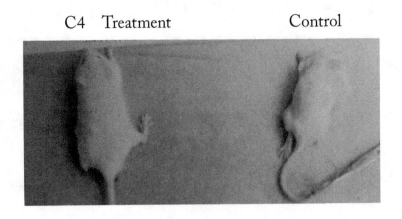

Tumor Thymus Spleen Kidney Liver

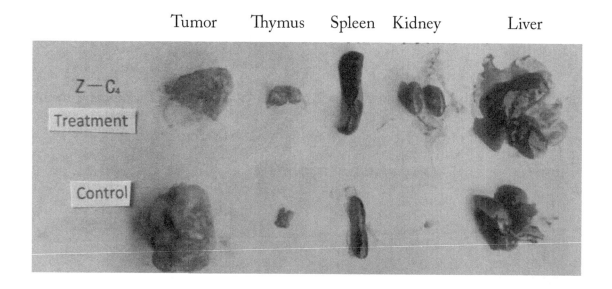

Z—C₄
Treatment

Control

C5 Treatment Control

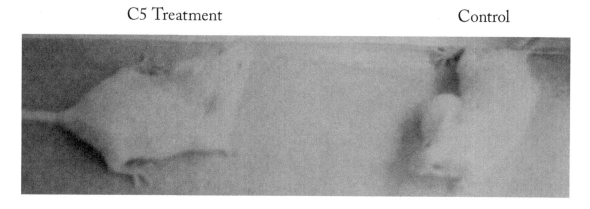

Tumor Thymus Spleen Kindey Liver

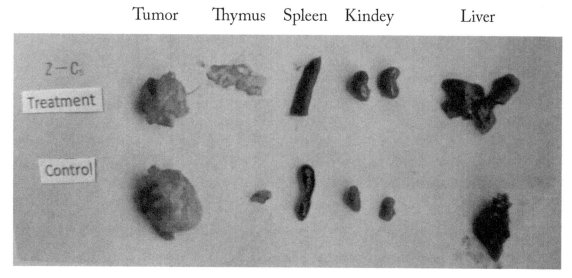

Z—C₅
Treatment

Control

Animal Model for Experimental Research on Anti-cancer Metastasis and Recurrence

Treatment of tumor-bearing group with S180 Sarcoma with ATCA

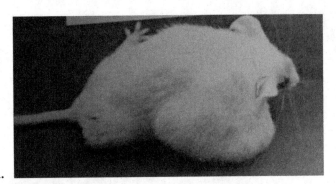

A.

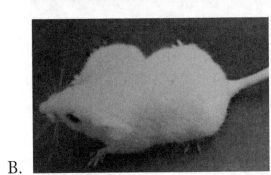

B.

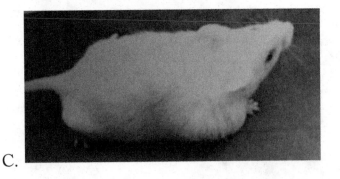

C.

Treatment of Cancer-bearing Mouse with H22 Liver Cancer with T.S.L

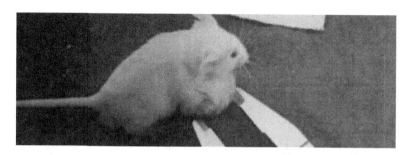

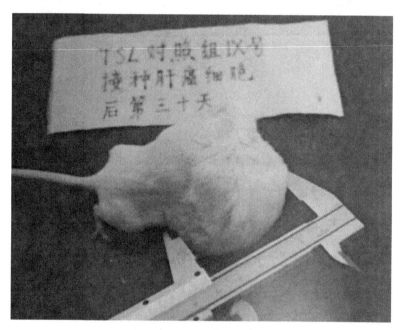

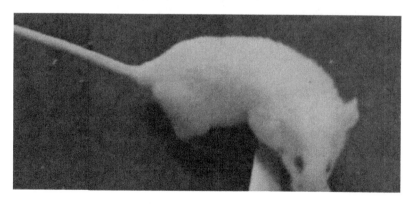

Observation of Inheritance of Cancer on Cancer-bearing Mouse through disemboweling to take the fetus after conception

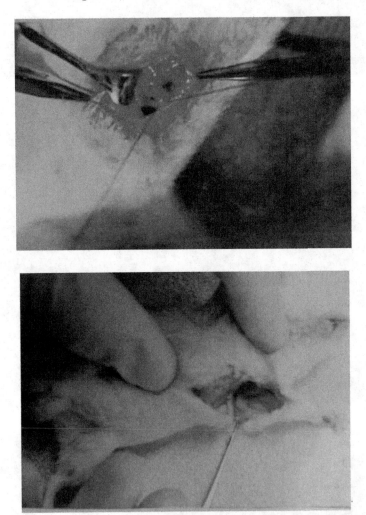

Transpanted the speciment into the omentum

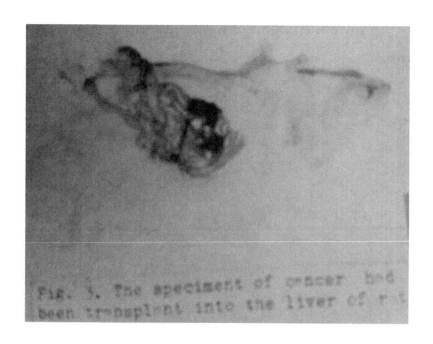

The speciment of cancer had been transplant into the liver of rat

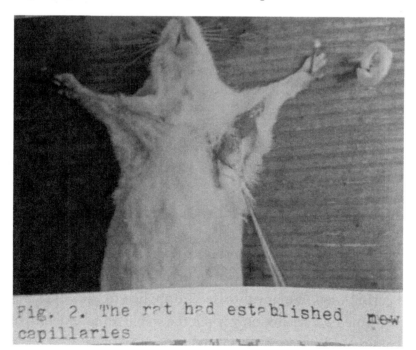

Thymus Atrophia of Cancer-bearing Mouse

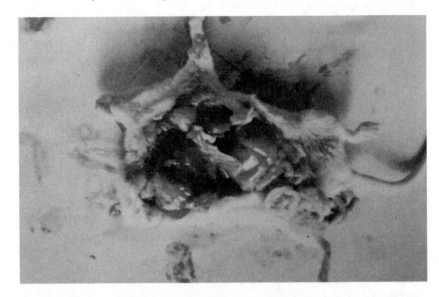

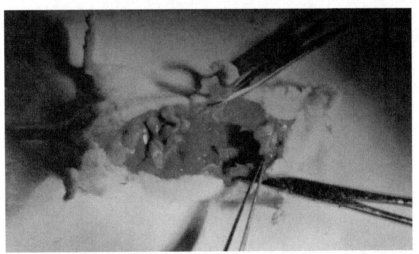

Experimental surgery play a very important role in developing the medical secience and it is one key to open up the out-of-bounds area of the medical science. The preventive and curing ways of many diseases are applied to the clinic and promote the development of the medical science only when the stable achievements have been made through the experimental research on animal for many times.

Animal Model for Experimental Research on Anti-cancer Metastasis and Recurrence

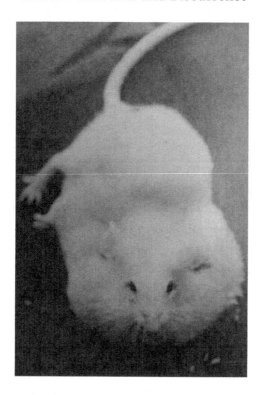

Cancer-bearing animal model with the cancerous block is exfoliative as a whole

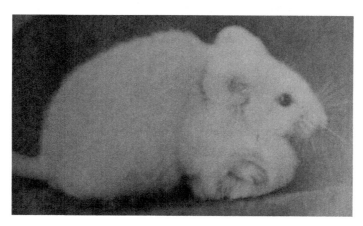

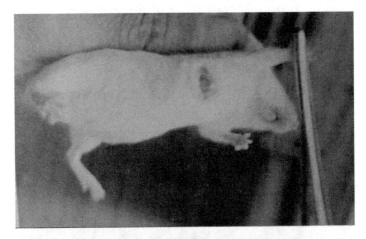

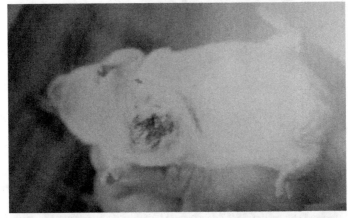

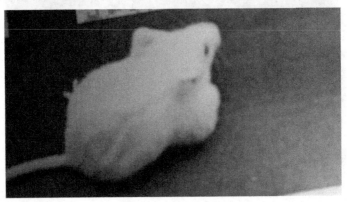

XZ-C 免疫调控抗癌中药治疗肝癌部分病例一览表

编号	姓名	病例号	性别	年龄	籍贯	职业	住址	诊断	诊断依据	确诊单位	特殊嗜好 吸烟年数	吸烟量	饮酒年数	饮酒量
1	施**	6101204	男	57	枣阳	农民	枣阳	肝癌	CT，MRI (98.6.22)	枣阳市医院	30年	一天1-2包	30年	一餐3-4两
2	兰**	6201222	男	35	大悟	教师	大悟	肝右叶巨块肝癌	CT(98.8)	大悟县医院协和医院			10年	
3	卢*	6201229	男	38	当阳	土地管理干部	当阳	右肝癌术后	B超CT (98.7)	协和医院	6-7年	少		
4	刘*	6201230	男	30	公安	工程师	公安	巨块型肝癌	B超CT (98.7.7)	公安县医院鄂州市医院	10多年	一日一包	10年	一餐2-3两
5	曾**	6301242	男	50	钟祥	农民	钟祥	原发性肝癌	CT(98.8)	钟祥市人民医院				
6	柯**	6301244	男	54	黄石	农行职员	黄石	肝癌	CT(98.8)	黄石医院协和医院	30多年	一日1-2包	10多年	一餐半斤
7	宋**	6301257	男	37	应城	小学校长	应城	巨块型肝癌	B超CT，MRI(98.7.1)	应城市人民医院协和医院				
8	杨**	6401263	男	51	鄂州	主治医师	鄂州	肝癌术后	B超CT (98.9)	鄂州市医院协和医院				
9	蒋**	6401264	男	57	河南	无线电厂电焊工	孝感	巨块型肝癌	B超 (98.2.10)	三江航天０六六基地红星医院协和	20年	一包	10多年	一餐一斤
10	张**	6401267	女	64	上海	会计师	武汉	肝胆胰癌肺转移	B超CT (98.9.25)	铁路医院协和医院				
11	李**	6401269	男	36	黄陂	农民	黄陂	左肝癌,胆囊壁受侵	B超. (98.7)	协和医院	10年余	2-3包		
12	三**	6401273	男	47	武汉	水泥厂工人	武汉	左肝癌术后复发肺转移	B超 (98.4)	同济医院	10年	一日2包	10年	常饮
13	杨**	6401277	男	46	通城	保卫科员	武汉	原发性肝细胞癌	B超CT (98.9.13)	武钢二医院协和医院	20年	一日12根	10年	
14	严**	6501295	女	56	天门	农民	天门	原发肝癌转移	B超CT，MRI(98.5)	协和医院				

Medical Records

XZ-C 免疫调控抗癌中药治疗肝癌部分病例一览表

编号	是否常吃 泡菜	腌菜	熏肉	干咸鱼	咸菜	香肠	油煎食品	辣椒	大蒜	洋葱	新鲜蔬菜	水果	霉变食物	是否常饮 绿茶	浓茶	其它	饮水方式	是否常吃 肉食	排骨汤	素食	工作情况 一般	紧张超负荷	性格情况 开朗	沉闷易怒	是否爱好运动	慢性疾病史	家族三代癌症病史	敷药止痛情况 消失	减轻	有效	敷药消肿块情况 肿块部位及大小	敷药后肿块缩小情况
1		√		√							√					√	井水	√肥肉						√		91年患胸膜炎,作穿刺抽出黄色液体	无			√	98.6.22检查肝内 2个占位1-3cm不等	
2	√	√			√			√			√			√			自来水					√		√		初中时患黄疸肝炎,肝功能正常,80年急性黄疸肝炎	父亲因食道癌去世				98.8.18右腹至11上腹扪及B 12×10cm cm² 98.8.30复检	
3								√	√		√			√			自来水							√	否	83年乙肝,91,96,97年现乙肝三阳	无					
4								√	√		√						自来水	√肥肉								乙肝阳性有流鼻血史	无				98.7.10CT 肝方叶2.5×2.5×3cm³肝右叶10×5×9cm³	
5	√	√		√	√			√						√			糖水				√	√				89年发现大量腹水查以血吸虫反复发生,先后查过HbsAg(+)有时阴性	三弟肝癌未切除广泛转移插管未起作用术后3个月于84年去世				98.8CT 肝右叶为8×10 cm²占位	
6								√	√		√						井水	√						√		查有血吸虫70年有肺结核治愈						
7									√		√			√			自来水				√	√		√	否	83年患乙肝治疗半年,一直迁延间断服药	无				98.7.1肝右叶8.7×7.1cm²大小	
8									√		√			√			井水							√		二月前检查有乙肝	父亲贲门癌于97年去世				98.9肝区肿块4.3×4.4cm²大小	
9								√	√			√		√			自来水	√肥肉	√		√	√			否	67年乙肝三阳住院三月治疗未转阴有肺结核已钙化胃溃疡	无				98.2.10B超肝右叶15.4×12cm²占位	
10							√		√		√	√					自来水				√			√		有糖尿病	无				98.9.29彩超肝右叶2.5×2.4cm²胰头3×3.1cm²	
11									√		√						自来水	√				√			√	有血吸虫病史七年前小三阳未治疗	无				98.8.3CT 左肝4.3×9.9cm²占位	
12									√								自来水								否	83年患急性黄疸肝炎,住院一月有时肝区痛有胆囊炎	父亲因肝癌去世					
13			√					√	√	√	√		√吃霉米一日				自来水	√			√	√	√	√	否	84年急性黄疸肝炎,住院一月,一月后又复发	无					
14		√									√						井水				√	√	√		否	60,70年代先后三次住院治疗血吸虫属晚期,胃糜烂:贫血胃粘膜脱垂	无					

Medical Records

XZ-C 免疫调控抗癌中药治疗肝癌部分病例一览表

编号	作过何种治疗				服药时间、种类及其疗效	备注
	手术方式	介入	放化疗	何时复发转移及部位大小		
1	不宜	98.8.5 至 9.15 作两次肝介入			98.7.14-9.22 服用 XZ-C$_{1,4,5,2}$ 号,XZ-C$_3$ 号外敷,服药后食欲精神好肝区疼痛明显,夜间痛不能眠,为剌痛 10AM-2PM 痛明显些,服药后疼痛明显减轻,介入后无任何不良反应,肝肿块由 3.2×3.9 cm^2 缩至 2.2×2.4 cm^2 大小	
2		98.8 月至 11 月作三次介入			98.8.14-12.25 服用 XZ-C$_{1,4,5}$ 号,XZ-C$_3$ 号外敷介入血管阻塞异常,血管服药后精神食欲好,日食一斤,行走活动如腑形,二次介入后不能起带人,右上腹包块比前软些,缩小些,由 12×10 cm^2 缩小至 11×8 cm^2 大小	床不能进食右上腹疼痛加重腰痛乏力
3	98.8.5 作右半肝切除				98.8.19-11.15 服用 XZ-C$_{1,4,5}$ 号服药后精神好,面色红润食欲好,如常人.	
4	不宜	98.7.21 置泵化疗四次			98.8.20-9.24 服用 XZ-C$_{1,4,5}$ 号,XZ-C$_3$ 号外敷化疗用药 Mitoniyan5Fu 肝服药后精神食欲好	素有右肿上结核硬结
5					98.9.7-11.28 服用 XZ-C$_{1,4,5}$ 号服药后,精神食欲较前好转,可以起床行走,走一里路,晨起锻炼,肝区有痛感,有时隐隐剌痛,轻度腹水征.	四弟肝癌作切除,术后两年去世有腹水,母亲肝硬化腹水病人腹水住血防医院四次,治血吸虫服吡喹酮三天疗法
6	98.8.20 行剖腹探查未能切除	98.8.30 作置泵于肝动脉二 次卡铂阿霉素		98.8.20 术中见肝内转移	98.9.8 至今服用 XZ-C$_{1,4,5}$ 号,服药后精神好转,食欲增加体重增加 8 斤,行走活动如常生活自理	
7	98.7.2 手术探查未能切除	98.7.27 及 8.27 作二次肝动脉药泵化疗		98.10.8 胸片右下肺转移,二个 1.2 cm^2 直径病灶	98.9.20-10.18 服用 XZ-C$_{1,4,5}$ 号服药后一般好,精神食欲好,98.7.27 第一次药泵化疗阿霉素顺铂 5-FU 消化道反应大, WBC↓2300,8.27 第二次化疗反应大 WBC↓1500病灶有缩小,9.19B 超 5.0×5.0 cm^2	98.7.1 突发下腹痛 7.2 肝破裂大出血急症手术,探查见肝癌破裂豆腐渣状未能切除,结扎肝 A
8	98.9.15 作肝方叶切除胆囊切除				98.9.25-11.30 服用 XZ-C$_{1,4,5}$ 号服药后精神食欲好,体力渐恢复,复查 AFP.CEA 均正常	
9	不宜	98.2.18 至 11 月作六次介入反应大		98.9.15CT 考虑胆囊转移可能	98.9.27-11.18 服用 XZ-C$_4$ 号,服药后自觉良好,疼痛症状消失,原来肝区胀痛,一直腰痛作第四次介入说不清话,动则痛,咳不痛,不动则不痛,每天抽筋样右肩不能动疼痛.	
10	不宜			98.9.30 胸片见肺转移	98.9.30-10.11 服用 XZ-C$_{1,4,5}$ 号退黄消水汤,服药后精神好些,原来全身肌肉酸痛,现在不痛了,腹胀,下肢肿	
11	不宜	98.8.7 及 9.21 二次介入,术后肝区胀痛			98.10.3-10.18 服用 XZ-C$_{1,4,5}$ 号服药后一般好,精神食欲好,行走活动如常面色红润,栓塞治疗后于 98.98 复查下,肝肿块大,为 8×6.8 cm^2 稍小	
12	98.4.30 作左肝切除	98.6.23 至 9.4 三次动静脉药泵注药		二次化疗后右肝转移10.19 胸片双肺转移	98.10.10-11.22 服用 XZ-C$_{1,4,5,2}$ 号,XZ-C$_3$ 号外敷鹅胆二乳抗癌消水汤服药后一般好,食欲好,右肩痛腹胀,呕吐咳嗽,呼吸困难尿少,大量腹水外敷后有些许好转	
13	98.9.29 作肝右叶切除	98.11.9 作介入,MMC+5FU		98.11.13 彩超复查肝左叶 1.5×7.3 cm^2 占位为术后复发	98.10.11-11.29 服用 XZ-C$_{1,4,5}$ 号服药后病情稳定,一般好,精神食欲好,行走活动如常	
14	不宜	98.10.6-10.31 5Fu+CF+HCPT 胞必性		98.5 月肝癌伴腹膜,胸周转移	98.10.31-12.7 服用 XZ-C$_{1,4,5}$ 号,XZ-C$_3$ 号外敷服药后面色较前好,仍疼痛,间断性有呕吐.	

Medical Records

Printed in the United States
By Bookmasters